SC Lehrich
610 421 8456

ADAPTING COGNITIVE THERAPY FOR DEPRESSION

Adapting Cognitive Therapy for Depression

Managing Complexity and Comorbidity

edited by **Mark A. Whisman**

THE GUILFORD PRESS

New York   London

© 2008 The Guilford Press
A Division of Guilford Publications, Inc.
72 Spring Street, New York, NY 10012
www.guilford.com

Printed in the United States of America

This book is printed on acid-free paper.

Last digit is print number: 9   8   7   6   5   4   3   2   1

The authors have checked with sources believed to be reliable in their efforts to provide
information that is complete and generally in accord with the standards of practice that are
accepted at the time of publication. However, in view of the possibility of human error or
changes in medical sciences, neither the authors, nor the editor and publisher, nor any other
party who has been involved in the preparation or publication of this work warrants that the
information contained herein is in every respect accurate or complete, and they are not
responsible for any errors or omissions or the results obtained from the use of such
information. Readers are encouraged to confirm the information contained in this book
with other sources.

Library of Congress Cataloging-in-Publication Data

Adapting cognitive therapy for depression : managing complexity and comorbidity / edited
by Mark A. Whisman.
    p. ; cm.
  Includes bibliographical references and index.
  ISBN-13: 978-1-59385-638-0 (hardcover : alk. paper)
  1. Depression, Mental—Treatment. 2. Neuroses—Treatment. 3. Cognitive therapy.
I. Whisman, Mark A.
  [DNLM: 1. Depressive Disorder—therapy. 2. Cognitive Therapy—methods. 3. Comorbidity.
WM 171 A221 2008]
  RC537.A247 2008
  616.85′2706—dc22

                                                        2007042203

To my parents,
Jack and Marie

ABOUT THE EDITOR

Mark A. Whisman, PhD, is Professor of Psychology and Director of Clinical Training at the University of Colorado at Boulder. He is a Founding Fellow of the Academy of Cognitive Therapy and a former Van Ameringen Scholar at the Beck Institute for Cognitive Therapy and Research. A major focus of Dr. Whisman's research has been cognitive models of depression, and the predictors and processes of change in cognitive therapy of depression. He has published over 80 journal articles and book chapters and has coedited one book (with Douglas K. Snyder, *Treating Difficult Couples: Helping Clients with Coexisting Mental and Relationship Disorders*). His research has been funded by the National Institute of Mental Health and by the National Alliance for Research on Schizophrenia and Depression. Dr. Whisman was formerly Associate Editor of *Contemporary Psychology* and has served on the editorial boards of *Journal of Consulting and Clinical Psychology, Journal of Family Psychology, Clinical Psychology: Science and Practice, Behavior Therapy,* and *Applied and Preventive Psychology.*

CONTRIBUTORS

Patricia A. Areán, PhD, Department of Psychiatry, University of California, San Francisco, San Francisco, California

Aaron T. Beck, MD, Department of Psychiatry, University of Pennsylvania, Philadelphia, Pennsylvania

Gregory K. Brown, PhD, Department of Psychiatry, University of Pennsylvania, Philadelphia, Pennsylvania

Robert M. Carney, PhD, Department of Psychiatry, Washington University School of Medicine, St. Louis, Missouri

Lee Anna Clark, PhD, Department of Psychology, University of Iowa, Iowa City, Iowa

Sandra J. Coffman, PhD, Private practice, and Department of Psychology, University of Washington, Seattle, Washington

John F. Curry, PhD, Department of Psychiatry and Behavioral Sciences, Duke Child and Family Study Center, Duke University, Durham, North Carolina

Sona Dimidjian, PhD, Department of Psychology, University of Colorado at Boulder, Boulder, Colorado

Keith S. Dobson, PhD, Department of Psychology, University of Calgary, Calgary, Alberta, Canada

Jacqueline E. Donnelly, MA, Department of Psychology and Neuroscience, Duke University Medical Center, Durham, North Carolina

David J. A. Dozois, PhD, Social Science Centre, Department of Psychology, University of Western Ontario, London, Ontario, Canada

Stefania Fabbri, PsyD, Center for Addiction Research and Education, Department of Psychiatry and Neurobehavioral Sciences, University of Virginia, Charlottesville, Virginia

Giovanni A. Fava, MD, Department of Psychology, University of Bologna, Bologna, Italy

Leilani Feliciano, PhD, Department of Psychiatry, University of California, San Francisco, San Francisco, California

C. Virginia Fenwick, PhD, Department of Psychiatry and Behavioral Sciences, Duke University Medical Center, Durham, North Carolina

Kenneth E. Freedland, PhD, Department of Psychiatry, Washington University School of Medicine, St. Louis, Missouri

Arthur Freeman, EdD, Department of Psychology and Counseling, Governors State University, University Park, Illinois

Anne Garland, RN, Nottinghamshire Healthcare NHS Trust, Nottingham Psychotherapy Unit, Nottingham, United Kingdom

Marjan Ghahramanlou-Holloway, PhD, Department of Medical and Clinical Psychology, Uniformed Services University of the Health Sciences, Bethesda, Maryland

Erin T. Graham, MS, Department of Psychology, University of Michigan, Ann Arbor, Michigan

Stefan G. Hofmann, PhD, Department of Psychology, Boston University, Boston, Massachusetts

Steven D. Hollon, PhD, Department of Psychology, Vanderbilt University, Nashville, Tennessee

Glenetta Hudson, PhD, Department of Psychology, University of Michigan, Ann Arbor, Michigan

Robin B. Jarrett, PhD, Department of Psychiatry, University of Texas Southwestern Medical Center, Dallas, Texas

Laura Kohn-Wood, PhD, Department of Psychology, University of Michigan, Ann Arbor, Michigan

Jennie Lacy, BA, Department of Psychology and Neuroscience, Duke University Medical Center, Durham, North Carolina

Christopher R. Martell, PhD, ABPP, Private practice, and Department of Psychiatry and Behavioral Sciences, University of Washington, Seattle, Washington

Ivan W. Miller, PhD, Department of Psychiatry and Human Behavior, Warren Alpert Medical School of Brown University and Butler Hospital, Providence, Rhode Island

Cory F. Newman, PhD, Center for Cognitive Therapy, University of Pennsylvania, Philadelphia, Pennsylvania

Michael W. Otto, PhD, Center for Anxiety and Related Disorders, Department of Psychology, Boston University, Boston, Massachusetts

Mark B. Powers, PhD, Department of Clinical Psychology, University of Amsterdam, Amsterdam, The Netherlands

Mark A. Reinecke, PhD, ABPP, Department of Psychology and Behavioral Sciences, Feinberg School of Medicine, Northwestern University, Chicago, Illinois

Clive J. Robins, PhD, ABPP, Department of Psychiatry and Behavioral Sciences, Duke University Medical Center, and Department of Psychology and Neuroscience, Duke University, Durham, North Carolina

Gwen E. Rock, MS, Department of Psychology, Philadelphia College of Osteopathic Medicine, Philadelphia, Pennsylvania

Jan Scott, MD, Institute of Psychiatry, London, United Kingdom

Alisa R. Singer, PhD, Early Psychosis Treatment Service, University of Calgary, Calgary, Alberta, Canada

Judith A. Skala, RN, PhD, Department of Psychiatry, Washington University School of Medicine, St. Louis, Missouri

Georgia Stathopoulou, MA, Department of Psychology, Boston University, Boston, Massachusetts

Lisa A. Uebelacker, PhD, Department of Psychiatry and Human Behavior, Warren Alpert Medical School of Brown University and Butler Hospital, Providence, Rhode Island

Jeffrey R. Vittengl, PhD, Division of Social Science, Truman State University, Kirksville, Missouri

Lauren M. Weinstock, PhD, Department of Psychiatry and Human Behavior, Warren Alpert Medical School of Brown University and Butler Hospital, Providence, Rhode Island

Marjorie E. Weishaar, PhD, Department of Psychiatry and Human Behavior, Warren Alpert Medical School of Brown University, Providence, Rhode Island

Mark A. Whisman, PhD, Department of Psychology, University of Colorado at Boulder, Boulder, Colorado

PREFACE

One of the most influential theories and treatments of depression is cognitive theory and cognitive therapy (CT) of depression (Beck, Rush, Shaw, & Emery, 1979). To date, there have been over 75 clinical trials evaluating the efficacy of CT for depression. Results from these studies indicate that CT is an effective treatment for major depression (Gloaguen, Cottraux, Cucherat, & Blackburn, 1998; Hollon, Thase, & Markowitz, 2002), and that it may have a prophylactic effect in reducing relapse and recurrence of depression (Hollon et al., 2002).

Despite its overall efficacy, however, not all depressed patients respond to standard CT for depression (Hamilton & Dobson, 2002; Whisman, 1993). Furthermore, most depressed patients present with complex sets of issues and problems that exacerbate, or are exacerbated by, their depressive symptoms. Although clinicians are likely to believe they can improve treatment success by modifying and supplementing standard CT for depression, there are few guidelines for clinicians to use in deciding whether, when, and how to modify standard treatment in working with different kinds of depressed patients.

This book was written to respond to that need. In these chapters, authors integrate clinical, theoretical, and empirical developments in presenting a unified set of clinical guidelines for adapting CT to different manifestations of depression. The focus of the book is on presentations of depression that are commonly encountered in everyday clinical practice, that are likely to be difficult or challenging to treat, and that call for modifying "standard" CT for depression.

The book is divided into four main sections. Part I provides an overview of, and delineates the most current methods for, conducting CT for
depression, including detailed discussions of assessment, case conceptualization, and treatment planning.

Part II focuses on the treatment of subtypes or subgroups of depressed
patients that are defined in terms of severity and historical features. The
treatment of a severely or chronically depressed patient poses a challenge to
even the well-seasoned clinician. Therefore, this section includes chapters on
adaptations of CT for severe, chronic, drug-resistant, partially remitted, and
recurrent depression.

Part III focuses on treating depression that co-occurs with other mental, physical, or interpersonal problems. Nearly three-fourths of people with
lifetime and nearly two-thirds of people with 12-month major depression
also met criteria for at least one other Axis I disorder during their lifetime
or the past year, respectively (Kessler et al., 2003). In addition, approximately
50–85% of depressed inpatients and 20–50% of depressed outpatients have
personality disorders (Corruble, Ginestet, & Guelfi, 1996). Depression has
also been found to co-vary with medical conditions (Stevens, Merikangas, &
Merikangas, 1995) and impaired interpersonal and social relationships
(Hirschfeld et al., 2000). Furthermore, compared to depressed individuals
without comorbid conditions, those with comorbid conditions have more
severe and persistent depression (Kessler et al., 1996) and are more likely to
seek mental health services (Kessler et al., 2003), suggesting that the
depressed people clinicians are likely to encounter are people with comorbid conditions. Moreover, most individuals with comorbid conditions seeking treatment for depression desire treatment for their comorbid conditions
(Zimmerman & Chelminski, 2003). The high rate of comorbidity suggests
that "pure" cases of depression not only are rare but also may be unrepresen-
tative of people with depression, particularly with respect to depressed individuals in treatment. The relative rarity of cases that meet criteria for a single
diagnosis of major depression suggests the need for a change in the way
depression is conceptualized and treated. The chapters in Part III cover
adaptations of CT for depression for some of the most common conditions
and disorders that co-occur with depression, including suicide, Axis I disorders (anxiety disorders, substance use disorders), personality disorders, medical conditions, and family and relationship problems.

Part IV focuses on the treatment of depression in special populations.
Research has shown that the manifestation, risk factors, and treatment of
depression vary among people who differ in race and ethnicity, sexual orientation, and age. For example, sociodemographic characteristics are associ-

ated with differential exposure to discrimination, which in turn is associated with elevated risk for depression (Kessler, Mickelson, & Williams, 1999). Consequently, Part IV focuses on adaptations of CT for depression in special populations, including racial and ethnic minorities; lesbian, gay, and bisexual women and men; adolescents; and older persons.

Each chapter begins with a brief overview and general conceptualization of the manifestation of depression covered in the chapter, along with a discussion of clinical assessment methods. The emphasis of each chapter, however, is on providing a detailed, practical discussion of treatment strategies, including recommended adaptations of standard CT for depression and recommendations regarding the use of medication. Each chapter also includes a case study to further illustrate the core aspects of the approach. Finally, each chapter ends with a summary of the empirical findings regarding the efficacy of the treatment for the manifestation of depression covered in the chapter.

Taken as a whole, this book provides readers with detailed and practical suggestions for conceptualizing, assessing, and treating different presentations of depression that are commonly encountered in clinical practice. Each of the chapters can be read as a compact treatment manual for a particular manifestation of depression. The adaptations of CT that are covered are both evidence based (i.e., empirically supported) and clinically flexible. Although the chapters differ in their recommendations, they share a common theoretical and philosophical model of psychopathology and change in psychotherapy: namely, a cognitive theory of psychopathology and therapy in which maladaptive information processing is central to understanding the onset, course, and treatment of depression (Clark, Beck, & Alford, 1999). It is this cognitive theory, and not whether an intervention is labeled a "cognitive" intervention (vs. a behavioral, interpersonal, or some other intervention), that "provides a unifying theoretical framework within which the clinical techniques of other established, validated approaches may be properly incorporated" (Alford & Beck, 1997, p. 112).

Clinicians and researchers from across the globe have contributed to the book, reflecting international developments in adapting CT for various presentations of depression. This book, therefore, comprises a wealth of information regarding the evolution of CT for depression over the past 30 years. The guidelines offered on adapting CT for the varying, and often challenging, presentations of depression commonly encountered in clinical practice not only should improve clinical outcome, but should also serve as a foundation for future developments in cognitive theory and therapy for depression.

REFERENCES

Alford, B. A., & Beck, A. T. (1997). *The integrative power of cognitive therapy.* New York: Guilford Press.

Beck, A. T., Rush, A. J., Shaw, B. F., & Emery, G. (1979). *Cognitive therapy of depression.* New York: Guilford Press.

Clark, D. A., Beck, A. T., & Alford, B. A. (1999). *Scientific foundations of cognitive theory and therapy of depression.* Hoboken, NJ: Wiley.

Corruble, E., Ginestet, D., & Guelfi, J. D. (1996). Comorbidity of personality disorders and unipolar major depression: A review. *Journal of Affective Disorders, 37,* 157–170.

Gloaguen, V., Cottraux, J., Cucherat, M., & Blackburn, I.-M. (1998). A meta-analysis of the effects of cognitive therapy in depressed patients. *Journal of Affective Disorders, 49,* 59–72.

Hamilton, K. E., & Dobson, K. S. (2002). Cognitive therapy of depression: Pretreatment patient predictors of outcome. *Clinical Psychology Review, 22,* 875–893.

Hirschfeld, R. M. A., Montgomery, S. A., Keller, M. B., Kasper, S., Schatzberg, A. F., Moller, H.-J., et al. (2000). Social functioning in depression: A review. *Journal of Clinical Psychiatry, 61,* 268–275.

Hollon, S. D., Thase, M. E., & Markowitz, J. C. (2002). Treatment and prevention of depression. *Psychological Science in the Public Interest, 3,* 39–77.

Kessler, R. C., Berglund, P., Demler, O., Jin, R., Koretz, D., Merikangas, K. R., et al. (2003). The epidemiology of major depressive disorder: Results from the National Comorbidity Survey Replication (NCS-R). *JAMA, 289,* 3095–3105.

Kessler, R. C., Mickelson, K. D., & Williams, D. R. (1999). The prevalence, distribution, and mental health correlates of perceived discrimination in the United States. *Journal of Health and Social Behavior, 40,* 208–230.

Kessler, R. C., Nelson, C. B., McGonagle, K. A., Liu, J., Swartz, M., & Blazer, D. G. (1996). Comorbidity of DSM-III-R major depressive disorder in the general population: Results form the U.S. National Comorbidity Survey. *British Journal of Psychiatry, 168,* 17–30.

Stevens, D. E., Merikangas, K. R., & Merikangas, J. R. (1995). Comorbidity of depression and other medical conditions. In E. E. Beckham & W. R. Leber (Eds.), *Handbook of depression* (2nd ed., pp. 147–199). New York: Guilford Press.

Whisman, M. A. (1993). Mediators and moderators of change in cognitive therapy of depression. *Psychological Bulletin, 114,* 248–265.

Zimmerman, M., & Chelminski, I. (2003). Clinical recognition of anxiety disorders in depressed outpatients. *Journal of Psychiatric Research, 37,* 325–333.

CONTENTS

I

FOUNDATIONS OF
COGNITIVE THERAPY
FOR DEPRESSION

1

COGNITIVE THERAPY FOR DEPRESSION

Keith S. Dobson

Cognitive therapy (CT) was first named and identified as a distinct type of treatment in an article in 1970 (Beck, 1970), in which Aaron Beck described CT, and distinguished it from behavior therapy, based on the increased attention paid to negative thinking in CT and the importance of core negative beliefs, also seen to be pivotal in the genesis of depression. In the mid-1970s, Beck and colleagues engaged in the first trial of this new form of treatment for depression (Rush, Beck, Kovacs, & Hollon, 1977; Rush, Hollon, Beck, & Kovacs, 1978). In a trial that compared the efficacy of CT relative to antidepressant medication, superior outcomes were reported for CT, particularly at the follow-up assessment. It is fair to say that these results caused a minor sensation in the fields of psychiatry and psychology: first, because the results presented a credible research trial that challenged the "gold standard" of medications for depression, and second, because they provided a manualized treatment that could, in principle, be evaluated and then disseminated. In the wake of the discussion about the research trial, the publication of *Cognitive Therapy of Depression* (Beck, Rush, Shaw, & Emery, 1979) led to widespread interest in CT. Indeed, although the book is now over 25 years old, it is still widely used as a training manual and stands as the definitive description of this treatment approach to depression.

This chapter provides a description of the fundamental aspects of CT for depression, including its typical course and the prototypical interventions used in this treatment model. Finally, toward the end of this chapter, some of the essential research outcomes associated with CT of depression are presented.

THE COGNITIVE THEORY OF DEPRESSION

CT rests on a theoretical model of human functioning that has been elaborated over the years. This model is based on a Realist epistemology (Dobson & Dozois, 2001; Held, 1995), which asserts that reality exists independent of human experience. At the same time, the model holds that humans are "natural scientists" and seek to make sense of the world and their experiences, through the development of broad, organizational cognitive constructs. The constructs were typically defined as "core beliefs" or "underlying assumptions" in early descriptions of CT, but over the years the term "schema" (Kovacs & Beck, 1978) has come to predominate in the literature. Regardless of the specific term, the general concept imparted is that all individuals, through a combination of forces (personal experience, parenting, peer relations, media messages, popular culture), develop global, enduring representations of themselves, people in their world, and the way that the world functions. These cognitive representations may be accurate or distorted, but for individuals who eventually become depressed, they are characteristically negative. The relationship between negative thinking and depression has been generally supported in research (cf. Clark, Beck, & Alford, 1999), even though there continues to be a discussion about whether or not depressed persons are more "realistic" than nondepressed persons, and that the nondepressed part of the population perhaps distorts perceptions in an unduly positive direction (Ackermann & DeRubeis, 1991; Dobson & Franche, 1989). Negative representations often establish expectations for the self, or the self in relation to others in the world, that increase the risk of depressive ways of thinking and behaving.

The cognitive model is often discussed as a diathesis–stress model (Monroe & Simons, 1991; Robins & Block, 1989), reflecting the idea that negative core beliefs, assumptions, or schemas represent diatheses, or vulnerabilities, that then interact with life stress to eventuate in a process leading to depression (see Figure 1.1). There is consistent evidence that depression often is predicted by significant negative life events (Monroe & Simons,

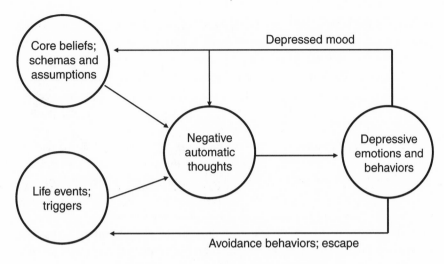

FIGURE 1.1. The cognitive model of depression.

1991). Some of these events are independent of the person's control, such as some interpersonal losses, but others may actually be inadvertently established or maintained by the depressed person him/herself (Davila, Hammen, Burge, Paley, & Daley, 1997; Joiner & Schmidt, 1998). For example, an individual who has developed a core belief of him/herself as a "loser," and as someone who cannot form an intimate relationship, may well avoid social situations or rebuff interpersonal advances. The resulting social isolation then becomes a life event that perpetuates the very negative belief of being an interpersonal "loser" that led to these behaviors in the first instance.

Regardless of whether the life events that interact with or trigger negative beliefs and assumptions are truly exogenous to the person, or whether in some unwitting way these events are the result of the depressed person's own actions, the cognitive model states that once the diathesis and stress have interacted, characteristically negative thinking emerges. This negative thinking may accurately reflect negative life events, but it is quite common in depression for this thinking to become negatively skewed, and possibly even to be at some variance with the actual events in the world. "Cognitive distortions," as they are called (Beck et al., 1979; J. S. Beck, 1995), can take a number of specific forms, including magnification of problems, minimization of success, jumping to conclusions, mind reading, black-and-white or absolutistic thinking, and labeling, among others. These distortion processes in turn lead to negative thinking in specific situations, or what may be termed "automatic thoughts." The term "automatic" refers to this thinking, because it is typified by reflexive and unquestioned appraisals based on the core beliefs that prompted them. Also, because negative thinking is congruent with depressed mood, these thought patterns are often seen as "reasonable" by the depressed person.

The cognitive model of depression further asserts that the negative automatic thoughts, or interpretations of situations, lead to specific feelings and behaviors. For example, the thought that one cannot take any positive action to solve problems leads to feelings of helplessness and a lack of action. The perception that one's problems will never improve can lead to feelings of hopelessness and escapist behaviors, including suicide. Finally, the model asserts that once a person starts to feel depressed, there is a feedback process, such that negative affect increases the probability of further negative thinking, and also reinforces negative beliefs and schemas. Feedback also occurs because depressive behaviors, such as avoidance and withdrawal, tend to increase the prospect of negative events through processes such as social isolation or social rejection (Coyne, 1976; Joiner, 2000).

The cognitive model of depression helps to explain why the typical complaints of depressed patients relate to their emotional experience and inability to cope with life's demands, because the emotional and behavioral aspects of depression are in some respects the "end" of the process of depression. The role of the cognitive therapist is to translate the problems of the patient who comes to treatment into a case formulation that explains the core beliefs or schemas that have interacted with life events to eventuate in the process leading to depression (Persons, 1989; Persons & Davidson, 2001; see also Whisman & Weinstock, Chapter 2, this volume). This case formulation then becomes the basis for deciding on strategic targets of change, with the goal of solving problems and reducing depression. Choosing which problems to address first in therapy is a matter of clinical experience and skill, but the case conceptualization guides this process.

ASSESSMENT

Although the focus of this chapter is on basic elements of the treatment of depression using CT, treatment invariably begins with an assessment process. The amount of information included in the assessment, its breadth and complexity, and its duration are determined by a number of factors, but the general features of the assessment plan include a diagnostic evaluation, measurement of the severity of problems, the development of a problem list, evaluation of the history of problems and past efforts to ameliorate these problems, consideration of patient strengths and resources, and assessment of other aspects of functioning that may be critical to develop a case formulation for the patient.

A large number of assessment tools exist for patients who present with a primary problem of depression. Dozois and Dobson (2002) provide an introduction to assessment of depression and the integration of assessment information into case formulation and planning (see also Whisman & Weinstock, Chapter 2, this volume). Another excellent resource is the book by Nezu, Ronan, Meadows, and McClure (2000), which provides a summary of major empirically based measures of depression. Clinicians who work in the general domain need to be conversant with the symptoms of depression and how these might be expressed in various cultural groups or specific populations. In addition, because depression often presents coincidentally with other conditions (e.g., anxiety disorders, substance use, personality disorders, suicide), the clinician who works in this domain should also know how to conduct assessments in these related areas and be ready to intervene or to refer, as appropriate.

GENERAL CHARACTERISTICS OF COGNITIVE THERAPY

Therapeutic Relationship

The therapeutic relationship has long been recognized as an important aspect of CT (Beck et al., 1979; J. S. Beck, 1995). CT is not something that is done *to* patients; it is a treatment that is done *with* them. Thus, CT emphasizes the development of a good working alliance between therapist and patient, and a collaborative partnership as the ideal way of working together. There are several ways in which the CT therapist tries to develop this type of relationship. First, the therapist enters the treatment process with an attitude of empathy and respect. Cognitive therapists recognize that depressed patients often come to treatment with a sense of personal failure and a need for help. The therapist conveys concern and caring, and an optimism that derives from both a general conviction that CT for depression is effective and competence with the approach. At the same time, another common perspective in CT is that the patient is the expert on his/her own life. Thus, though the cognitive therapist has knowledge and expertise, the patient's opinions need to be understood and respected, because it is he/she who has to implement any therapy ideas in the context of his/her life.

Psychoeducation

One important way that cognitive therapists develop a collaborative relationship is through the process of psychoeducation. Cognitive therapists generally want their patients to understand the treatment plan and, as far as they are able, to participate actively in establishing the course of treatment. A number of educational materials that highlight the model, value, and clinical utility of CT for depression have been developed for patients, including self-help books (Burns, 1980; Greenberger & Padesky, 1995; Young & Klosko, 1994), web-based materials (Academy of Cognitive Therapy, 2006), and computerized programs (Wright et al., 2002). Thus, in addition to the information that the therapist imparts over the course of therapy, a number of other methods exist to provide this information. It is often helpful to ask patients how they optimally learn new ideas (e.g., reading, video or audio materials, or direct experience), so that the therapist can tailor the delivery of psychoeducation to the patient's best advantage.

Psychoeducation is often a particular feature of early CT sessions. It is common during the initial session for the therapist to hear about difficulties or problems that fit fairly well into the CT model. These situations present the opportunity for the therapist to inform the patient about the role of thinking in depression, and possibly even to draw out a model of the patient's problem, using a diagram similar to Figure 1.1. This may also be an appropriate time to ask the patient whether he/she would like to read about the model. I like to assign Chapters 1 to 4 of *Feeling Good* (Burns, 1980) to interested patients, if they believe this is a reasonable task at this stage of therapy and for their level of depression.

Psychoeducation also takes place throughout the course of therapy. One of the defining characteristics of cognitive therapists is that they suggest to their patients what techniques or methods might be helpful to overcome depression, then obtain patients' reactions to these suggestions. Only if both therapist and patient think that the method might be helpful do they then collaboratively figure out how best to implement this idea, and work together to set appropriate homework. Through this process, the therapist needs to be able to describe the rationale for the techniques that he/she is proposing. This process also compels the patient to be more active in the treatment process, because he/she needs to think through what methods will and will not be effective, and to assume a role in the treatment implementation.

Homework

One of the hallmark features of CT for depression is the use of homework (Beck et al., 1979). Cognitive therapists generally believe that what happens between treatment sessions is *more* important than what goes on within the session (Kazantzis & Deane, 1999; Kazantzis, Deane, Ronan, & L'Abate, 2005; Tompkins, 2004). Thus, whereas the sessions are essential for identifying problems and teaching strategies to deal with these problems, it is the implementation of these strategies in the patient's actual life that represents successful treatment. Certainly, most cognitive therapists would maintain that "insight" attained within a session is relatively meaningless, unless it can be translated into a concrete and specific implementation plan. Furthermore, it has been demonstrated that early completion of homework is a predictor of positive outcome in CT for depression (Startup & Edmonds, 1994), so it is critical to assign homework, to monitor it, and to evaluate its intended and actual outcomes. CT therapists purposely assign some homework in the first session (whether it be reading or other tasks described below), in part for the value of being able to assess the patient's ability to carry through on agreed assignments. This assessment also serves as a model for following up on assigned work, and may also lead to a discussion about how to maximize the chances of homework completion (Detweiler & Whisman, 1999).

THE STRUCTURE OF A TYPICAL SESSION

Although the *content* of CT for depression varies dramatically from patient to patient, the *process* of therapy is relatively similar. Sessions typically last 50 minutes and are scheduled on a weekly basis, although it is not uncommon at the beginning of the treatment process (i.e., the first 3 or 4 weeks) to schedule two sessions a week for more severely depressed patients. Session scheduling and session time frames can be used flexibly, though. With more depressed patients, it may be more productive to have relatively shorter sessions more frequently at the beginning of treatment, then move toward a weekly schedule of sessions as the depression begins to lift. Also, it is fairly common for the assignments between one session and the next to become somewhat more elaborate and to need time for implementation as the treatment develops. In such a case, it may be that scheduling sessions too frequently does not permit the patient enough time to complete homework, and may be somewhat unproductive. Clinical judgment is required to ensure that sessions are frequent enough that positive momentum is maintained, but not so frequent that the patient feels that the steps between one session and the next are too small, or that therapy is too slow. Of course, issues such as holidays, financial considerations, or the limits imposed on therapy by managed care or insurance repayment programs, can also place restrictions on the ability to have regular sessions. Because of these practical considerations, it is important at the outset of treatment to discuss with the patient the approximate length of time that treatment takes (20–24 sessions in research trials, for outpatient depression), as well as the costs associated with treatment.

A typical CT session can be conceptualized as having three phases: a beginning, the "work," and wrapping up. Each part is discussed below, although it should be noted that the therapist might move forward or backward across these phases, if indicated. For example, one part of the beginning of each session is to set the agenda—to identify the topics to be discussed that session—before actually dealing with each in turn. Sometimes it turns out that a given topic is larger than anticipated at the beginning of the session, however, so therapist and patient should both feel comfortable renegotiating the agenda, if it becomes clear that it is not manageable within the available time frame.

The beginning part of a CT session itself has several components. Particularly in the earliest phases of CT for depression, therapists typically have patients complete a depression inventory, such as the Beck Depression Inventory—Second Edition (BDI-II; Beck, Steer, & Garbin, 1988); see also Nezu et al., 2000) prior to the start of the session. Thus, the beginning of the session consists of a check-in on functioning. Significant symptom changes are noted, and the causes of these changes might form part of the content of the session agenda, if it seems helpful. Indeed, cognitive therapists often capitalize on happenstance events that have a dramatic effect on the patient's functioning (negative and positive), because understanding these events helps them to develop the case conceptualization, to teach the CT model to the patient, to introduce new techniques, to develop the collaborative relationship, or simply to encourage to reflection about progress made during treatment.

In addition to the use of a questionnaire, CT therapists typically conduct a "mood check" with their patients, which comprises a 0- to 100-point rating of depression, with 0 as *Best ever,* and 100 as *Most depressed ever.* The mood check is a very "quick and dirty" assessment device, but it can be used to track mood across time, even within sessions. Also recommended, especially in the early stages of treatment for depression, is regular assessment of possible hopelessness and suicidality. If the therapist uses BDI-II as a presession measure, items 2 (pessimism) and 9 (suicidal thoughts or wishes) may be quickly reviewed to look for changes on these dimensions. Cognitive therapists who work with depressed patients should know not only local laws and ethical requirements about suicide but also the risk factors for suicidality, how to assess suicide risk, and how to use available resources effectively to mitigate suicide risk.

Following a brief review of the patient's functioning, and in the absence of a suicidal crisis that may warrant attention in its own right, the next part of the beginning phase of a CT session most often deals with the homework. General success or problems with the assigned homework are reviewed, and the lessons learned may be briefly stated, or the assignment itself might be put on the agenda for further discussion. Certainly, if the homework was not completed, if there were major problems with its implementation, or if there was a major benefit from the homework, it is likely to be put on the formal agenda.

The therapist also inquires whether the patient has brought any particular issue to the session that he/she wants to discuss. This issue might be something learned over the course of therapy, a recent difficulty, or an impending problem. The issue is named, then put on the list of agenda topics. In addition, the therapist may have items that he/she wants to put on the agenda. For example, it may be an appropriate point in the course of therapy for the therapist to introduce a particular technique, and if so, the therapist can introduce this idea at the beginning of the session and formally ask to schedule part of the session for this purpose.

Having identified the possible topics for the agenda, the therapist typically briefly reviews the list out loud, and asks the patient whether the agenda is reasonable for the time available. If not, it may be necessary either to limit discussion of some topics purposely or to drop them from the agenda completely for that session, to permit more time for more important topics. Generally, about two or three items is a good limit for a single session. A topic eliminated from one session is most often carried over to the next session, when the therapist asks the patient if it is a continuing concern. A common strategy used by cognitive therapists is to ask the patient for his/her perception of the most important topic in terms of reducing depression, and to start with that topic. Other topics can be similarly ordered by importance. General principles demonstrated through this strategy include spending the most time where there is likely maximal benefit, working on issues of high import to the patient, and collaboration between therapist and patient.

The second phase of a CT session consists of "the work." This phase involves turning to each agenda item in sequence, examining the issues/problems that are present, and using CT techniques to help the patient to understand better the dynamics of the problem, and to try to overcome the problem. The therapist needs to transition from an assessment mode as each new topic is introduced and discussed, to an intervention mode, once some useful technique becomes apparent. Knowing what to ask about and how to collect useful assessment information are skills that requires considerable experience, just as knowing when to stop the assessment and start the intervention is a matter of skill and practice. Furthermore, a wide range of techniques can, in principle, be employed in CT, and the skillful selection of techniques is perhaps one of the most challenging aspects of CT. Doing all

of these things, while fostering a collaborative and efficient working therapeutic relationship, is a complex endeavor that requires considerable interpersonal skill, knowledge of the CT model, training, and experience.

The actual content of "the work" phase of a CT varies depending on
the patient's level of depression; his/her progress in treatment; the case conceptualization; and the presence of acute stressors, comorbid problems, and
other factors. Examples of typical content in CT for depression are offered
below. From a process perspective, though, it is important to note that as
each content issue is discussed, and as therapist and patient come to some
resolution, they will most often work together to develop a homework
assignment in which the patient implements the ideas discussed in the session in his/her actual life. Important questions for the therapist to consider
when assigning homework follow:

1. Is the general nature and purpose of the homework clear to both
   the therapist and patient?
2. Is the homework planned for a specific time and place?
3. Will it be obvious when the homework is/is not completed?
4. Have possible deterrents or impediments to completing the homework been evaluated and problem-solved, if necessary?
5. Did the patient make an active commitment to attempt the homework?
6. Are the expected benefits of the homework clear to both patient
   and therapist? (Kazantzis et al., 2005).

Towards the end of the session, the therapist should note that time is
winding down (or that the issues put on the agenda have been discussed).
With the patient's participation, he/she should review the entire session,
including the main themes, as well as the specific homework assignments
that have emerged. The therapist may invite the patient to summarize the
session, because this process both involves the patient and helps the therapist
to ensure that what he/she sees as the key elements are appreciated by the
patient. Such reviews can sometimes also identify that the patient has mis-
construed or reinterpreted the work done in the session, and so provides an
opportunity for the therapist not only to use this information in the case
conceptualization but also to correct these misperceptions. For example, if a
patient failed to do homework, and the therapist includes the homework on
the agenda and further inquires at length about the patient's reasons for not
completing the homework, it is possible that in the session review the
patient may have the idea, "You are disappointed with me because I didn't

do my homework." The therapist may use this type of misunderstanding (assuming the therapist is in fact not disappointed) to find out whether he/she did something to signal such a reaction to the patient, whether the patient is oversensitive to the issue of criticism, or to show how the patient tends to perceive disappointment or rejection from others based on minimal information.

Sometimes the summary and homework review reveal that the plan is too ambitious. In such cases it is better to reduce the overall homework to maximize the chances for successful completion of those items that are left on the list (Detweiler & Whisman, 1999). One way to accomplish this goal is to keep certain key issues as homework, but place everything else in a "bonus" category, that is clearly conceptualized as extra, and not part of the key homework. It is also often a good idea to have the homework written down, because this action reinforces the activities to the patient. Other benefits of writing include the ability to make sure the homework is clearly understood and to serve as a memory aid to the patient between sessions. Homework can be recorded in lots of different ways, including on index cards, on sheets of paper, on Post-it notes, in a binder, on an electronic organizer, in a computer file, on a voice recorder, or in a therapy notebook. The therapist should ask the patient about his/her preferred method, because it is the one that maximizes chances for him/her to attempt the homework. The therapist should also record the homework in his/her therapy notes, to be able to inquire about this aspect of therapy at the beginning of the next session.

Before the patient leaves, it is helpful to ask briefly if he/she has any other reactions to the session. A positive predictor of treatment response in CT for depression is early completion of homework (Burns & Nolen-Hoeksema, 1991), so if the patient expresses some enthusiasm for attempting the homework, the therapist can reinforce this reaction. Patient reactions to sessions may also be used to gauge whether any therapy relationship issues need to be addressed in future sessions. For example, a recent patient of mine indicated that she was "a control freak" and wanted to be in charge of most relationships. Being in a potentially "one down" position as patient was a challenge to her sense of autonomy and control, so I was careful to involve her fully in all major decisions. Even so, the patient reported discomfort with therapy at the end of one session, because she felt "stupid" and "incompetent" learning about new ways to approach her life issues. This report helped me to build the case conceptualization and also allowed us to discuss the issue openly, and circumvent a potential impediment to treatment.

THE TYPICAL COURSE OF THERAPY

Although the description of the *process* of CT sessions is important to learn and to use in treating depression, none of the processes I have discussed really address the *content* of the treatment of depression, or what I described earlier as "the work" phase of treatment. Unfortunately, there is no single "cookbook" or formula for treating depression. Every patient is unique and presents with his/her particular history, past efforts to overcome depression, comorbid problems, schemas, and current resources. What is presented below, therefore, is more of an overall guide to typical phases of CT for depression (cf. Beck et al., 1979; J. S. Beck, 1995, 2005; Gilbert, 2001; see also Beutler, Clarkin, & Bongar, 2000).

One way to conceptualize the overall treatment of depression is as a series of three loosely connected phases. These phases tend to have different treatment targets; therefore, they require somewhat different intervention techniques or methods. It is important to note, however, that these are not lockstep phases, because the targets of intervention in one domain may continue for some time into therapy, even while other areas of intervention are introduced. Furthermore, if the course of treatment is not steadily in the positive direction, it may in some cases be necessary to "go back" to issues and interventions used earlier in the process of treatment.

Figure 1.2 is an attempt to show how these phases of treatment roughly relate to symptom change in a "typical" case of depression. Approximately the first one-third of treatment is focused on behavioral change; the middle one-third of treatment, on negative automatic thoughts; and the final one-third of treatment is focused on the assessment and modification of core beliefs and schemas. Typically, the first phase of treatment is associated with the greatest reduction in depressive symptomatology, because over half of the changes in symptomatology takes place within the first six sessions of treatment. The second phase of treatment is usually associated with more gradual but continued reduction in levels of depression. Patients typically transition from meeting the diagnostic criteria for major depression to no longer meeting such criteria during this middle phase of treatment. By implication, the third phase of treatment is largely conducted with a patient whose depression has recently remitted. Here, the focus shifts to understanding the genesis of the most recent or of other, past episodes of depression, examining vulnerabilities for future relapse or recurrence, and providing interventions that emphasize relapse prevention. Each of these phases is described in turn below, along with a description of some of the typical interventions.

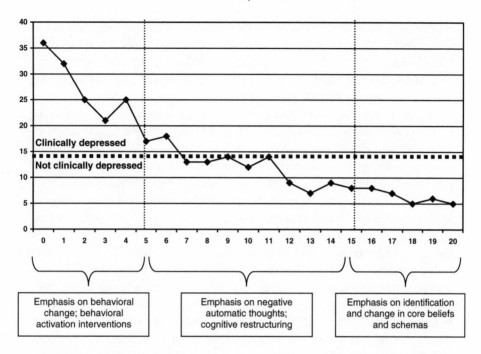

FIGURE 1.2. Hypothetical progress in CT for depression (based on BDI-II scores), and targets of intervention.

The Early Phase of Treatment

The first aspects of CT for depression emphasize increasing the engagement of the patient in his/her environment and restoring functioning as quickly as possible. Decreased motivation, low energy, and tendencies toward avoidance or social withdrawal are all primary features of depression that need to be addressed if other cognitive work is to be effective. The goals of this phase of CT, though, are not only to increase activity and reduce depression levels but also to begin using various activities to generate a CT conceptualization of the case.

Some common methods are used in working with depressed patients in the earliest phase of CT. For example, most therapists want to understand the patient's typical day: how active he/she is during the day; his/her sleep cycles; and any unusual patterns in the patient's arousal or activity patterns. The therapist can gain this information by inquiring about a typical day, or a recent specific day, but such information is subject to presentational biases on the part of the patient, his/her embarrassment about activity patterns, depression–related distortions, memory problems, or simple forgetting some activities. For these reasons, cognitive therapists commonly ask patients to complete an activity schedule as homework following the first session. This assignment may be used more systematically to record patients' activities, because it requests that they indicate major activity in 1-hour time slots throughout each day. Some therapists also ask patients to indicate activities that are associated with mood changes, so that they can see which activities have positive or negative associations for patients. Another possible strategy is to ask patients to track events associated with mastery (success, accomplishment) or pleasure (fun, enjoyment), both to determine the frequency of such activities in patients' lives and to see whether their occurrence is associated with changes in the patients' moods. Indeed, activity schedules can be used to track any type of event or activity that the therapist and patient think might be related to changes in mood.

In addition to the benefits of monitoring the relationship between activities and mood, use of a more structured activity scheduling exercise offers three other advantages. First, it is an explicit example of the use of homework in CT, which the therapist should have described as a key part of the treatment. Second, it offers an "incidental" way to assess the patient's ability to enact agreed to homework. As described earlier, one of the principles relative to homework is that the therapist should always inquire about it at the start of the next session. As such, the assignment of activity monitoring in the first session can be a fairly easy way to socialize the patient into the process of homework. Third, the evaluation of activities is a natural precursor to scheduling specific activities that use the same activity schedule method.

Activity scheduling is typically done as a graded activity. As such, the first scheduled activities are simple tasks that can be accomplished in fairly discrete time periods. These may be "stand-alone" events or activities (e.g., pay the bills), or they might constitute the first steps in an elaborate, multistage process that needs to be planned over a series of weeks (e.g., systematic financial planning and budget setting). Either way, the activities need to be perceived as relevant to the patient's overall goals. They also need to be sufficiently challenging to the patient, at his/her current level of depression, to be seen as a success experience, but not so daunting as to prove impossible. It is relatively common for depressed patients (especially in the early stages of treatment) to perceive that they need to accomplish a lot, to set unreasonable goals as a consequence, then become frustrated and "give up." The therapist's role is to help the patient set reasonable goals, and to stage activity scheduling to be successful.

Activity scheduling provides an opportunity to examine patients' tendencies to predict future outcomes and to judge past ones. A common part of activity scheduling is to ask patients to predict their likely ability to do the assigned activity, as well as the likely outcome if they do so. If the patient makes a negative prediction, the therapist can ask some questions to determine whether this prediction represents a negative bias or might have some factual basis. If there is a good reason for concern, then therapist and patient can scale down or reconsider the homework it in its entirety. Sometimes the exercise of predicting the outcome of homework reveals an impediment to completion of the homework. If so, patient and therapist can problem solve the issues that are implicated, and either reassign or revise the homework. For example, sometimes it becomes clear through these discussions that the patient lacks some required social skill or other behavioral competence to do an assignment, and behavioral coaching or instruction may be necessary as a prerequisite to assigning the activity. Sometimes, a patient may have the apparent skill to complete the homework, but predicts no benefits, even if they exist. In such cases, the therapist can reevaluate with the patient whether this prediction is valid or yet another example of depressive thinking that needs to be evaluated against the experience of actually doing the homework. Another advantage of having the patient predict the likely success of behavioral assignments is that these predictions can then be contrasted with the patient's success with the homework assignment. It is fairly common for depressed patients to succeed with homework (if it is skillfully set), but then to minimize its value or their role in its successful completion. If this tendency toward minimization occurs, it is important for the therapist to ensure that the "facts" are established, so that the patient is compelled to give him/herself the deserved credit for homework completion. Also, if a patient is identified as someone who does not make internal attributions for success, this tendency can be incorporated into the next behavioral assignment, with the therapist acting as a kind of "guard" against minimization or externalization of successes. Importantly, a discovered tendency to minimize can be used as part of the emerging case conceptualization. For example, it is likely that a patient who predicts difficulties in life's tasks and/or minimizes success has some general sense of inadequacy or incompetence. Discovery of the domains in which these issues emerge help to sharpen the therapist's understanding of the patient's particular vulnerabilities and depressive schemas.

In addition to behavioral activation, another general technique in the early phase of CT is problem solving, which is particularly useful when the nature of the problem(s) a patient brings to therapy seem to be based more on verifiable events and less on negative core beliefs. For example, an immigrant coping with the stresses and strains of life in a new country, who shows signs of depression due to this adjustment, may be better served by a focus on language training and connection with social service agencies than by a focus on negative thinking. Activity scheduling is often a part of the successful treatment of patients with real-life stressors, but the focus on negative thinking is likely to be less than that in patients with fewer objective stressors.

Often specific symptoms or problems commonly associated with depression respond well to focused behavioral interventions. Sleep disturbance, for example, can often be ameliorated with several behavioral rules, such as the development of a regular sleep cycle, a change in bedtime habits, use of the bed only for sleep and sex, not permitting naps, or a change in the sleep environment (e.g., removing televisions or other distractions, ensuring the bedroom is as quiet and dark as possible), but cognitive interventions are also helpful (cf. Harvey, 2005). Low appetite can often be improved by setting regular meals, disallowing snacking, improving the quality of the food ingested (e.g., fewer carbohydrates), and spending more time with food preparation (as opposed to eating fast foods). Low energy can be addressed through a gradual increase in physical activity, recognizing and adjusting to normal diurnal rhythms of the body, planning for improved food and nutrient intake, and better sleep. Paying attention to negative predictions or beliefs in each domain and overcoming these cognitive sets as problem(s) improve often are important parts of treatment.

The Middle Phase of Treatment

Once the patient is more active and involved in his/her environment, the focus of therapy quickly shifts to cognitive assessment and restructuring. The term "cognitive restructuring" refers to a large number of interventions that generally focus on situation-specific (as opposed to underlying, broad, or trait-like) negative thinking. As noted earlier, depressed patients can perceive the world accurately or in a distorted fashion (Beck et al., 1979; J. S. Beck, 1995; Clark et al., 1999), and the identification of a variety of cognitive distortions and the use of clinical tools to challenge distorted *automatic thoughts* (ATs) are hallmark features of CT. As such, a significant part of CT for depression is spent educating patients about this process and helping them to recognize negative ATs and to evaluating them in real time, so that the spiraling effect of these thought patterns is disrupted.

The role of negative ATs in depression is usually discussed in the first session, when the therapist provides a broad overview of CT. Therefore, when the therapist is prepared to actually identify and work with a specific negative AT, the patient has already been introduced to the concept. At the point in treatment when the therapist begins to work on cognitive restructuring, it is often particularly useful to teach the patient to ask at the time he/she notice a shift in mood, "What was going through my mind?" (J. S. Beck, 1995). This question helps the patient to recognize that ATs mediate emotional and behavioral responses to life events. Some therapists also assign reading, which can help the patient to recognize this process (Burns, 1980; Greenberger & Padesky, 1995). If it seems appropriate, some therapists may also reprint and review with the patient a list of common cognitive distortions (J. S. Beck, 1995, p. 119).

A common intervention in CT for depression is use of the Dysfunctional Thoughts Record (DTR; see Figure 1.3; note that other variations exist). Once the patient has been introduced to the concept of negative ATs and has recognized its possible relevance to him/herself, the therapist suggests a more formal written record of these processes, to help both patient and therapist to examine this process more fully. The therapist introduces the DTR, and encourages the patient to start to write down both events that trigger negative reactions, such as negative ATs, and such as negative emotional and behavioral reactions themselves. After practicing with the DTR in session, the patient is given the homework assignment of completing the DTR between sessions, when he/she notices an increase in depression (or other negative moods). Subsequent sessions are spent reviewing the DTR, including problems with its completion, and helping the patient to increase his/her understanding of the nature of, and associations among, problematic or triggering events, ATs, and changes in mood and behavior.

Once the patient has some fluency with the DTR, and can consistently collect this type of information, it is possible to move to the step of intervening with these thoughts. Interventions generally involve the patient reconsidering his/her negative thoughts based on three sets of questions generally framed as "What's the evidence?," "Is there an alternative?," and "So what?" In some cases, one of these questions has the most utility, but it is useful to introduce each line of questioning, so that the patient has the full set of skills before the end of treatment. Each question is discussed briefly below.

The "What's the evidence?" question requires the patient systematically to evaluate the facts, data, or evidence related to each thought. Implicit in this question is a stance that cognitive therapists do not accept a thought as true simply because it has occurred. The idea that "a thought is not a fact" is in fact itself a metamessage that supports a more detailed analysis of negative thinking. Sometimes a problem has a high degree of evidentiary support,

Date and Time	Situation	Automatic Thoughts	Emotional Responses	Behavioral Responses	Cognitive Distortions	Alternative Thoughts	Alternative Responses

Note. To generate alternative thoughts, consider the following:
1. The evidence that supports or refutes the original automatic thoughts,
2. Whether any other more reasonable or alternative thoughts are possible in the situation, or
3. Whether the original meaning or importance of the situation is the only possible way to think about it.

FIGURE 1.3. The Dysfunctional Thought Record.

which may suggest the need for a more problem-solving orientation relative to these negative thoughts. In depression, though, it is common for patients to exaggerate or overstate the negative aspects of an event, or to minimize the positive aspects. In these cases, examining the evidence that supports and refutes the original negative AT can be very helpful, both to expose patients to this line of inquiry about their thinking and to generate a realistic appraisal of the positive and negative features of an event or situation.

Sometimes the process of examining the evidence related to a negative thought reveals that the patient clearly does not have much evidence on which to base his/her negative AT. Mind reading and jumping to negative conclusions, two common distortion patterns seen in depression, are typically based on insufficient evidence. Such revelations can lead to the assignment of behavioral experiments as homework to establish more fully the "facts" related to the negative thoughts. Such homework increases the patient's contact with his/her environment and provides a more realistic basis on which to deal with problems.

The second question, "Is there an alternative?" requires the patient to consider whether there is an alternative thought or explanation to the original thought. This alternative sometimes become obvious once the evidence related to an AT has been examined. Thus, if the patient's original negative thoughts can be demonstrated to be out of alignment with the "facts," then a more realistic alternative can be generated (note, however, that the cognitive therapist aims not for an alternative that is distorted in a positive direction, but for one that is in keeping with the available information).

In other cases the situation is ambiguous and open to alternative interpretations, thus making it possible to generate a series of alternative interpretations or ATs. A therapist pointing out the choice of alternative thoughts is itself sometimes revelatory to patients, and the exercise of generating these alternatives often takes the "sting" out of the first, typically depressive, cognition. Some patients report that with the recognition of alternatives, the original thought is just one of many, that has no special priority or valence. In other cases, the patient may benefit from being asked how someone else might interpret the situation. The therapist can also offer some alternative ideas, although he/she must always be sure to evaluate whether patients accept or reject these alternatives, and why. When the interpretation of the event remains unclear, the therapist might design homework to collect the necessary evidence, then weigh these alternative ideas and see which one best fits the facts.

The third question used to explore negative ATs is "So what?" It requires patients to explore the meaning they have assigned to the AT, and to determine whether this is the only possible meaning. For example, a depressed student who fails an examination might jump to the conclusion that his academic career is doomed, and that this dismal career path confirms his inadequacy. He might be asked to reconsider whether the meaning he has attached to this interpretation is valid, however. In effect, the therapist is asking him to step outside his usual way of viewing things, to say to himself, "So what if I failed this exam?", and to realize that he does not have to jump to the conclusion that because he has failed, he has no academic future or career prospects. It should be recognized that this is a difficult question, though, because it requires the patient to adopt a different perspective on his/her difficult situation. Asking this question is almost like asking the patient to suspend his/her usual beliefs about the world and to determine whether the meanings he/she first applied to the event are valid.

The "So what?" question should not be employed too early in the treatment of depression, because it often exposes the patient's core beliefs or meaning structures. If this work is done too early in therapy, it may confirm for the patient the hopelessness of his/her situation *and* core beliefs. Depressed patients often struggle with accepting alternative thoughts that are not consistent with being depressed, so patients may perceive the "So what?" question as the reflection of an uncaring or misunderstanding thera- pist, if it is employed before the client–therapist relationship has time to solidify. Even when examining specific negative ATs, the "So what?" ques- tion is typically used only after the first two sessions of therapy have been completed, because addressing this question too early can lead to a kind of rigid defense of the original ATs. Also, changing negative ATs based on the first two questions is somewhat more straightforward than an examination of the meanings a patient has assigned to an event.

The Final Phase of Treatment

The cognitive model of depression assumes that individuals who become depressed generally have schemas or core beliefs that make them vulnerable to precipitating events (Young, Klosko, & Weishaar, 2003). More generally, according to the cognitive model, everyone has schemas that are the heri- tage of early experience, cultural and media messages, peer relationships, a history of mental health or disorder, and other developmental issues. Hypothetically, every person has his/her own areas of schema vulnerability. These vulnerabilities remain "latent," however, unless activated by relevant or matching triggers. For example, a perfectionist is theoretically vulnerable to depression if he/she experiences failure or lack of perfection, but he/she does not demonstrate depression as long as his/her perfectionistic goals are met.

As I noted earlier, by the time that an intervention addressing core beliefs takes place in CT, the patient often is no longer clinically depressed. Rather, he or she is most likely a recently recovered depressed patient, or "in remission" (American Psychiatric Association, 2000). Many patients continue to exhibit residual symptoms (Gollan, Raffety, Gortner, & Dobson, 2005; Paykel et al., 2005), and the gradual elimination of these symptoms remains an important goal of treatment, if possible. At the same time, the focus of therapy often naturally shifts to an examination of broader themes that have emerged over the course of treatment, to the identification of risk factors that led the patient to develop depression, and to a consideration of relapse prevention. Within the CT framework, this work is accomplished through the assessment and intervention addressing core beliefs.

Assessment of core beliefs may be accomplished with a number of methods. Often, patients' beliefs emerge through consideration of the distressful situations they describe. For example, if a patient consistently reports thoughts about being judged harshly by others, it is fairly easy to identify a core belief related to concerns about inadequacy and/or a harsh social environment. Sometimes, patients realize these themes themselves and spontaneously report them to the therapist. Other times, the therapist sees the patient's interpretive consistency across situations and can offer a tentative interpretation of this behavior as a reflection of an underlying or core belief. One strategy to accomplish this type of awareness is through a review of the various types of events that have led to similar distressful reactions over the course of therapy. Patient and therapist can engage in a mental "factor analysis" to look for common meanings ascribed to these events and that bind them together.

A specific technique developed to determine the broader implications that a patient assigns to difficult situations is called the "downward arrow technique" (Burns, 1980). This technique begins with the identification of a set of negative thoughts related to a specific situation. Rather than examining the evidence or generating alternative thoughts to dispute these negative ATs, however, the therapist asks the patient to entertain the thought for the moment that his/her negative thoughts are realistic and that no alternative thoughts exist. The therapist then asks the patient to generate the logical conclusion from this idea; in effect, the therapist asks, "So what if these thoughts were true?," but without any effort to resist negative thoughts that might emerge. For example, a gay male patient wanted to form a new intimate relationship, but after an initial date, the other man refused to provide his phone number. The patient automatically thought, "He has rejected me." The patient was asked to consider what it meant if he was actually rejected, and he quickly responded that he was likely never to see the man again. When asked to consider the implication of this second "fact," the patient said it meant that he would likely be alone again for a while. He generalized the implication of this "fact" to mean that he likely would never be in another relationship, which meant he could never be fully happy in his life, and that he was probably an unlovable person. Thus, through the examination of the "downward" implications of a single rejection event, it became clear that this patient's underlying belief was one of unlovability, even though part of his prescription for lifetime happiness was being in a loving relationship.

The downward arrow technique can be employed in real–life situations and is effective when used with reference to recent, acutely distressing situations. It can also be employed in hypothetical situations, however: "What would it mean to you if . . . ?" The therapist can also conduct a downward arrow analysis of a real, recent life event, then modify it slightly in the patient's imagination to see whether the same or different implications are generated. The strategy of generating hypothetical circumstances similar to actual events is an efficient way to identify subtle aspects of core beliefs, without waiting for these events to actually occur. Yet another, more risky, strategy for identifying core beliefs is to design homework to test out their possible operation. In the previous example, it might have been possible to get the male patient to agree to attempt another date, while paying attention to any activation of anxiety or fear of rejection that might be underpinned by a belief of unlovability. Through the examination of such repeated events, the activity of core beliefs can be exposed.

All of these strategies are effective in the assessment or identification of core beliefs that operate across a number of specific situations or events in the patient's life. It is worth noting that the timing of these assessments is a critical clinical decision. It is relatively easy to use the downward arrow, for example, particularly if the patient is already somewhat distressed and the negative automatic thoughts are accessible. Typically, though, the technique ends with the patient recognizing that he/she has a negative core belief. Thus, if this technique is used too early in the course of therapy, before the patient has some resiliency, and/or his or her depression levels have already been ameliorated to some extent, the patient may possibly feel worse after the technique. On the other hand, if the therapist waits until the treatment has progressed too far, the patient may have difficulty accepting the "So what?" question at face value, and may not be able to generate the negative interpretations that might have emerged earlier in the course of therapy. Thus, it is a matter of some skill to use this type of technique early enough in treatment that some of the patient's negative thinking is still accessible, but not too early to expose a raw belief that might be overwhelming to the patient.

Once negative beliefs have been identified, the therapist needs to help the patient to complete his/her own case conceptualization. This understanding is essential to any belief change that the therapist might attempt. One strategy is for the therapist to share with the patient the case conceptualization that he/she has generated. This model may be drawn in the form of Figure 1.1, if that would be helpful to the patient. Other diagrammatic ways to represent the cognitive case conceptualization (e.g., J. S. Beck, 1995) review early historical factors related to the emergence of core beliefs, the life assumptions that the patient has adopted (typically in the form of conditional assumptions, as in "If I am unlovable, then I need to stay out of relationships"), and the situations seen in therapy that conform to the conceptualization.

In addition to the clinically derived case conceptualization methods described earlier, it is also possible to use questionnaires to identify core beliefs. Three such measures include the Dysfunctional Attitudes Scale (DAS; Beck, Brown, Steer, & Weissman, 1991), the Sociotropy–Autonomy Scale (SAS; Bieling, Beck, & Brown, 2004; Clark & Beck, 1991), and the Schema Questionnaire (SQ; Young & Brown, 1990). The DAS yields endorsements of a series of potentially dysfunctional attitudes, written in the form of conditional statements. It has been factor-analyzed into two main dimensions, related to Performance Evaluation and Approval by Others (Cane, Olinger, Gotlib, & Kuiper, 1986). The SAS was created specifically to assess sociotropic (interpersonally dependent) and autonomy-related (achievement) beliefs, and this factor structure has also been supported in research (Clark & Beck, 1991). The SQ was rationally developed to measure 11 different types of schemas, and is related to Young's schema therapy–focused version of CT (Young & Brown, 1990; Young et al., 2003). The SQ has the clinical utility to differentiate among these schematic dimensions (Schmidt, Joiner, Young, & Telch, 1995). It yields a rich assessment of core beliefs/schemas and can be used as an adjunct to the clinical derivation of schemas to buttress or challenge the emerging case formulation.

Once the conceptualization of the core beliefs has been accomplished, and patient and therapist concur about their roles in the development of dysfunctional thinking, behavior, and emotional patterns, the question shifts to one of change. This process starts with the identification of a reasonable alternative belief to the dysfunctional one that has been identified. It is critical that this alternative belief be one that is attainable and desired by the patient. Therapist and patient can discuss the advantages and disadvantages of both the original and alternative beliefs from the perspective of short- and long-term consequences. Often this analysis reveals certain historical and/or short-term advantages but long term disadvantages of the dysfunctional beliefs, including increased risk of depression. The alternatives typically have better long-term consequences but often entail short-term discomfort and anxiety, changes in social relations, and even a "personal revolution," if the degree and type of change is dramatic.

If the patient remains committed to change after the discussion of the implications of changing core beliefs, then a number of techniques can be adopted, including public declarations of the intent to change, clarifying the "old" and "new" ways to think and act (or even to dress and talk), or changing relationships and the personal environment so that they are more consistent with the new schema that is being cultivated. One particularly powerful change method, the "as if" technique, involves discussing how a patient would think and act if he/she had truly internalized the new belief, then structuring behavioral homework "as if" the patient had actually done so. This technique potentially allows the patient to discover that he/she can live life using the new beliefs. It also has a reasonable probability of engendering negative reactions from others in the social environment, so these reactions must be anticipated. Part of this planning may include discussion of assertive ways for the patient to communicate his/her desire for change and the need to modify others' cognitions or beliefs about him/her.

Sometimes the discussion of the implications of schema change leads a patient to reconsider the advisability of changing his/her schemas. For example, a patient who has previously seen herself as incompetent and has developed interpersonal relationships that support this belief (i.e., in which others also view her as incompetent) may wish to change this self-schema. Although such a change has definite benefits for her, it also carries the risk of interpersonal stress and rejection from people in her current social circle. Thus, there is a "cost" associated with schema change, even if the long-term benefits are quite positive. From my perspective, it is entirely the patient's right to step away from schema change. The therapist's obligations in such an instance are not only to validate the patient's right to make that decision but also to discuss the implications of this decision, including the risk of relapse. The clinical focus then becomes one of accepting and coping with ongoing negative beliefs. In such cases, it is also important to encourage the patient's continued use of the behavioral activation and cognitive restructuring techniques learned earlier in therapy.

Termination of CT for depression typically involves a review process, as well as a planning phase. The review includes the case conceptualization, and the various techniques that the patient learned and used over the course of therapy. This review clarifies the extent to which initial treatment goals have been attained, and whether any goals remain. Sometimes, this review leads to the renegotiation of continued therapy for a short period of time, around a discrete goal, but more often it leads to a discussion of how life is an ongoing process that always involves change. Another typical process is planning for the future and anticipation of possible relapse (Bieling & Antony, 2003). This part of the termination process includes discussion about strategies to achieve ongoing goals, how to deal with ongoing or anticipated problems, how to recognize the early warning signs of depression, and how to keep the techniques the patient learned over the course of therapy active in his/her life. In the latter regard, one possible strategy is the use of a "self-session," in which the patient chooses a time to sit down and identify current issues, review cognitive and behavioral strategies to deal with these issues, and assign his/her own homework. Self-sessions also serve as a bridge to treatment termination, if the final sessions are spaced out over time.

It is often helpful to arrange one or more follow-up appointments (i.e., booster sessions) in the weeks following treatment discontinuation to see whether any new issues have emerged and to reinforce the lessons of treatment. Cognitive therapists typically predict risk of relapse or recurrence of depression and often have permissive rereferral policies that are predicated on the idea that learning new techniques takes time and practice, and that their role is not to "cure" the patient but to aid him/her in skills development and use. Because it is also not possible to anticipate all eventualities over the course of a single treatment process, sometimes a few booster sessions can be an effective way to supplement a course of CT for depression.

REVIEW OF EFFICACY RESEARCH

The Place of CT as an Empirically Supported Therapy for Depression

CT for depression has been subjected to a large number of investigations, some of which have examined CT in its own right, whereas others have compared CT to alternative treatments. The earliest comparative trial contrasted the efficacy of CT and that of tricyclic medication, and found that the two treatments had roughly equivalent outcomes (Rush et al., 1977, 1978). This early success lead to a number of trials, the most notable of which was the Treatments of Depression Comparative Research Program (TDCRP; Elkin et al., 1989) sponsored by the National Institute of Mental Health (NIMH). This large, multisite study compared CT to another short-term psychotherapy, interpersonal therapy (IPT; Klerman, Weissman, Rounsaville, & Chevron, 1984), and to tricyclic medications. Whereas the overall treatment outcomes were roughly equivalent, patients with higher initial depression severity who were assigned to CT did relatively less well than patients assigned to either IPT or medication. This "treatment × severity interaction" has led to the popular idea that CT is mostly effective for mild–to–moderate levels of depression, and to treatment guidelines that also reify this idea, such as those by the American Psychiatric Association (*www.psych.org/psych_pract/treatg/pg/mdd2E_05-15-06.pdf*).

The conclusion regarding the treatment equivalency of CT and other treatments, and the recommendation that CT be used only for mild-to-moderate depression are both called into question by other, more recent data. Two meta-analyses of CT for depression have now been completed (Dobson, 1989; Gloaguen, Cottraux, Cucherat, & Blackburn, 1998). Both analyses used the BDI as an outcome measure and compared CT to four other types of treatments: waiting list/no treatment; behavior therapy, pharmacotherapy, and other psychotherapies. The absolute effect size for CT compared to no treatment was 1.86 in the Dobson (1989) study, and the approximate average effect size for the other comparisons was 0.50, indicating that patients treated with CT were half a standard deviation lower on the BDI at posttest compared to other treatments. Gloaguen et al. (1998) reported that the comparison between CT and no treatment remained large, and that whereas CT still demonstrated a statistically significant advantage over both pharmacotherapy and other psychotherapies, the effect size was smaller than earlier reported. Notably, the comparison between CT and behavior therapy failed to show an advantage for either treatment. Finally, Gloaguen et al. presented the follow-up data for the comparisons between CT and pharmacotherapy, and concluded that naturalistic follow-up relapse rates over approximately a 1- to 2-year follow-up period were about half the rates reported for medication conditions.

The treatment × severity interaction effect discussed earlier was subjected to a further "mega-analysis" (DeRubeis, Gelfand, Tang, & Simons, 1999). This study combined the raw data from four independent comparative trials of CT and pharmacotherapy (including the NIMH TDCRP data), and despite several ways of examining the data, failed to find the interaction effect. DeRubeis et al.'s argument, based on their analyses with more statistical power and more sophisticated data methods, was that the treatment × severity interaction did not in fact exist, and that these treatments were equally efficacious in both less and more severely depressed patients. These predictions have subsequently been borne out in two recent studies. One of these studies was completed at two sites and only employed more severely depressed patients (DeRubeis et al., 2005; Hollon et al., 2005). Results indicated roughly equivalent outcomes between CT and selective serotonin reuptake inhibitor (SSRI) medications in the short term, but significantly better survival (i.e., less depression relapse/recurrence) in the group previously treated with CT as opposed to that treated with antidepressant medication. These results have been replicated in a more recent trial (Dimidjian et al., 2006; Dobson et al., 2007).

Mechanisms of Change and Predictors of Outcome in CT for Depression

Given the success of CT for depression, a number of ancillary questions arise, including questions related to how CT exerts its influence and whether the treatment is more or less appropriate for clients with known characteristics. The first of these questions was examined by mediational analyses and the examination of therapy processes related to outcome. Results of these studies include the observation that early completion of homework is associated with better clinical outcome (Startup & Edmonds, 1994); that attention to the specific techniques of CT are associated with more change than are the nonspecific aspects of treatment (DeRubeis & Feeley, 1990; Feeley, DeRubeis, & Gelfand, 1999); and that patients with a sudden but sustained decrease in depression severity scores tend to have better long-term outcomes than patients with more gradual but equal outcomes (Tang & DeRubeis, 1999; Tang, DeRubeis, Beberman, & Pham, 2005). These studies, as well as many others that explore the assumptions of the cognitive model of depression (Clark et al., 1999), reveal aspects of how to optimize treatment outcomes.

Experimental analyses of the effective components of CT of depression are rare. The major study to date used an incremental dismantling strategy and randomly assigned depressed outpatients to receive 20 sessions of behavioral activation (BA) interventions, 20 sessions of BA and cognitive restructuring interventions, or 20 sessions of the full CT treatment (Gortner, Gollan, Dobson, & Jacobson, 1998; Jacobson et al., 1996). All three conditions had equal outcomes in this study, both in the acute phase of treatment, and in the 2 years of follow-up. Taken literally, the results of this study indicate that adding cognitive interventions to the BA components of therapy do not enhance short-term outcome or reduce relapse; in other words, they call into question the clinical utility of the cognitive interventions in CT! Although these results raise provocative questions about the mechanisms of change in CT for depression, replication is needed to understand the full implications of these results.

The other approach that has explored clinically relevant questions about CT has examined predictors of outcome. It has generally been demonstrated that patients with more severe initial depression, as well as those with more chronic depression, do worse than less severely or less chronically depressed patients in CT for depression (Hollon & Beck, 1994; Hollon, Thase, & Markowitz, 2002), but other patient predictors of outcome have been notoriously difficult to establish (Hamilton & Dobson, 2002). It has also been difficult to establish therapist predictors of outcome (Hollon & Beck, 1994). Although therapist adherence to CT techniques appears to predict outcome, the rated competence of CT therapists has only been demonstrated to have a positive relationship to outcome in a few studies (Jacobson et al., 1996; Shaw et al., 1999; Trepka, Rees, Shapiro, Hardy, & Barkham, 2004). Further study of these questions, and perhaps improved instrumentation, is needed to understand more fully these issues.

CONCLUSIONS

This chapter has provided a description of the cognitive model of depression and the typical process of CT for depression. The typical behavioral, cognitive restructuring, and assumptive interventions employed in CT are associated with clinical outcomes that are as strong as those in any other treatment in depression, and potentially with stronger long-term effects that pharmacotherapy (Hollon, Stewart, & Strunk, 2006). It also appears that CT is effective across the range of depression severity, so it can be used in different clinical settings. Furthermore, given the concerns about side effects of some antidepressant medications, some treatment guidelines now recommend the use of CT or related models as the preferred treatment in less severe cases of depression (National Institute for Clinical Excellence, 2006). Despite the overall value of CT and the fact that it is generally recognized as an empirically supported therapy (Chambless & Ollendick, 2001), about one-third of patients fail to respond to this treatment model. Furthermore, relapse rates of about 25% at 1 year following treatment suggest that there is more to learn about treatment failure and relapse.

I concluded the chapter with a brief description of some of the research related to the CT model and therapy. Much remains to be known about CT for depression. We still do not know as much as would be ideal about the treatment factors associated with positive outcome in CT for depression. Additional dismantling and process studies are needed to explore these dimensions. Finally, we know relatively little about patient predictors of outcome in CT for depression. Although higher levels of initial depression severity, more chronicity, and more comorbidity are predictors of more negative outcomes, much more research is needed to explore factors such as depression subtypes or other factors that may affect patients' short- and long-term responses to this treatment model. Also, the field desperately needs studies that examine the predictors of outcome in CT relative to other evidence-based treatments. In summary, the field has at this point in the history of established its overall efficacy, but it now needs to address issues related to its effectiveness (Nathan, Stuart, & Dolan, 2000), and its efficacy relative to other empirically supported treatments for depression.

REFERENCES

Academy of Cognitive Therapy. (2006). *Information for patients about depression*. Accessed October 21, 2006, from *www.academyofct.org/folderid/1094/sessionid/ {bc1F26BC-b39e-44ad-a7f1-369E3275c8cd}/pagevars/library/infomanage/guide. htm.*

Ackermann, R., & DeRubeis, R. J. (1991). Is depressive realism real? *Clinical Psychology Review, 11*, 565–584.

American Psychiatric Association. (2000). *Diagnostic and statistical manual of mental disorders* (4th ed., text rev.). Washington, DC: Author.

Beck, A. T. (1970). Cognitive therapy: Nature and relation to behavior therapy. *Behavior Therapy, 1*, 184–200.

Beck, A. T., Brown, G., Steer, R. A., & Weissman, A. N. (1991). Factor analysis of the Dysfunctional Attitudes Scale in a clinical population. *Psychological Assessment, 3*, 478–483.

Beck, A. T., Rush, A. J., Shaw, B. F., & Emery, G. (1979). *Cognitive therapy of depression*. New York: Guilford Press.

Beck, A. T., Steer, R. A., & Garbin, H. G. (1988). Psychometric properties of the Beck Depression Inventory: Twenty-five years of evaluation. *Clinical Psychology Review, 8*, 77–100.

Beck, J. S. (1995). *Cognitive therapy: Basics and beyond.* New York: Guilford Press.

Beck, J. S. (2005). *Cognitive therapy for challenging problems.* New York: Guilford Press.

Beutler, L. E., Clarkin, J. F., & Bongar, B. (2000). *Guidelines for the systematic treatment of the depressed patient.* New York: Oxford University Press.

Bieling, P. J., & Antony, M. M. (2003). *Ending the depression cycle: A step-by-step guide for preventing relapse.* Oakland, CA: New Harbinger.

Bieling, P. J., Beck, A. T., & Brown, G. K. (2004). Stability and change of sociotropy and autonomy subscales in cognitive therapy of depression. *Journal of Cognitive Psychotherapy, 18*, 135–148.

Burns, D. (1980). *Feeling good.* New York: Morrow.

Burns, D. D., & Nolen-Hoeksema, S. (1991). Coping styles, homework compliance, and the effectiveness of cognitive-behavioral therapy. *Journal of Consulting and Clinical Psychology, 59*(2), 305–311.

Cane, D. B., Olinger, L. J., Gotlib, I. H., & Kuiper, N. A. (1986). Factor structure of the Dysfunctional Attitude Scale in the student population. *Journal of Clinical Psychology, 42*(2), 307–309.

Chambless, D., & Ollendick, T. H. (2001). Empirically supported psychological interventions: Controversies and evidence. *Annual Review of Psychology, 52,* 685–716.

Clark, D. A., & Beck, A. T. (1991). Personality factors in dysphoria: A psychometric refinement of Beck's Sociotropy–Autonomy Scale. *Journal of Psychopathology and Behavioral Assessment, 13,* 369–388.

Clark, D. A., Beck, A. T., & Alford, B. A. (1999). *Scientific foundations of cognitive theory and therapy of depression.* Hoboken, NJ: Wiley.

Coyne, J. C. (1976). Toward an interactional description of depression. *Psychiatry, 39,* 28–40.

Davila, J., Hammen, C., Burge, D., Paley, B., & Daley, S. E. (1997). Poor interpersonal problem solving as a mechanism of stress generation in depression. *Journal of Abnormal Psychology, 104*(4), 592–600.

DeRubeis, R. J., & Feeley, M. (1990). Determinants of change in cognitive therapy for depression. *Cognitive Therapy and Research, 14*(5), 469–582.

DeRubeis, R. J., Gelfand, L. A., Tang, T. Z., & Simons, A. D. (1999). Medications versus cognitive behavioral therapy for severely depressed outpatients: Mega-analysis of four randomized comparisons. *American Journal of Psychiatry, 156,* 1007–1013.

DeRubeis, R. J., Hollon, S. D., Amsterdam, J. D., Shelton, R. C., Young, P. R., Salomon, R. M., et al. (2005). Cognitive therapy vs medications in the treatment of moderate to severe depression. *Archives of General Psychiatry, 62,* 409–416.

Detweiler, J. B., & Whisman, M. A. (1999). The role of homework assignments in cognitive therapy for depression: Potential methods for enhancing adherence. *Clinical Psychology: Science and Practice, 6,* 267–282.

Dimidjian, S., Hollon, S. D., Dobson, K. S., Schmaling, K. B., Kohlenberg, R. J., Addis, M. E., et al. (2006). Randomized trial of behavioral activation, cognitive therapy, and antidepressant medication in the acute treatment of adults with major depression. *Journal of Consulting and Clinical Psychology, 174,* 658–670.

Dobson, K. S. (1989). A meta-analysis of the efficacy of cognitive therapy for depression. *Journal of Consulting and Clinical Psychology, 57,* 414–419.

Dobson, K. S., & Dozois, D. J. A. (2001). Historical and philosophical bases of the cognitive-behavioral therapies. In K. S. Dobson (Ed.), *Handbook of cognitive-behavioral therapies* (2nd ed., pp. 3–39). New York: Guilford Press.

Dobson, K., & Franche, R.-L. (1989). A conceptual and empirical review of the depressive realism hypothesis. *Canadian Journal of Behavioural Science, 21,* 419–433.

Dobson, K. S., Hollon, S. D., Dimidjian, S., Schmaling, K. B., Kohlenberg, R. J., Gallop, R., et al. (2007). *Randomized trial of behavioral activation, cognitive therapy, and antidepressant medication in the prevention of relapse and recurrence of major depression in adults.* Unpublished manuscript, University of Calgary.

Dozois, D. J. A., & Dobson, K. S. (2002). Depression. In M. M. Antony & D. H. Barlow (Eds.), *Handbook of assessment and treatment planning for psychological disorders* (pp. 259–299). New York: Guilford Press.

Elkin, I., Shea, M. T., Watkins, J. T., Imber, S. D., Sotsky, S. M., Collins, J. F., et al. (1989). NIMH treatment of depression collaborative research program: I. General effectiveness of treatments. *Archives of General Psychiatry, 46,* 971–983.

Feeley, M., DeRubeis, R. J., & Gelfand, L. A. (1999). The temporal relation of adherence and alliance to symptom change in cognitive therapy for depression. *Journal of Consulting and Clinical Psychology, 67*(4), 451–459.

Gilbert, P. E. (2001). *Overcoming depression* (2nd ed.). New York: Oxford University Press.

Gloaguen, V., Cottraux, J., Cucherat, M., & Blackburn, I. (1998). A meta-analysis of the effects of cognitive therapy in depressed outpatients. *Journal of Affective Disorders, 49,* 59–72.

Gollan, J., Raffety, B., Gortner, E., & Dobson, K. (2005). Course profiles of early- and adult-onset depression. *Journal of Affective Disorders, 86,* 81–86.

Gortner, E. T., Gollan, J. K., Dobson, K. S., & Jacobson, N. S. (1998). Cognitive-behavioral treatment for depression: Relapse prevention. *Journal of Consulting and Clinical Psychology, 66*(2), 377–384.

Greenberger, D., & Padesky, C. A. (1995). *Mind over mood: Change how you feel by changing the way you think.* New York: Guilford Press.

Hamilton, K. E., & Dobson, K. S. (2002). Cognitive therapy of depression: Pretreatment patient predictors of outcome. *Clinical Psychology Review, 22,* 875–894.

Harvey, A. G. (2005). A cognitive theory and therapy for chronic insomnia. *Journal of Cognitive Psychotherapy, 19,* 41–59.

Held, B. S. (1995). *Back to reality: A critique of postmodern theory in psychotherapy.* New York: Norton.

Hollon, S. D., & Beck, A. T. (1994). Cognitive and cognitive-behavioral therapies. In A. E. Bergin & S. L. Garfield (Eds.), *Handbook of psychotherapy and behavior change* (4th ed., pp. 428–466). New York: Wiley.

Hollon, S. D., DeRubeis, R. J., Shelton, R. C., Amsterdam, J. D., Salomon, R. M., O'Reardon, J. P., et al. (2005). Prevention of relapse following cognitive therapy vs. medications in moderate to severe depression. *Archives of General Psychiatry, 62,* 417–422.

Hollon, S. D., Stewart, M., & Strunk, D. (2006). Enduring effects for cognitive behavior therapy in the treatment of depression and anxiety. *Annual Review of Psychology, 57,* 285–315.

Hollon, S. D., Thase, M., & Markowitz, J. C. (2002). Treatment and prevention of depression. *Psychological Science in the Public Interest, 3,* 39–77.

Jacobson, N. S., Dobson, K. S., Truax, P. A., Addis, M. E., Koerner, K., Gollan, J. K., et al. (1996). A component analysis of cognitive-behavioral treatment for depression. *Journal of Consulting and Clinical Psychology, 64*(2), 295–304.

Joiner, T. E. (2000). Depression's vicious scree: Self-propagating and erosive processes in depression chronicity. *Clinical Psychology: Science and Practice, 7,* 203–218.

Joiner, T. E., & Schmidt, N. B. (1998). Excessive reassurance-seeking predicts depressive but not anxious reactions to acute stress. *Journal of Abnormal Psychology, 107*(3), 533–537.

Kazantzis, N., & Deane, F. P. (1999). Psychologists' use of homework assignments in clinical practice. *Professional Psychology: Research and Practice, 30*(6), 581–585.

Kazantzis, N., Deane, F. P., Ronan, K. R., & L'Abate, L. (Eds.). *Using homework assignments in cognitive behavioral therapy.* New York: Routledge.

Klerman, G. L., Weissman, M. M., Rounsaville, B. J., & Chevron, C. S. (1984). *Interpersonal psychotherapy of depression.* New York: Basic Books.

Kovacs, M., & Beck, A. T. (1978). Maladaptive cognitive structures in depression. *American Journal of Psychiatry, 135*, 525–533.

Monroe, S., & Simons, A. (1991). Diathesis–stress theories in the context of life stress research: Implications for the depressive disorders. *Psychological Bulletin, 110*(3), 406–425.

Nathan, P. E., Stuart, S. P., & Dolan, S. L. (2000). Research on psychotherapy efficacy and effectiveness: Between Scylla and Charybdis? *Psychological Bulletin, 126*, 964–981.

National Institute for Clinical Excellence. (2006). *Compilation—Issue 10: Mental health.* Retrieved October 15, 2006, from *www.nice.org.uk/download.aspx?o= 272364.*

Nezu, A. M., Ronan, G. F., Meadows, E. A., & McClure, K. S. (2000). *Practitioner's guide to empirically based measures of depression.* Dordrecht, The Netherlands: Kluwer.

Paykel, E. S., Scott, J., Cornwall, P. L., Abbott, R., Crane, C., Pope, M., et al. (2005). Duration of relapse prevention after cognitive therapy in residual depression: Follow-up of controlled trial. *Psychological Medicine, 35*, 59–68.

Persons, J. B. (1989). *Cognitive therapy in practice: A case formulation approach.* New York: Norton.

Persons, J. B., & Davidson, J. (2001). Cognitive-behavioral case formulation. In K. S. Dobson (Ed.), *Handbook of cognitive-behavioral therapies* (pp. 86–110). New York: Guilford Press.

Robins, C. J., & Block, P. (1989). Cognitive theories of depression viewed from a diathesis–stress perspective: Evaluations of the models of Beck and of Abramson, Seligman, and Teasdale. *Cognitive Therapy and Research, 13*(4), 297–314.

Rush, A. J., Beck, A. T., Kovacs, M., & Hollon, S. (1977). Comparative efficacy of cognitive therapy and pharmacotherapy in the treatment of depressed outpatients. *Cognitive Therapy and Research, 11*(1), 17–37.

Rush, A. J., Hollon, S. D., Beck, A. T., & Kovacs, M. (1978). Depression: Must psychotherapy fail for cognitive therapy to succeed? *Cognitive Therapy and Research, 2*(2), 199–206.

Schmidt, N. B., Joiner, T. E., Young, J. E., & Telch, M. J. (1995). The Schema Questionnaire: Investigation of psychometric properties and the hierarchical structure of a measure of maladaptive schemas. *Cognitive Therapy and Research, 19*, 295–322.

Shaw, B. F., Elkin, I., Yamaguchi, J., Olmsted, M., Vallis, T. M., Dobson, K. S., et al. (1999). Therapist competence ratings in relation to clinical outcome in cognitive therapy of depression. *Journal of Consulting and Clinical Psychology, 67,* 837–846.

Startup, M., & Edmonds, J. (1994). Compliance with homework assignments in cognitive-behavioral psychotherapy for depression: Relation to outcome and methods of enhancement. *Cognitive Therapy and Research, 18*(6), 567–580.

Tang, T. Z., & DeRubeis, R. J. (1999). Sudden gains and critical sessions in cognitive-behavioral therapy for depression. *Journal of Consulting and Clinical Psychology, 67*(6), 894–904.

Tang, T. Z., DeRubeis, R. J., Beberman, R., & Pham, T. (2005). Cognitive changes, critical sessions, and sudden gains in cognitive-behavioral therapy for depression. *Journal of Consulting and Clinical Psychology, 73,* 168–172.

Tompkins, M. A. (2004). *Using homework in psychotherapy: Strategies, guidelines and forms.* New York: Guilford Press.

Trepka, C., Rees, A., Shapiro, D. A., Hardy, G. E., & Barkham, M. (2004). Therapist competence and outcome of cognitive therapy for depression. *Cognitive Therapy and Research, 28,* 143–157.

Wright, J. H., Wright, A. S., Salmon, P., Beck, A. T., Kuykendall, J., Goldsmith, L. J., et al. (2002). Development and initial testing of a multimedia program for computer-assisted cognitive therapy. *American Journal of Psychotherapy, 56*(1), 76–86.

Young, J. E., & Brown, G. (1990). *Young Schema Questionnaire.* New York: Cognitive Therapy Center of New York.

Young, J. E., & Klosko, K. S. (1994). *Reinventing your life.* New York: Plume.

Young, J. E., Klosko, K. S., & Weishaar, M. E. (2003). *Schema therapy: A practitioner's guide.* New York: Guilford Press.

$$\boxed{2}$$

INITIAL ASSESSMENT, CASE CONCEPTUALIZATION, AND TREATMENT PLANNING

Mark A. Whisman
Lauren M. Weinstock

With the trend toward manualization of psychosocial interventions, there have been increased attempts to clarify a distinction between the "essence" of a treatment and its specific components (Abramowitz, 2006); that is, along with certain techniques that make up an intervention, it is important that there exist an empirically based theoretical rationale to guide the treatment. This approach is at the heart of evidence-based practice generally, and of cognitive therapy (CT; Beck, Rush, Shaw, & Emery, 1979) for depression specifically. CT is grounded in an empirical and conceptual model that implicates certain underlying and maladaptive cognitive schemas as risk factors for depression onset and maintenance (Clark, Beck, & Alford, 1999). Building upon this model, the aim of the therapist is to work collaboratively with the patient to identify and modify negative cognitions, using specific strategies such as automatic thought monitoring and cognitive restructuring. As such, cognitive therapists utilize a "nomothetic template" that comprises well-defined theoretical and practical considerations in their clinical approach (Persons, 2006).

It is important to emphasize that this nomothetic template does not exclude an individualized approach to CT. Indeed, using the CT model as a guide, it is important that clinicians assess the unique presenting problems and generate for each patient an individualized case conceptualization representing a hypothesis about the mechanisms that underlie the patient's problems. Such hypotheses provide clues to the clinician as to what may be most relevant or clinically useful for the patient, and guide selection of specific CT techniques to be used in the treatment. Furthermore, as therapy proceeds, the case conceptualization provides a framework for hypothesis testing, and for refinement and revision of the treatment plan. Thus, CT rooted in such a case conceptualization benefits from being both personalized and flexible, within a coherent empirical and theoretical framework.

As discussed throughout this volume, there are many ways to adapt or tailor CT to treat various presentations of depression more effectively. In this chapter, we focus on the use of assessment-driven case conceptualization as a guiding force in deciding when and how to adapt treatment to the needs of individual patients. Specifically, we first provide an overview of initial assessment, then discuss how assessment data can be incorporated into cognitive case conceptualization; finally, we propose ways in which this conceptualization can be used to guide decisions regarding modification of CT for depressed individuals based upon their presentation.

INITIAL ASSESSMENT

In many clinical settings, an initial assessment is performed to obtain useful information in the development of a specific treatment plan. Information from an initial assessment is useful not only in understanding the patient but also in identifying the problems and issues that need to be addressed in treatment, and formulating recommendations about the most effective way to address these problems.

Several types of assessment methods can be used to conduct an initial assessment of a patient presenting with depression. A comprehensive review of available measures is beyond the scope of this chapter, and the reader is referred to Nezu, Ronan, Meadows, and McClure (2000) for a review of assessment measures of depression. We would like to draw attention to three areas that we believe are particularly important to assess in formulating a treatment plan. First, it is important to assess for co-occurring conditions that may impact treatment planning. For example, it is important to assess for co-occurring Axis I disorders; it has been reported that nearly three-fourths of people with lifetime depression and nearly two-thirds of people with 12-month major depression also meet criteria for at least one other Axis I disorder during their lifetime or in the past year, respectively (Kessler et al., 2003). Clinicians can comprehensively assess Axis I disorders using a diagnostic measure such as the Structured Clinical Interview for DSM-IV Axis I Disorders (SCID-I), a semistructured interview that includes questions relating to specific symptoms that determine differential diagnoses. There are several versions of the SCID-I, including a shorter Clinician Version (SCID-CV; First, Spitzer, Gibbon, & Williams, 1996) and a longer Research Version (SCID-I-RV), which in turn has several versions. The SCID-CV covers the Axis I diagnoses most commonly seen in clinical practice, and excludes the subtypes and specifiers found in the longer SCID-I-RV. It is designed to be completed in a single sitting, and its administration takes 45–90 minutes, depending on the skill and experience of the clinician, the complexity of the psychiatric history, and the ability of patients to describe their psychopathology succinctly. In situations in which the clinician does not have time to administer the full SCID-I, specific modules may be administered to assess for the occurrence of specific disorders. The importance of structured interviews in the assessment of Axis I disorders come from research comparing comorbidity rates, as determined by unstructured clinical interviews and structured research diagnostic interviews, which suggests that comorbidity is underdetected in unstructured interviews routinely used in clinical practice (Zimmerman & Mattia, 1999).

Structured interviews such as the SCID-I provide important information for not only for identifying the presence of other Axis I disorders but also determining age of onset, and the history and number of prior episodes of depression and other conditions. Such information is necessary to determine whether the patient has a chronic and/or recurrent depression, and whether a comorbid condition emerged before, simultaneous with, or after the onset of depression. In addition to Axis I problems, the SCID-I includes important questions about the patient's physical health and social functioning, because depression has been found to covary with medical conditions (Stevens, Merikangas, & Merikangas, 1995), and impaired interpersonal and social relationships (Hirschfeld et al., 2000). If the patient reports health problems or impaired social functioning, then the clinician may want to conduct a more formal assessment that includes severity of impairment, as described below.

Whereas the SCID-I is useful in assessing Axis I disorders and alerting clinicians about the presence of comorbid medical conditions and social problems, it does not assess for the presence of Axis II disorders. The importance of assessment of Axis II conditions comes from findings that approximately 50–85% of depressed inpatients and 20–50% of depressed outpatients have personality disorders (Corruble, Ginestet, & Guelfi, 1996). There are many interview and self-report instruments for Axis II disorders, and the interested reader is referred to Widiger and Samuel (2005) for an overview of these instruments. The use of self-report measures to alert clinicians to the potential presence of Axis II disorders may be particularly useful in clinical settings, because completion of such measures requires minimal clinician time; semistructured interviews may then be used to verify the presence of Axis II disorders.

A second area of assessment is the patient's degree of functional impairment and subjective distress. Information about degree of severity may be important in generating hypotheses regarding prognosis, intensity, and length of treatment. Symptom measures, also useful for monitoring outcome, are measured from session to session, as well as from pre- to posttreatment. The many measures for assessing depression include, for example, the widely used Beck Depression Inventory—Second Edition (BDI-II; Beck, Steer, & Brown, 1996). In interpreting the BDI-II, a score ≤ 13 indicates minimal depression; 14–19, mild; 20–28, moderate; and ≥ 29 indicates severe depression. In addition to measuring depression, therapists may periodically want to assess symptom severity of co-occurring disorders for which the patient meets criteria, as well as to identify significant elevations in symptoms of disorders for which the patient does not meet diagnostic criteria (i.e., subthreshhold elevations). In addition, for the patients who report physical health problems or impaired social functioning, self-report data may be used to evaluate severity of impairment, as well as the impact of treatment. Although a review of applicable measures is beyond the scope of this chapter, the interested reader is referred to Maruish (1999) for a description of measures for treatment planning and outcome assessment.

A third area of assessment concerns the assessment of theory-specific mechanisms of change. As applied to CT for depression, this involves assessment of cognitions. For example, a therapist may wish to assess the degree to which a patient endorses dysfunctional attitudes or automatic thoughts, or the extent to which a patient makes cognitive errors. Unlike the situation with symptom-based measures, relatively few guidelines for interpreting scores on cognitive measures of psychopathology may have resulted in clinicians being less likely to use them in clinical practice. However, Dozois, Covin, and Brinker (2003) have provided normative data on six self-report indices of depression-related cognitions, including measures of automatic thoughts, cognitive errors, and dysfunctional attitudes. The means and standard deviations for the commonly used cognitive measures obtained from this article are presented in Table 2.1.

**TABLE 2.1. Normative Data on Cognitive
and Personality Vulnerabilities for Depression**

Measure	Mean	SD
Automatic Thoughts Questionnaire—Positive[a]	99	13
Automatic Thoughts Questionnaire—Negative[a]	53	18
Adolescents	64	21
Adults	53	18
Older persons	42	14
Women	54	19
Men	48	16
Beck Hopelessness Scale[a]	3	3
Cognitive Bias Questionnaire[a]	2	2
Cognitive Error Questionnaire[a]	17	12
Dysfunctional Attitude Scale[a]	119	27
Adolescents	135	32
Adults	115	27
Older persons	117	24
Revised Sociotropy–Autonomy Scale		
Sociotropy scale	64	16
Solitude scale	26	6
Independence scale	45	8
Revised Personal Style Inventory		
Sociotropy scale	95	16
Autonomy scale	84	14

[a]Data reported in Dozois, Covin, and Brinker (2003).

As discussed by Dozois et al. (2003), normative data on depressive cognitions can be clinically useful in at least three ways. First, normative data can help to determine the extent to which a patient's score on a given cognitive measure falls outside the normal range of that measure in severity or frequency; that is, normative data on these cognitive measures can be used to create standardized scores, the most common of which are T-scores. The following equation can used in computing a T-score from a patient's raw score (X), the mean of the normative data (M), and the standard deviation of the normative data (SD):

$$T = 50 + 10[(X - M)/SD]$$

For example, if an adult patient had a raw score of 168 on the Dysfunctional Attitude Scale (DAS), substituting this score and the normative data provided in Table 2.1 in the foregoing formula would produce a T-score of 70:

$$T = 50 + 10[(168 - 115)/27] = 50 + 10(2) = 50 + 20 = 70$$

T-scores have a mean of 50 and a standard deviation of 10. Thus, a *T*-score of 70 means that a score is 2.0 standard deviations above the mean. Therefore, whereas a raw score of 168 on the DAS means virtually nothing by itself, knowing that it corresponds to a *T*-score of 70 is informative insofar as it tells the clinician that the patient's score on this scale is 2.0 standard deviations above the mean of the normative data. In interpreting *T*-scores, values between 40 and 60 (i.e., ±1 standard deviation from the mean) are generally considered to fall within the normal range, whereas scores > 60 can be considered clinically elevated. In particular, *T*-scores above 65 or 70 are considerably elevated, because they correspond to 1.5 and 2.0 standard deviations above the mean, respectively.

As discussed by Dozois et al. (2003), a second use of normative data (as translated into *T*-scores) is in providing directions for intervention. For example, a clinician can compare a patient's *T*-scores on two measures to determine the patient's relative elevations across different cognitive variables. Such comparisons can usefully determine which specific types of depression-related cognitions are most elevated. For example, this information may be used to help the therapist determine whether it may be most useful to target reducing negative automatic thoughts or increasing positive automatic thoughts. Comparing *T*-scores across measures is based on the assumption that such scores have similar meaning from one measure to the next, which is valid, however, only if the scales involve similar distributions. Future research is needed to evaluate this assumption with respect to cognitive assessment measures.

As discussed by Dozois et al. (2003), a third use of normative data (as translated into *T*-scores) is to assist clinicians in deciding when to terminate treatment. For example, based on the perspective that cognitive change is important in preventing relapse and recurrence, a clinician might decide to continue treatment until a patient's scores on the DAS fall within the normative range (e.g., within 1 standard deviation from the normative mean).

Before leaving the topic of clinical applications of cognitive assessment, it should be noted that the impact of using such measures to guide treatment planning has not been tested empirically; that is, the recommendations to use these data in selecting cognitive domains to target for treatment, or to continue treatment until a certain level of end-state functioning is reached, are theoretical positions that need to be evaluated in future research.

Once the cognitive therapist has collected assessment information, he or she is ready to organize this information in developing a conceptualization of the patient. We turn now to an overview of case conceptualization in CT of depression.

CASE CONCEPTUALIZATION IN CT

Before considering ways we might consider using cognitive case conceptualization to modify CT for differing presentations of depression, it is important to provide a general overview of the existing cognitive case conceptualization for depression. Although there are a number of models firmly based in cognitive theory, we rely primarily on Persons's (1989) case formulation approach in this overview.

Overt Difficulties

According to Persons's (1989) case formulation model, psychological problems are considered at two levels, the first of which represents a patient's overt difficulties. These problems may take the form of cognitions, behaviors, or moods. Specifically, at the cognitive level, overt difficulties may take the form of negative automatic thoughts, such as "I'm stuck—I'll never get this promotion," or other forms, such as images. At the behavioral level, overt difficulties may take the form of nonverbal behaviors (e.g., withdrawal from activities, self-injury, or substance abuse), verbal behaviors (e.g., excessive reassurance seeking, negative feedback-seeking, or suicidal threats), or physiological responses (e.g., agitation, fatigue, or insomnia). Finally, overt difficulties may take the form of negative or unpleasant mood states, such as sadness, fear, or guilt.

Although patients are typically more likely to be aware of and to attend to overt difficulties at the level of distressed mood (J. S. Beck, 1995; Persons, 1989), overt difficulties in one area likely reflect overt difficulties in other areas. For example, depressed mood might be accompanied by negative automatic thoughts, such as "I can't do this," and related problematic behaviors, such as procrastination. Thus, Persons argues that problems in cognitions, behaviors, and mood are *synchronous*. Following from this notion of synchrony, cognitions, behavior, and mood are also conceptualized as *interdependent*; that is, it is likely that change in one overt problem area is likely to result in change in the other problem areas. Indeed, this idea forms an important tenet in CT, which is based on the assumption that changes in maladaptive information processing are central to understanding changes in depression (Clark et al., 1999). Furthermore, this hypothesis is supported by research demonstrating that interventions targeted at producing change in one system are also associated with change in other systems (Persons, 1995). For example, in their component analysis of CT for depression, Jacobson and colleagues (1996) found that a strictly behavioral therapy was nevertheless associated with significant changes in dysfunctional attitudes from pre- to posttreatment. Similarly, from pre- to posttreatment, a strictly cognitive intervention was associated with significant changes in behavior, as evidenced by increases in pleasant events.

Underlying Mechanisms

At the presumed root of a patient's overt difficulties lie the underlying psychological mechanisms, which represent the second level of Persons's (1989) case formulation model. Indeed, an underlying psychological mechanism represents a problem or deficit that causes or contributes to an individual's overt difficulties. According to the cognitive theory of depression (Clark et al., 1999), maladaptive schemas are the underlying psychological mechanisms for depression and associated difficulties. The specific content of these schemas represents one's core beliefs: one's most central ideas about the self, others, and the world (J. S. Beck, 1995). These schemas may be represented as conditional beliefs, such as "If I put others' needs before my own, they will love me," or unconditional beliefs, such as "I am a worthless person." Furthermore, the underlying psychological mechanisms may represent other deficits, such as a lack of problem-solving skills (Nezu, Wilkins, & Nezu, 2004).

In considering potential underlying mechanisms of depression, Beck (1983) identified two cognitive–personality styles that are hypothesized to reflect distinct underlying themes associated with major depression— "sociotropy," or excessive need for approval from others, and "autonomy," or excessive concern about independent achievement. Sociotropy and autonomy correspond to the core beliefs of unlovability and worthlessness, respectively, which are the two broad categories of core beliefs associated with psychopathology (J. S. Beck, 1995). Cognitive theory proposes that individuals whose underlying schemas reflect themes of sociotropy develop symptoms of depression in response to rejection or other interpersonal difficulties, whereas individuals whose underlying schemas reflect themes of autonomy may develop depressive symptoms in response to failure events or exposure to obstacles that prevent goal achievement. Research to date has yielded partial and inconsistent support for the congruency hypothesis; there is also some evidence that sociotropy represents a general vulnerability to depressive symptoms in the face of both interpersonal and achievement stressors (Clark et al., 1999). Conceptual and methodological shortcomings in existing research make it difficult to draw firm conclusions regarding these cognitive–personality styles and depression onset. However, the two broad dimensions of sociotropy/unlovability and autonomy/worthlessness may provide a useful conceptual model for understanding a patient's under-lying belief systems.

Integrating Overt Difficulties and Underlying Mechanisms

According to Persons's (1989) case formulation model, overt difficulties and underlying mechanisms are closely linked. Indeed, just as underlying nega-tive beliefs may influence one's cognitions, behavior, and mood, overt diffi-culties may serve to reinforce one's underlying beliefs. Yet, in contrast to overt difficulties, which may be relatively accessible to patients and amenable to assessment by clinicians, it is more difficult to access and identify these underlying core beliefs. As such, it is important to emphasize that formula-tions of the underlying psychological mechanisms should be considered working hypotheses to be evaluated over the course of therapy.

EXPANDING CASE CONCEPTUALIZATION FOR COMPLICATED PRESENTATIONS OF DEPRESSION

In this section, we highlight several conceptual considerations that may be useful in guiding the case conceptualization with different presentations of depression, including those that might be difficult or challenging to treat with standard CT for depression. The following generalizations about dif-ferent presentations of depression may be useful in generating hypotheses to consider in formulating a case conceptualization for a particular individual.

Parameters of Depression

As previously noted, it is important to evaluate the severity, history, and per-sistence of depression. These are important parameters to evaluate, because they may provide important information regarding the cognitive factors tar-geted in treatment. According to the *severity–persistence* hypothesis of the cognitive theory of depression, the "extent of negative self-referent cogni-tion, reduced positive thinking, and negativity processing bias are linearly related to depression severity and persistence" (Clark et al., 1999, p. 168). This means that patients with more severe or more long-standing and per-sistent depression should have more frequent and pervasive negative self-referent automatic thoughts and more prominent negative processing biases. As reviewed by Clark et al., there is considerable empirical support for this hypothesis. As applied to CT for depression, the implication of this perspective is that negative cognition is likely to be particularly pronounced among these types of patients (i.e., patients with severe or persistent depression may be defined, in part, by the degree of endorsement of negative cognition). Furthermore, it is important to consider parameters related to history of illness, such as number of prior major depressive episodes, evidence of extended periods of residual symptomatology, or whether the patient has experienced multiple failed treatment attempts. Indeed, such historical parameters may impact the patient's level of hopelessness and expectations for treatment.

Comorbid Conditions

Earlier in this chapter we made the case that it is important to assess for co-occurring conditions in working with depressed patients. A number of different models have been proposed to account for comorbidity among psychiatric disorders, and the reader who is interested in systematic reviews of these models is referred to Krueger and Markon (2006). Although a full review of these models is beyond the scope of this chapter, we discuss several of the most commonly studied models of comorbidity. Specifically, given that the focus of the chapter is case conceptualization in CT for depression, we discuss the application of these models to cognitive factors in depression. However, it should be noted that Beck (1991) clearly asserts that cognitive theory does not claim that depression is *caused* by negative cognitions, noting instead that depression is caused by a combination of biological, genetic, familial, developmental, personality, and social factors. Whereas cognitive theory is compatible with other models of vulnerability for depression, the theory proposes that these other factors are important in that they activate latent maladaptive schemas, which are the cognitive mechanism by which depression develops. Thus, we focus our discussion on implications of comorbidity models as they may influence the activation of the cognitive mechanisms (i.e., maladaptive schemas) of depression. Diagrams of these three models are provided in Figure 2.1.

The first model of comorbidity is a *correlated liabilities* model, in which both depression and comorbid conditions have their own liability or vulnerability factors, but the liability or vulnerability factors are correlated (i.e., an increase in risk factors for one condition is associated with an increase in risk factors for the other condition). As applied to the cognitive theory of depression, the correlated liabilities model suggests that depression and co-occurring clinical conditions each have their own cognitive vulnerability. Such a perspective is consistent with one of the basic tenets of cognitive theory, namely, the cognitive *content specificity hypothesis*. According to this

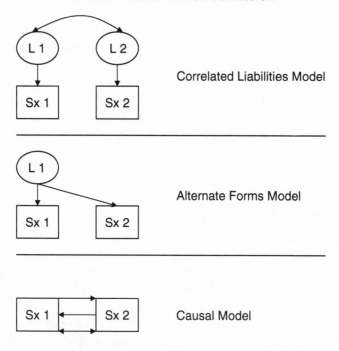

FIGURE 2.1. Representations of hypothetical associations between latent liability factors (L) and observed symptoms (Sx) for disorders 1 and 2.

perspective, psychological disorders are distinguished by the form and content of their associated dysfunctional cognitions, beliefs, attitudes, and processes: "The key differences among the neuroses are revealed in the *content* of the aberrant thinking rather than in its form" (Beck, 1976, p. 82). The thought content associated with depression is believed to center on significant losses, particularly with reference to the loss of something considered essential to one's happiness. This can be contrasted with disorders such as mania, which is associated with an exaggerated positive view of self, world, and the future, or anxiety, which is associated with threat or danger. As reviewed elsewhere, there is considerable support for the content specificity hypothesis in terms of depression and anxiety (R. Beck & Perkins, 2001), although there has been less research evaluating specificity between depression and other disorders. Furthermore, although the content specificity hypothesis was originally proposed to account for differences in Axis I disorders, it has more recently been applied to Axis II disorders as well; that is, each personality disorder is hypothesized to have its own set of idiosyncratic beliefs and attitudes, which in turn give rise to the idiosyncratic behavioral patterns associated with that specific personality disorder (Beck, Freeman,

Davis, & Associates, 2003). Support for this perspective comes from research indicating that each personality disorder does indeed have a unique set of dysfunctional beliefs, and that these belief systems tend to be correlated with one another (Beck et al., 2001).

As applied to CT for depression with comorbid conditions, the cognitive content specificity hypothesis predicts that in some situations, a patient presenting with depression and a comorbid condition would have dysfunctional cognitions associated with not only depression but also the content of each of the comorbid conditions. Thus, it would be expected that the cognitive content of a person with comorbid depression and anxiety would include both loss and threat, whereas that of a person with depression and a narcissistic personality disorder would include both loss and views of self as inferior and others as superior, hurtful, and demeaning. The implication of this model is that in such situations, CT with a patient with comorbid conditions may require more targeting of additional beliefs than would be the case for someone with "pure" depression.

It should be noted that the cognitive content specificity hypothesis was advanced to account for the differences between disorders, not to explain the comorbidity that occurs between disorders. However, we believe that this perspective can be expanded to account for comorbidity as well. Specifically, whereas each disorder may indeed have its own unique cognitive content, people who endorse one set of such beliefs are also likely to endorse other sets of beliefs. In other words, the degree or magnitude of endorsement of cognitive vulnerabilities for one disorder is likely to be correlated with the degree or magnitude of endorsement of cognitive vulnerabilities for another disorder. Therefore, comorbidity between depression and another condition in some situations might occur because the specific, underlying cognitive vulnerabilities for the two conditions are themselves correlated, which is what the correlated liabilities model of comorbidity hypothesizes. Support for this perspective comes from research finding correlations between cognitive contents associated with depression and anxiety (R. Beck & Perkins, 2001) and among the cognitive contents of different personality disorders (Beck et al., 2001).

The second comorbidity model is an *alternate forms* model, in which depression and comorbid conditions are alternate manifestations of a single liability or vulnerability factor. According to this model, comorbid conditions share a single vulnerability factor. A common example of an alternate forms model that is advanced to account for the comorbidity between depression and anxiety is the recently updated tripartite model—the revised integrative hierarchical perspective (Mineka, Watson, & Clark, 1998). This model hypothesizes that depression and anxiety share a common higher-order vulnerability of trait negative affectivity and the related personality trait of neuroticism. Results from population-based samples suggest that the personality trait of neuroticism may indeed help to account for the co-occurrence of depressive and anxiety disorders (e.g., Weinstock & Whisman, 2006).

As applied to the cognitive model of depression, there may be cognitive vulnerability factors that give rise both to depression and to comorbid conditions. As previously discussed, Beck (1983) identified two cognitive–personality dimensions—sociotropy and autonomy—that are believed to be important in understanding depression onset, symptomatology, and treatment response. The introduction of these two dimensions represents a shift in the evolution of cognitive vulnerabilities for depression, because cognitive theory for depression before this time focused more on specific, idiosyncratic negative schemas (Clark et al., 1999). Although they were initially proposed as vulnerabilities to depression, research has shown that sociotropy and autonomy are also associated with other Axis I disorders, including anxiety (e.g., Alford & Gerrity, 1995) and bulimia (e.g., Hayaki, Friedman, Whisman, Delinsky, & Brownell, 2003); with personality disorders (e.g., Ouimette, Klein, Anderson, Riso, & Lizardi, 1994); and with other clinical conditions that co-occur with depression, such as problematic interpersonal relationships (e.g., Lynch, Robins, & Morse, 2001). Thus, emerging evidence that sociotropy and autonomy may represent broad-based cognitive vulnerabilities that give rise to depression and other clinical conditions would be consistent with the alternate forms model of comorbidity.

As applied to CT for depression with comorbid conditions, the alternate forms model of comorbidity suggests that in some situations, comorbid conditions and depression have a common, underlying cognitive vulnerability. For example, a highly sociotropic patient, who believes that he or she is unlovable, might worry about forming and maintaining relationships, avoid situations in which interpersonal rejection is possible, and experience distress when an interpersonal relationship ends. In this example, comorbid generalized anxiety disorder, social phobia, and depression could all be alternate manifestations of the same underlying cognitive vulnerability of sociotropy and the core belief of being unlovable. The implication of this model is that treating the common underlying cognitive mechanism should help reduce both depression and the comorbid condition(s).

In a final comorbidity model, the *causation model*, one condition has a direct influence on the development of another condition, or the two can directly influence each other in a reciprocal fashion. In discussing causation models, it is important to consider the temporal ordering of onset of depression relative to other conditions. In a large, representative community survey, Kessler et al. (1996) found that lifetime cases of depression were most often secondary to other Axis I disorders, with anxiety disorders being the most common primary disorders associated with secondary depression. Interestingly, they also found that secondary depression was more severe and persistent than primary or pure depression. Although temporal precedence does not in itself imply causation, these findings are important in suggesting that depression may in many cases be secondary to other Axis I psychiatric disorders. Similarly, other clinical conditions have also been shown to precede and, therefore, potentially to be related causally to depression. For example, depression is secondary to many medical conditions (Stevens et al., 1995), and there is evidence that adverse social relationships, such as marital discord, are predictive of depression onset (e.g., Whisman & Bruce, 1999).

As applied to cognitive theory of depression, relatively few causation models have been advanced to account for the comorbidity between depression and other conditions. One notable exception is a model proposed by Alloy, Kelly, Mineka, and Clements (1990) to account for the comorbidity between depression and anxiety. According to this model, depressive and anxiety disorders share a cognitive vulnerability of expectation of uncontrollability (i.e., an expectation of helplessness), but depression occurs only when helplessness turns into hopelessness. Specifically, this model suggests that people who expect to be helpless in controlling important future outcomes, but are unsure of their helplessness, exhibit anxiety. If they then become convinced of their helplessness, but are still uncertain about the future likelihood of negative events, they experience mixed anxiety and depression. Finally, if the perceived probability of future negative events becomes certain, then helplessness becomes hopelessness, and they exhibit depression.

As applied to CT for depression with comorbid conditions, the causation model of comorbidity suggests that in some situations, comorbid conditions may be a cause of depression (i.e., primary), whereas in other situations they could be a consequence of depression (i.e., secondary). As such, this model suggests that treating the primary condition may enhance the impact of treatment for the secondary condition. For example, if interpersonal problems (e.g., relationship or marital problems) are conceptualized as occurring before the onset of depression, addressing these problems (e.g., with couple or family therapy) may make it easier to address other factors in CT for depression.

There are other comorbidity models in addition to these three models. For example, it may be that comorbidity is a separate disorder (or a subtype of one of the disorders), with a liability or vulnerability that is independent of either disorder. Because these models do not easily map onto the cognitive theory of depression, they are not discussed here.

In summary, there are at least three ways of conceptualizing comorbidity that may occur between depression and other conditions. Each model has its own implications for how CT may be conducted to deal most effectively with depression and co-occurring conditions.

Demographic Characteristics

A third factor to consider in developing the case conceptualization concerns demographic characteristics of patients, including age, race/ethnicity, and sexual orientation. First, there may be demographic differences in the prevalence, expression, and acceptability of different symptoms of depression. For example, cultural variations in the stigma associated with depression and other mental health problems may be important to consider in conceptualizing a depressed individual's view of him/herself. Furthermore, there may be differences across groups in the presentation of depression symptomatology. For example, although the data are somewhat mixed (Salokangas, Vaahtera, Pacriev, Sohlman, & Lehtinen, 2002), there is some evidence that, in comparison to men, women may more frequently endorse somatic symptoms of depression (Silverstein, 1999). Second, there may be demographic differences in the experiences and stressors that precipitate an episode of depression. For example, discrimination might be more common among older; minority; or gay, lesbian, bisexual, or transgender individuals. Discrimination may in turn increase the likelihood of someone experiencing depression and other mental health problems (Kessler, Mickelson, & Williams, 1999). Third, because different developmental and historical events may lead people from different demographic groups to develop different expectancies and beliefs about themselves, their world, and their future, these belief systems need to be incorporated within the conceptualization and treatment plan. For example, an older depressed individual may have internalized age stereotypes into her view of herself (e.g., viewing depression as part of the inevitable decline and decrepitude associated with aging) or may be more likely than younger individuals to believe that depression is a sign of weakness, either of which could keep her from engaging in stimulating and reinforcing activities; such beliefs may need to be addressed before the person is able to make other life changes that would help to reduce his/her depression (Laidlaw, Thompson, & Gallagher-Thompson, 2004).

DIAGRAMMING THE COGNITIVE
CASE CONCEPTUALIZATION AND PRESENTING IT
TO THE PATIENT

To aid in the development of the cognitive case conceptualization, it may be useful for clinicians to diagram the conceptualization. Such a diagram can be useful in organizing the information available about the patient. J. S. Beck (1995) provided a Cognitive Conceptualization Diagram that we believe is particularly useful in mapping information about the patient. This diagram includes spaces for depicting the relationship between automatic thoughts, and emotional and behavioral reactions, as well as the relationship between automatic thoughts and deeper level beliefs, such as conditional assumptions and core beliefs.

Recently, J. S. Beck (2005) recommended expanding the Cognitive Conceptualization Diagram in working with patients whose complex difficulties include displays of therapy-interfering behaviors; that is, patients' beliefs and compensatory behavioral strategies are likely to occur in therapy just as they occur in other areas of their lives. For example, patients who rarely take risks or try new behaviors because of fear of failure may have a difficult time with homework that requires them to test out their beliefs by engaging in novel behavior. Similarly, patients who compensate for their belief that they are unlovable by trying to please others are likely to try to please therapists by following through with whatever homework is assigned, regardless of its perceived or actual benefit. Specifying problematic situations that occur in therapy, and identifying the automatic thoughts, emotional and behavioral reactions, and compensatory strategies that accompany these situations, may be useful for challenging or complex presentations of depression. Furthermore, J. S. Beck discussed ways of working with challenging behavior in CT that occurs in sessions (e.g., challenges involved in setting goals, structuring sessions, or modifying beliefs) and between sessions (e.g., challenges involved in solving problems and doing homework). Using the case conceptualization in anticipating and responding to such challenges is likely to improve outcome in working with depressed patients.

Whereas J. S. Beck's (1995) Cognitive Conceptualization Diagram is likely to be helpful in working with many depressed patients, including people with severe, chronic, or treatment-resistant depression, it does not specifically address co-occurring conditions. To aid in diagramming case conceptualization for patients with comorbid conditions, we have provided in Figure 2.2 a Case Conceptualization Diagram for Comorbid Conditions modeled after J. S. Beck's (1995) Cognitive Conceptualization Diagram.

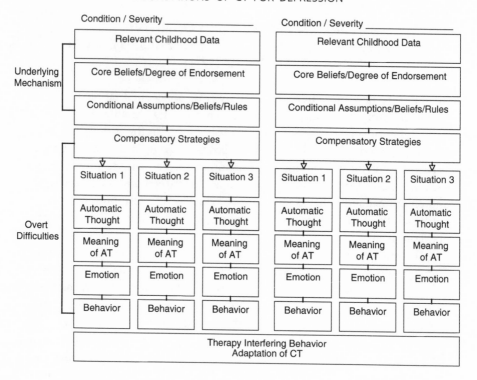

FIGURE 2.2. Case Conceptualization Diagram for Comorbid Conditions.

However, to minimize the complexity of the diagram, we have chosen not to include the sections on conditional assumptions, compensatory strategies, and meaning of automatic thoughts. Furthermore, we have added Persons's (1989) terminology of underlying mechanisms and overt difficulties, so that the diagram is consistent with our earlier discussion of case conceptualization.

Following the recommendations of J. S. Beck (1995), the therapist begins diagramming the case conceptualization by providing several examples of typical situations in which the patient becomes upset. The therapist then fills in the automatic thought elicited by each situation, and the patient's subsequent emotional and behavioral responses. From these typical automatic thoughts, the therapist hypothesizes the likely deeper level (i.e., core) beliefs. Finally, therapist and patient work together in generating hypotheses to understand the origins of relevant childhood and developmental experiences that may have contributed to the development and maintenance of these core beliefs.

To address issues of comorbidity, the Case Conceptualization Diagram for Comorbid Conditions includes space for completing two parallel sets of overt difficulties representing the situations, automatic thoughts, emotions, and behaviors for each of the two conditions; additional diagrams may be used for additional conditions. Completing the diagrams in tandem encourages the therapist to consider ways the comorbid condition(s) may be associated with depression. For example, if each of the two conditions is conceptualized as having its own underlying cognitive mechanism (i.e., the associated liabilities model of comorbidity), then the therapist completes the underlying mechanism section for each disorder and draws a line connecting the two underlying mechanisms (cf. top panel in Figure 2.1). In comparison, if the two conditions are conceptualized as arising from a common underlying cognitive mechanism (i.e., the alternate forms model of comorbidity), then the therapist draws a line from one underlying mechanism to both sets of overt difficulties (cf. middle panel in Figure 2.1). Finally, if one condition is conceptualized as having caused the other condition, then a directional arrow is drawn from one condition to the other, depicting unilateral or bilateral direction of effect (cf. bottom panel in Figure 2.1). In each conceptualization, the simultaneous completion of multiple diagrams serves to encourage the therapist to generate hypotheses about how the conditions are related.

As in the case of the original diagram, the Case Conceptualization Diagram for Comorbid Conditions is "introduced to the patient as an explanatory device, designed to help make sense of the patient's current reactions to situations" (J. S. Beck, 1995, p. 143). The conceptualization is presented as a series of hypotheses, and the patient provides input as to the accuracy of the conceptualization. Based on the view that the more authentic and collaborative the understanding that develops between the patient and the therapist, the better the outcome is likely to be (Persons, 1989), completing the cognitive conceptualization together as a collaborative exercise should promote better outcome. As such, this diagram is useful for helping both therapist and patient develop a working, common understanding of the patient.

In addition to providing hypotheses about relationships among the patient's problems, the case conceptualization should ultimately provide information regarding selection of an appropriate treatment modality (e.g., individual, couple, or family therapy) and specific intervention strategies, and the pacing of therapy. Case conceptualization may also provide information about other contextual factors that are relevant to treatment (e.g., the therapeutic relationship). Finally, it should be noted that case conceptualization is not fixed at the beginning (or at any stage) of therapy. Although it begins with an initial assessment, conceptualization does not end with this assessment. Instead, case conceptualization is viewed as a fluid, working hypothesis of the person, which is revised as additional information becomes available.

Because case conceptualization is so closely linked to the treatment plan, the utility of the conceptualization is evaluated by the outcome of the intervention that follows from it. Therefore, if an intervention based on the conceptualization is successful, the conceptualization is supported. In comparison, if an intervention based on the conceptualization is unsuccessful or ineffective, then the conceptualization is not supported. In this case, the conceptualization would need to be modified and alternative interventions implemented. We turn now to a discussion of ways in which standard CT may be adapted in treating different presentations of depression.

ADAPTING CT IN TREATING VARIOUS PRESENTATIONS OF DEPRESSION

Having discussed assessment and conceptualization, we turn our attention to ways of tailoring CT for various presentations of depression. In this section, we present a framework for ways in which treatment can be adapted; specific recommendations for adaptations of CT for specific presentations of depression are covered in the remaining chapters in this volume.

Adapting the Parameters of Treatment Delivery of CT for Depression

Based on the case conceptualization, a therapist might choose to modify the parameters under which CT is administered. Specifically, a therapist might choose to modify the length of treatment. For example, strong endorsement of negative schemas associated with severe depression might require that treatment be extended to provide a greater number of opportunities for testing out alternative belief systems. Similarly, the therapist might decide that patients who only partially respond to treatment require periodic follow-up sessions to help ensure that they are practicing the skills learned in therapy and thereby maintaining their gains. Alternatively, based on the case conceptualization, the therapist might choose to modify the time between sessions. For example, to help get a suicidal patient through a crisis might require more frequent sessions than the typical weekly session.

Adapting the Style of Presentation of CT for Depression

Another potential way to modify treatment concerns the style or manner of conducting CT; that is, there may be individual differences in preference and responsiveness to different types of CT interventions. For example, the underlying personality characteristics of sociotropy and autonomy are believed to be associated with how depressed individuals respond to different aspects of treatment. This has been labeled the *differential treatment hypothesis* (Clark et al., 1999). According to Beck (1983), patients who are high in sociotropy prefer and are more responsive to interventions that emphasize support, helping, and emotional closeness. It is hypothesized that these individuals likely prefer an informal and closer relationship with their therapist and may rely on him/her to help them solve their problems. In comparison, patients who are high in autonomy prefer and are more responsive to goal-directed, task-focused, and problem-oriented interventions. It is hypothesized that these individuals likely prefer a more formal, detached relationship with their therapist, and respond to a collaborative relationship in setting the agenda, selecting topics for each session, and assigning homework.

To be able to adapt CT in response to the differential treatment hypothesis, clinicians need to administer a measure of sociotropy and autonomy. To aid in interpretation of such measures, we have provided normative data on two of the most commonly used measures of these constructs—the Revised Sociotropy–Autonomy Scale (SAS; Clark & Beck, 1991) and the Revised Personal Style Inventory (PSI-II; Robins et al., 1994). To obtain normative data on these measures, we used PsycINFO to identify articles that cited the original reference for the measure, then, similar to the methodology used by Dozois et al. (2003), included data from studies that were written in English and based on the original standardized format of the measure, that involved samples not based on cutoff scores, and that excluded people with serious physical or mental health problems. The resulting means and standard deviations for this scale are provided in Table 2.1.

As with the data on cognitive measures, normative data can be used to compute T-scores that evaluate a patient's relative elevations on sociotropy versus autonomy, which in turn provides information used to modify treatment to match the person's dominant (i.e., highest scoring) personality style. For example, raw scores of 110 on the Sociotropy and Autonomy scales of the PSI-II, although equal at the level of raw scores, translate into a T-score of 60 on sociotropy:

$$T = 50 + 10[(110 - 95)/16] = 50 + 10(1) = 50 + 10 = 60$$

and a *T*-score of 70 on autonomy:

$$T = 50 + 10[(110 - 84)/14] = 50 + 10(2) = 50 + 20 = 70$$

Because the *T*-score is higher (by a full standard deviation) for autonomy than for sociotropy, a patient with these scores might be expected to benefit from problem-oriented interventions and actively collaborate with the therapist in structuring therapy.

Research on the differential treatment hypothesis has focused on whether sociotropy and autonomy are associated with differential treatment response to pharmacotherapy or group versus individual CT (Clark et al., 1999). As such, there is little empirical evidence to indicate whether tailoring treatment focus and therapist style based on a patient's level of sociotropy or autonomy is associated with a patient's preference and response to CT for depression, although this would be an important and clinically informative area for future research.

In addition to modifying the therapist's style and mode of interacting with patients, another aspect of CT for depression that may be modified is the way the treatment is presented to patients. For example, it may be important to change the cognitive rationale provided to certain types of patients. Along these lines, it has been suggested that a cognitive rationale focusing on negative aspects of self-appraisal is inappropriate for older persons experiencing a first episode of late-onset depression, because it does not adequately address the functional roles that positive beliefs have had in maintaining self-esteem over a lifetime (James, Kendell, & Katharina, 1999).

Adapting the Emphasis or Focus of CT for Depression

Another direction for modifying CT for depression is to emphasize or to place a greater focus on one or more specific aspects of CT of depression. For example, Beck et al. (1979) hypothesized that greater severity of depression requires greater use of behavioral strategies in CT. Therefore, whereas behavioral interventions might be included in working with many depressed individuals, they may make up a larger percentage of sessions for people who are more severely depressed.

Another area in CT for depression that is important in working with various manifestations of depression is different emphases on the therapeutic relationship. Whereas a good therapeutic relationship is viewed as necessary but not sufficient in conducting CT for depression (Beck et al., 1979), the therapeutic relationship may assume a greater role in working with certain types of depressed patients. For example, using the therapeutic relationship as a testing ground for modifying cognitions might be particularly helpful for people with chronic or persistent depression, or for people with personality disorders or dysfunctional personality traits (Beck et al., 2003; Young, Klosko, & Weishaar, 2003).

Augmenting Standard CT for Depression

A final method for adapting CT for depression is to supplement standard treatment with additional treatment interventions. From a theoretical perspective, interventions that are compatible with the cognitive theory of depression (i.e., the theory that maladaptive information processing is central to understanding the onset, course, and treatment of depression; Clark et al., 1999) can be appropriately considered to be cognitive in nature; that is, it is compatibility with cognitive theory, and not whether an intervention is labeled a "cognitive" intervention (vs. a behavioral or interpersonal intervention), that "provides a unifying theoretical framework within which the clinical techniques of other established, validated approaches may be properly incorporated" (Alford & Beck, 1997, p. 112). From this perspective, many different types of intervention that could be added to standard CT for depression might be useful in modifying maladaptive information processing.

Adapting standard CT for depression with supplemental interventions generally proceeds in one of two directions. First, a therapist might use additional clinical techniques in targeting other problems in a sequential fashion. For example, a clinician working with a patient who presents with comorbid depression and a substance use disorder might first decide to treat the depression, then the substance use disorder, in a sequential fashion. In deciding upon the order of treatment, the clinician may want to begin with the problem that is most distressing to the patient. Another approach to sequencing of treatment strategies is to begin with the problem that is seen as primary (i.e., occurring prior to other problems) and subsequently moving to secondary problems once the primary problem is successfully treated. For example, if a patient has developed an addiction to a medication prescribed to help with insomnia he/she experiences as part of depression, it may be most useful to treat the depression first, then the substance use disorder. Alternatively, if marital conflict is seen as contributing to a patient's depression, it may be beneficial first to reduce the amount of conflict (e.g., reduce the frequency or intensity of criticism from a spouse) before targeting the patient's beliefs about the meaning of such conflict in CT for depression.

In comparison to sequential treatment, there may be occasions in which treatment interventions are provided simultaneously within a given session or across several sessions. For example, in a case in which depression and anxiety are equally distressing to the patient, targeting the two conditions might alternate from one session to the next. Thus, sessions focusing on CT interventions targeting symptoms of depression could be alternated with sessions focusing on CT interventions targeting symptoms of anxiety.

A third approach to supplementing standard CT for depression involves developing a treatment that specifically addresses a particular manifestation of depression. Thus, unlike a treatment that focuses on independent forms of intervention that are presented in a successive or alternating fashion, such a modification reflects the development of a different treatment protocol that is delivered for a particular manifestation of depression. For example, depressed individuals who are suicidal may be one example of a manifestation of depression that requires its own type of CT protocol. In this case, the treatment shares the theoretical underpinning of CT for depression, as well as some common interventions, but the resulting protocol may be different enough to be considered its own treatment.

CONCLUSIONS

In this chapter we have presented a model for the assessment and case conceptualization of depression that focuses on different manifestations of depression. Specifically in assessing depressed patients, cognitive therapists are encouraged to consider depression parameters (e.g., severity, persistence), comorbid conditions (Axis I and II disorders, medical conditions, social functioning), and aspects associated with different demographic variables. Information gathered from this assessment can then be integrated by the clinician in formulating his/her case conceptualization.

We have also discussed how case conceptualization can be used in treatment planning, including ways to adapt standard CT in working with various presentations of depression. We have provided a general discussion of the parameters that might be modified or adapted in working with depressed patients in clinical practice; specific recommendations for specific presentations of depression are covered in the remaining chapters of this book. We hope that the assessment-driven case conceptualization described in this chapter aids in treatment planning and results in improved outcomes for treating depression in everyday practice.

REFERENCES

Abramowitz, J. S. (2006). Toward a functional analytic approach to psychologically complex patients: A comment on Ruscio and Holohan. *Clinical Psychology: Science and Practice, 13*, 163–166.

Alford, B. A., & Beck, A. T. (1997). *The integrative power of cognitive therapy.* New York: Guilford Press.

Alford, B. A., & Gerrity, D. M. (1995). The specificity of sociotropy–autonomy personality dimensions to depression vs. anxiety. *Journal of Clinical Psychology, 51,* 190–195.

Alloy, L. B., Kelly, K. A., Mineka, S., & Clements, C. M. (1990). Comorbidity of anxiety and depressive disorders: A helplessness–hopelessness perspective. In J. D. Maser & C. R. Cloninger (Eds.), *Comorbidity of mood and anxiety disorders* (pp. 499–543). Washington, DC: American Psychiatric Press.

Beck, A. T. (1976). *Cognitive therapy and the emotional disorders.* Madison, CT: International Universities Press.

Beck, A. T. (1983). Cognitive therapy of depression: New perspectives. In P. J. Clayton & J. E. Barrett (Eds.), *Treatment of depression: Old controversies and new perspectives* (pp. 265–290). New York: Raven Press.

Beck, A. T. (1991). Cognitive therapy: A 30–year retrospective. *American Psychologist, 46,* 368–375.

Beck, A. T., Butler, A. C., Brown, G. K., Dahlsgaard, K. K., Newman, C. F., & Beck, J. S. (2001). Dysfunctional beliefs discriminate personality disorders. *Behaviour Research and Therapy, 39,* 1213–1225.

Beck, A. T., Freeman, A., Davis, D. D., & Associates. (2003). *Cognitive therapy of personality disorders: Second edition.* New York: Guilford Press.

Beck, A. T., Rush, A. J., Shaw, B. F., & Emery, G. (1979). *Cognitive therapy of depression.* New York: Guilford Press.

Beck, A. T., Steer, R. A., & Brown, G. K. (1996). *Beck Depression Inventory–II manual.* San Antonio, TX: Psychological Corporation.

Beck, J. S. (1995). *Cognitive therapy: Basics and beyond.* New York: Guilford Press.

Beck, J. S. (2005). *Cognitive therapy for challenging problems: What to do when the basics don't work.* New York: Guilford Press.

Beck, R., & Perkins, T. S. (2001). Cognitive content-specificity for anxiety and depression: A meta-analysis. *Cognitive Therapy and Research, 25,* 651–663.

Clark, D. A., & Beck, A. T. (1991). Personality factors in dysphoria: A psychometric refinement of Beck's Sociotropy–Autonomy Scale. *Journal of Psychopathology and Behavioral Assessment, 13,* 369–388.

Clark, D. A., Beck, A. T., & Alford, B. A. (1999). *Scientific foundations of cognitive theory and therapy of depression.* Hoboken, NJ: Wiley.

Corruble, E., Ginestet, D., & Guelfi, J. D. (1996). Comorbidity of personality disorders and unipolar major depression: A review. *Journal of Affective Disorders, 37,* 157–170.

Dozois, D. J. A., Covin, R., & Brinker, J. K. (2003). Normative data on cognitive measures of depression. *Journal of Consulting and Clinical Psychology, 71*, 71–80.

First, M. B., Spitzer, R. L., Gibbon, M., & Williams, J. B. W. (1996). *Structured Clinical Interview for DSM-IV Axis I Disorders, Clinician Version (SCID-CV)*. Washington, DC: American Psychiatric Press.

Hayaki, J., Friedman, M. A., Whisman, M. A., Delinsky, S. S., & Brownell, K. D. (2003). Sociotropy and bulimic symptoms in clinical and nonclinical samples. *International Journal of Eating Disorders, 34*, 172–176.

Hirschfeld, R. M. A., Montgomery, S. A., Keller, M. B., Kasper, S., Schatzberg, A. F., Moller, H.-J., et al. (2000). Social functioning in depression: A review. *Journal of Clinical Psychiatry, 61*, 268–275.

Jacobson, N. S., Dobson, K. S., Truax, P. A., Addis, M. E., Koerner, K., Gollan, J. K., et al. (1996). A component analysis of cognitive-behavioral treatment for depression. *Journal of Consulting and Clinical Psychology, 64*, 295–304.

James, I. A., Kendell, K., & Katharina, R. F. (1999). Conceptualizations of depression in older people: The interaction of positive and negative beliefs. *Behavioural and Cognitive Psychotherapy, 27*, 285–290.

Kessler, R. C., Berglund, P., Demler, O., Jin, R., Koretz, D., Merikangas, K. R., et al. (2003). The epidemiology of major depressive disorder: Results from the National Comorbidity Survey Replication (NCS-R). *Journal of the American Medical Association, 289*, 3095–3105.

Kessler, R. C., Mickelson, K. D., & Williams, D. R. (1999). The prevalence, distribution, and mental health correlates of perceived discrimination in the United States. *Journal of Health and Social Behavior, 40*, 208–230.

Kessler, R. C., Nelson, C. B., McGonagle, K. A., Liu, J., Swartz, M., & Blazer, D. G. (1996). Comorbidity of DSM-III-R major depressive disorder in the general population: Results form the US National Comorbidity Survey. *British Journal of Psychiatry, 168*, 17–30.

Krueger, R. F., & Markon, K. E. (2006). Reinterpreting comorbidity: A model-based approach to understanding and classifying psychopathology. *Annual Review of Clinical Psychology, 2*, 111–133.

Laidlaw, K., Thompson, L. W., & Gallagher-Thompson, D. (2004). Comprehensive conceptualization of cognitive behaviour therapy for late life depression. *Behavioural and Cognitive Psychotherapy, 32*, 1–11.

Lynch, T. R., Robins, C. J., & Morse, J. Q. (2001). Couple functioning in depression: The roles of sociotropy and autonomy. *Journal of Clinical Psychology, 57*, 93–103.

Maruish, M. E. (1999). *The use of psychological testing for treatment planning and outcomes assessment* (2nd ed.). Mahwah, NJ: Erlbaum.

Mineka, S., Watson, D., & Clark, L. A. (1998). Comorbidity of anxiety and unipolar mood disorders. *Annual Review of Psychology, 49*, 377–412.

Nezu, A. M., Ronan, G. F., Meadows, E. A., & McClure, K. S. (2000). *Practitioner's guide to empirically based measures of depression*. Dordrecht, The Netherlands: Kluwer Academic.

Nezu, A. M., Wilkins, V. M., & Nezu, C. M. (2004). Social problem solving, stress, and negative affect. In E. C. Chang, T. J. D'Zurilla, & L. J. Sanna (Eds.), *Social problem solving: Theory, research, and training* (pp. 49–65). Washington, DC: American Psychological Association.

Ouimette, P. C., Klein, D. N., Anderson, R., Riso, L. P., & Lizardi, H. (1994). Relationship of sociotropy/autonomy and dependency/self-criticism to DSM-III-R personality disorders. *Journal of Abnormal Psychology, 103*, 743–749.

Persons, J. B. (1989). *Cognitive therapy in practice: A case formulation approach.* New York: Norton.

Persons, J. B. (1995). Are all psychotherapies cognitive? *Journal of Cognitive Psychotherapy, 9*, 185–194.

Persons, J. B. (2006). Case-formulation driven psychotherapy. *Clinical Psychology: Science and Practice, 13*, 167–170.

Robins, C. J., Ladd, J., Welkowitz, J., Blaney, P. H., Kutcher, D., & Diaz, R. (1994). The Personal Style Inventory: Preliminary validation studies of new measures of sociotropy and autonomy. *Journal of Psychopathology and Behavioral Assessment, 16*, 277–300.

Salokangas, R. K., Vaahtera, K., Pacriev, S., Sohlman, B., & Lehtinen, V. (2002). Gender differences in depressive symptoms: An artifact caused by measurement instruments? *Journal of Affective Disorders, 68*, 215–220.

Silverstein, B. (1999). Gender difference in the prevalence of clinical depression: The role played by depression associated with somatic symptoms. *American Journal of Psychiatry, 156*, 480–482.

Stevens, D. E., Merikangas, K. R., & Merikangas, J. R. (1995). Comorbidity of depression and other medical conditions. In E. E. Beckham & W. R. Leber (Eds.), *Handbook of depression* (2nd ed., pp. 147–199). New York: Guilford Press.

Weinstock, L. M., & Whisman, M. A. (2006). Neuroticism as a common feature of the depressive and anxiety disorders: A test of the revised integrative hierarchical model in a national sample. *Journal of Abnormal Psychology, 115*, 68–74.

Whisman, M. A., & Bruce, M. L. (1999). Marital distress and incidence of major depressive episode in a community sample. *Journal of Abnormal Psychology, 108*, 674–678.

Widiger, T. A., & Samuel, D. B. (2005). Evidence-based assessment of personality disorders. *Psychological Assessment, 17*, 278–287.

Young, J. E., Klosko, J. S., & Weishaar, M. E. (2003). *Schema therapy: A practitioner's guide.* New York: Guilford Press.

Zimmerman, M., & Mattia, J. I. (1999). Psychiatric diagnosis in clinical practice: Is comorbidity being missed? *Comprehensive Psychiatry, 40*, 182–191.

II

COGNITIVE THERAPY
FOR COMPLEX DEPRESSION

3

SEVERE DEPRESSION

Sona Dimidjian
Christopher R. Martell
Sandra J. Coffman
Steven D. Hollon

In the treatment of major depression, severity has emerged as one of the more controversial variables with respect to the performance of cognitive therapy (CT). Empirical studies investigating the efficacy of CT with severely depressed patients have yielded mixed findings, and recent data suggest the possibility that when CT works for more severely depressed patients, its success may be attributable to the importance of the behavioral strategies.

In this chapter we propose a series of guidelines for the practice of CT with moderate to severely depressed patients. Guidelines pertinent to conceptualization and assessment, as well as treatment intervention, are discussed; in particular, adaptations of standard CT for use with this population are emphasized. A case illustration is included to highlight key strategies in case conceptualization and intervention. In a concluding section we review the findings from clinical trials CT that have included moderately to severely depressed patients and highlight implications of these data for clinical practitioners.

CONCEPTUALIZATION OF SEVERE DEPRESSION

The severity of a major depressive disorder is generally defined according to the number of symptoms present, the severity of the symptoms, and the associated functional impairment or distress (American Psychiatric Association, 1994). According to criteria in the fourth edition of the *Diagnostic and Statistical Manual of Mental Disorders* (DSM-IV), mild depression is indicated by the presence of five or six symptoms, mild functional impairment, or the ability to function normally with significant effort. Severe depression is indicated by the presence of most of the symptoms of a major depressive episode and clear functional impairment. Up to 15% of severely depressed individuals also die by suicide (American Psychiatric Association, 1994); readers are strongly encouraged to consult specific guidelines regarding the assessment and management of suicidality (e.g., Ghahramanlou-Holloway, Brown, & Beck, Chapter 7, this volume). Moreover, severe depression may also be accompanied by psychotic symptoms; however, such presentations are not the focus of this chapter. Moderate depression is indicated by symptom severity and impairment that falls between the levels of mild and severe. Severity of depression is also commonly defined according to scores obtained on self-report or interview-based measures; the most common severity assessment tools are reviewed below.

In general, the conceptualization of severe depression follows the same general framework for case conceptualization of standard CT. To the extent that severe depression may be associated with increased comorbidity and psychosocial impairment, it may be important to highlight the importance of these factors in the patient's experience of depression. The case illustration below provides an extended example of discussion of the cognitive model of depression with a more severely depressed patient.

ASSESSMENT OF SEVERE DEPRESSION

For patients who have been diagnosed with major depressive disorder according to DSM-IV criteria, both interview- and self-report based measures are available for the assessment of depressive severity. The Beck Depression Inventory—Second Edition (BDI-II; Beck, Steer, & Brown, 1996) is perhaps the most widely used self-report measure. Beck et al. report the following ranges for depressive symptom severity: minimal (0–13), mild (14–19), moderate (20–28), and severe (29–63). Among the most widely used interview-based measures is the Hamilton Rating Scale for Depression (HRSD; Hamilton, 1960); scores on the 17-item version range in increasing severity from 0 to 69. In many clinical studies, scores of 20 or greater indicate moderate to severely depressed patients, and scores of 14 to 19 indicate less severely depressed patients. Other studies have used cutoffs of 25 or 28 to demarcate purely high-severity subgroups using the HRSD.

TREATMENT OF SEVERE DEPRESSION

Several areas of emphasis in the course of CT for more severely depressed patients are recommended, including heavy emphasis on the use of behavioral strategies, increased frequency of contact and continuity between sessions (including emphasis on between-session practice), collaborative presentation of the treatment model, attention to the therapeutic relationship, and consideration of concurrent pharmacotherapy. Finally, ongoing monitoring of one's competence in CT is recommended.

Behavioral Strategies

Behavioral Component of CT

The seminal formulation of CT suggested a strong emphasis on the use of behavioral strategies with more severely depressed patients (Beck, Rush, Shaw, & Emery, 1979). As Beck and colleagues (1979) noted:

> The behavioral techniques are clearly indicated with severely depressed patients. An individual with severe depression commonly has considerable difficulty focusing on more abstract conceptualizations. His attention span may be limited to well-defined concrete suggestions. Research findings in the area suggest "success" experiences on concrete behavioral tasks are most effective in breaking the vicious cycle of demoralization, passivity and avoidance, and self-disparagement. (p. 140)

And, as discussed in greater detail below, research by our group has suggested that purely behavioral treatments demonstrate comparable or possibly superior outcomes to CT among more severely depressed patients (Dimidjian et al., 2006; Jacobson et al., 1996).

When working with severely depressed patients, therefore, therapists are advised not to abandon prematurely the behavioral strategies in favor of the more purely cognitive interventions. Key behavioral interventions in CT include activity monitoring and scheduling, mastery and pleasure ratings, and graded task assignments. These strategies are used with more severely depressed patients in a format similar to that used with less depressed patients; however, therapists may need to pace interventions at a level that is appropriate to the patient's degree of depression. The aim of these strategies is to increase patient activity, specifically, those activities associated with mastery and pleasure, while decreasing activities found to be associated with depression (Beck et al., 1979). This early focus on behavior change is important to increase the patient's readiness for more direct exploration and evaluation of cognition. Activity monitoring and scheduling assignments can also be used to elicit and address patient beliefs about activity. Specifically, early behavior change can be critical in providing some of the early evidence required to evaluate specific depressive and hopeless thoughts (e.g., "I fail at everything, nothing will help me. I've tried everything. What is the point?"). Such thoughts may be targeted directly in the course of planning and debriefing behavioral homework assignments. Thus, although early homework assignments in CT for patients with more severe depression are heavily behavioral, discussion of these assignments during sessions often integrates a behavioral and cognitive focus.

In general, patients are initially asked to complete monitoring assignments in which they keep track of their moods and activities, and specific experiences of mastery or pleasure. Typically, patients are invited to record specific activities each hour of the day and to rate their level of depression on a 10-point scale that is associated with each activity. Therapists working with patients with particularly acute depression associated with significant functional impairment may move quickly to activity scheduling assignments. They may ask patients, "What might you do tomorrow if you were not depressed?" Then, using graded task assignment (as discussed below), therapists may ask patients to schedule small, specific behaviors to complete prior to the next contact with the therapist. Later, monitoring assignments can be superimposed on tasks that patients have been doing as they work to follow the scheduled activities.

Completed activity logs are then reviewed in session; discussion of these logs frequently emphasizes activities or interactions that are associated with increased depression. In addition, the logs provide essential information about the patient's daily schedule, including sleep, nutrition, and social isolation. The practice of keeping the schedule also helps to activate patients and begins training them to notice and label moods, and the specific relationships between activities and moods. Activity scheduling strategies involve inviting patients to plan specific activities during sessions and/or to plan activities each night for the following day. Therapists may emphasize that it is common for people not to accomplish everything that they plan, and tasks that are left undone can be scheduled for another day.

The use of graded task assignment is particularly important with more severely depressed patients, who may believe that even seemingly simple tasks are impossible to complete. The aim of graded task assignment is to program success into scheduled activities. Rather than trying to accomplish a large task all at once, tasks are broken down into component parts. As each successive step is completed, the patient has a success experience and makes concrete progress toward solving problems or developing a more fulfilling daily routine. Moreover, the patient gathers evidence that he/she can succeed at something, which may provide evidence against negative and overgeneralized beliefs about the self.

To the degree that severity also overlaps with hopelessness, it is also essential that therapists address this skillfully early in treatment. Therapists must take care not to get caught in the patient's despair, which may be associated with unwillingness to try new approaches and strategies. Therapists can provide hope and repeatedly encourage an experimental approach by inviting the patient to try a variety of strategies to improve mood and by emphasizing the importance of repeated, small steps. Although flexibility and persistence are core features of standard CT, with more severely depressed and hopeless patients, modeling both may be particularly important. At the same time, it is necessary to do so in a way that does not rely on false promises or guarantees; the essence of encouraging experiments is to find out whether something works, not simply to assume that it will. It is important that the patient learn to test things out rather than to assume the worst (or the best) in advance of action.

The Behavioral Activation Approach

Early work by Jacobson and colleagues (1996) suggested that the behavioral component of CT performed as well as the full CT package in the treatment of major depression. This work led to the evolution of the behavioral component of CT into a stand-alone treatment approach, called simply behavioral activation (BA; Jacobson, Martell, & Dimidjian, 2001; Martell, Addis, & Jacobson, 2001). This approach is based heavily on the behavioral component of CT, but, it also includes additional clinical innovations and a purely behavioral rather than a cognitive conceptualization that draws heavily from early behavioral work of Ferster (1973) and Lewinsohn (1974). The additional strategies and conceptualization of the BA approach may be of value in informing the practice of CT with more severely depressed patients.

In BA, behavior change is pursued for its direct impact on mood; it is not assumed that it is necessary to change thinking to treat depression.

Moreover, when utilizing the activity schedule, BA therapists emphasize the function of the patient's activity. In other words, activity serves many purposes. Staring out the window on a rainy day as one waits for a loved one to come home to a lovely dinner is different than staring out the window at the rain as one thinks about the dreariness of life. The form of the behavior is similar (i.e., staring out the window), but the function differs. The emotional outcome is quite different: in the first case, hopeful anticipation of the loved one's return; in the second, hopeless despair.

The BA therapist generates hypotheses about the function of the patient's activity and notes particularly behaviors that function as avoidance; these behaviors are hypothesized to maintain or exacerbate depression and, as such, are the initial targets of treatment. Depressed patients often engage in behaviors that may provide some temporary relief and yet have negative long-term consequences for mood and quality of life. Staying in bed, for example, may be reinforced by the relief of not having to address problems at work or in one's family. Therapy focuses on monitoring the short- and long-term consequences of such behaviors, and using graded task assignment and activity scheduling to interrupt avoidance patterns and increase activation. Essentially, patients learn to approach and engage rather than to avoid and withdraw. The acronym TRAP (Trigger, Response, Avoidance Pattern) can be used to teach patients to recognize situations that lead to negative feelings (or thoughts) to which the patients respond with avoidance behavior. Although, from a cognitive perspective, avoidance behavior may result from patients' negative beliefs (e.g., "What is the point of trying?"), the BA therapist does not address the validity of such beliefs directly. Instead, the emphasis in BA remains on the function or consequences of patient behavior, and as such, is very consistent with a focus on the "utility" of thoughts or behaviors in CT (e.g., asking "What is the utility of thinking that way?" as opposed to "What is the validity of that thought?").

We are not advocating that therapists do away with cognitive components in the treatment of severely depressed patients. Certainly, our results (described below) supporting the promise of the BA approach do not negate a cognitive conceptualization; approaching rather than avoiding an aversive situation may indeed provide important evidence to contradict patients' negative or global beliefs. However, our data and clinical experience suggest that in treatment of severely depressed patients, it may be ill-advised to rush through the behavioral component of CT in an effort to devote the majority of clinical time to addressing beliefs directly. Particularly in the context of time limited treatment, it may be more efficacious for therapists to concentrate on more concrete goals and to use simpler, more specific behavioral interventions for a longer period of time (Coffman, Martell,

Dimidjian, Gallop, & Hollon, 2007). In a sense, CT therapists may do more for their severely depressed patients by trying to cover less over the course of treatment. The importance of a systematic, graded, and prolonged focus on monitoring and scheduling activities is highlighted in the treatment of more severely depressed patients.

Frequency and Continuity of Sessions

Maintenance of continuity and consistency across sessions is also particularly important when treating more severe depression. Typical research protocols with such patients have specified the use of twice-weekly sessions for the first half of a 4-month protocol (DeRubeis et al., 2005; Dimidjian et al., 2006). Frequent sessions early in the course of treatment can maximize patient engagement with treatment and ensure success with initial homework assignments. In addition, such frequency helps the therapist to monitor the severity of the patient's depression on an ongoing basis and to intervene early if the patient's condition deteriorates or does not improve. If twice-weekly sessions are not pragmatic given financial or scheduling considerations, it may be advisable to schedule brief, check-in phone contacts with patients. Moreover, with respect to the duration of treatment, in one study in which patients were randomly assigned either to brief (8 weeks) or extended (16 weeks) CT, results suggested that more severely depressed patients improved significantly more with extended treatment (Shapiro et al., 1994).

Although assigning homework is a standard part of CT, it may be particularly important with more severely depressed patients. Given the importance of producing rapid and significant change with more severely depressed patients, assignment of regular homework is strongly advised. Toward this end, homework should be reviewed consistently each session and tailored to ensure that patients experience success.

Collaborative Presentation of the Treatment Model and Ongoing Attention to the Therapeutic Relationship

Attention to patient reactions to the cognitive model may be particularly important when therapists work with severely depressed patients. Among the patients who received CT in our recent trial, those who did poorly were more likely to be severely depressed and to have significant problems with their primary support group when they began treatment (in addition to having greater functional impairment; Coffman et al., 2007). The specific support group problems that were common to these patients included death of a family member, health problems in the family, and family disruption such as separation, divorce, and estrangement. For patients with such problems the sensitivity of the presentation of the cognitive model may be particularly critical. By emphasizing the meaning that patients attach to situations, the cognitive model highlights that problems reside not only in the environment but also in the beliefs and biases that affect individuals' information processing. To the extent that severity of depression is associated with significant interpersonal stress, therapists must take particular care to ensure that patients do not experience the cognitive conceptualization as either blaming or dismissive of the realities of the life problems they experience. Therapists are advised to ask patients for direct feedback about their understanding of the cognitive model and to elicit any patient concerns or negative reactions.

Moreover, breaches in the alliance may be particularly likely when therapist and patient explore cognitions about interpersonal problems (Hayes, Castonguay, & Goldfried, 1996). These findings suggest that particular skill may be needed to address interpersonal problems such that the therapist empathizes with the patient's experience, yet does not validate irrational beliefs and faulty attributions. The importance of the therapeutic relationship has been stressed in CT generally and in the treatment of complex patients with personality disorders specifically (Beck et al., 1979; Beck, Freeman, & Associates, 1990; Kohlenberg & Tsai, 1994; Safran & Segal, 1990). Given the high degree of overlap between severity and interpersonal difficulty, it is often helpful to include greater attention to the therapist–patient relationship than may be the case in standard CT for less severely depressed patients. For example, early in therapy, it may be prudent for the therapist to discuss the possibility that the patient may feel criticized, judged, or dismissed by the therapist at some point during their work together. The therapist can invite the patient to work collaboratively with him/her to watch for and discuss any possible instances. Identifying in session the patient's automatic thoughts about the therapist or therapy also provides an important opportunity to explore and evaluate such thoughts.

In summary, attention to the patient's reaction to the cognitive model, and to the development and maintenance of the therapeutic relationship over time, is central in working with more severely depressed patients. The frequent association between severity of depression and significant social support problems creates a context in which patients may experience the therapist's focus on cognitive change as problematic. It is important for the therapist to inquire about this possibility and to address it directly, openly, and nondefensively when it does occur.

Concurrent Use of Pharmacotherapy

Finally, it is recommended that therapists consider and discuss with their patients the option of concurrent pharmacotherapy. Although not all patients wish to take medication and many cannot tolerate the accompanying side effects, studies to date suggest a modest advantage of combined pharmacotherapy and psychotherapy. Although these studies have not focused specifically on severely depressed patients, they have included sizable numbers of such patients in their samples. In general, studies of combined treatments suggest an increase in response rates of approximately 10–15% (Hollon, Thase, & Markowitz, 2002).

When conducting CT with a patient who is taking an antidepressant, it is advisable to inquire regularly about the patient's experience of the medication, including possible side effects, beliefs about usage, and so forth. In addition, therapists who are not prescribing medication themselves are advised to make periodic contact with the prescribing physician for continuity of care. Maintaining a team approach with a severely depressed patient ensures that everyone is informed of progress and compliance, and provides an opportunity for individuals involved in the case to consult with one another. It is also important to monitor and to inquire about patient attributions for change, and in particular to assess and explore any patient beliefs that suggest all positive change is due to medication and ignore behavioral or cognitive change that may accompany or follow medication use.

Competence in CT

The guidelines we have presented are intended to increase the efficacy of CT with severely depressed patients. The manner in which therapists adhere to such guidelines is also likely to have a significant influence on treatment outcome. In a recent study comparing medication and CT with more severely depressed patients, experienced CT therapists demonstrated outcomes that were comparable to those achieved with antidepressant medication; however, medication significantly outperformed CT therapists who were less experienced (DeRubeis et al., 2005). These findings are consistent with an earlier multisite trial, in which sites whose therapists had greater expertise in CT demonstrated better outcomes (Elkin et al., 1989; Jacobson & Hollon, 1996). Together these results suggest that when working with more severely depressed patients, the level of practitioner competence is particularly critical. The most widely used measure for assessing competence in CT, the Cognitive Therapy Scale (Young & Beck, 1980), has documented reliability when used by expert raters (Dobson, Shaw, & Vallis, 1985; Vallis, Shaw, & Dobson, 1986). Generally, scores of 40 and above are considered to be within the range of competent CT.

With respect to methods for increasing one's competence, therapists may want to consider the following possibilities. First, ongoing monitoring of competence is highly recommended and can be achieved through consultation with colleagues or expert trainers in CT. Information about CT training and consultation can be obtained by contacting the Academy of Cognitive Therapy. In a recent study, Sholomskas et al. (2005) compared the influence of multiple training methods on the effectiveness of trainees' demonstration of particular strategies in role plays. Results suggested a clear advantage for participation in a didactic seminar plus 3 hours of individual case supervision, compared to simply reading the manual, or reading the manual plus participation in Web-based training. Second, more experience in the specific provision of CT is helpful in maximizing therapist competence, particularly treatment early in one's training of patients who demonstrate high "suitability" for CT (James, Blackburn, Milne, & Reichfelt, 2001). As therapists gain CT experience treating a greater number of patients, their ability to apply CT strategies flexibly may increase; thus, they may achieve competence with a greater variety of patients.

CASE ILLUSTRATION

Alex, a 58-year-old, divorced European American woman, entered treatment for major depressive disorder with a score of 41 on the BDI and a score of 24 on the HRSD. On both of these measures, she also endorsed feeling that life was not worth living, although she denied any specific thoughts of suicide or wish to die. She also had a history of significant weight problems, which had worsened recently; she was concerned about her lack of physical conditioning and her obesity, both of which made it difficult for her to engage in even routine physical activity. Alex also met criteria for avoidant personality disorder, symptoms of which began in her youth and contributed to her current social isolation.

Treatment began with a discussion of Alex's reasons for seeking treatment and her experience of her current depression. Alex reported that her depression had begun approximately 2 years earlier, when her son David died from a debilitating chronic illness. Alex had provided care for David for several years prior to his death. Although she had been employed before that point, Alex was currently unemployed and had many financial concerns. She had moved in with her adult daughter, who supported her financially;

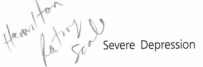

although Alex reported feeling grateful for this support, she also noted that her dependence likely contributed to her unhappiness. She was socially isolated and sad about her lack of regular contact with friends. Alex also reported one previous episode of depression that had occurred 20 years earlier, triggered by early marital problems; she and her husband experienced significant conflict during their 10-year marriage, which ultimately ended in divorce.

At the end of the first session, the therapist asked Alex to read the booklet *Coping with Depression* for a homework assignment. The therapist also discussed with Alex a plan for scheduling sessions during the next few weeks, suggesting that they meet twice a week.

> "We've found that it's helpful to meet frequently when you are more depressed, so that you can become more active. Then you can more quickly begin to start the process of changing any thinking patterns that may be related to your depression. Meeting more frequently also helps to counter any challenges you encounter. We find that this progress helps to undermine the discouragement that many depressed people experience when starting to learn some of the strategies in this therapy. Once you are feeling a little better and have more practice with the tools, we can move to weekly sessions, and ultimately to periodic booster sessions. By then you'll have many new skills and, hopefully, a new outlook on life and yourself, which will help with any future relapse of depression. How does that sound to you?"

Alex agreed to this approach, although she expressed some concerns about getting to therapy sessions twice a week.

The second session began with further discussion of the CT model and Alex's reaction to the *Coping with Depression* booklet. Alex's thoughts and feelings about this homework assignment provided a valuable starting place for a discussion of the treatment model and an overview of therapy. Alex began by reporting some confusion about the model.

> ALEX: I think I get that connection between thoughts and feelings at times. But does that mean that all of my sadness and is just because of my thinking? I mean, are you saying it's all in my head? I thought that is what the book was saying, but then my daughter read it, and she thought it was right on target and was really excited for me to be doing this.
>
> THERAPIST: How did you feel when you thought that this therapy was saying "it's all in your head"?

ALEX: Well, I guess I felt pretty lousy. I felt like maybe I was just making myself miserable.

THERAPIST: I am so glad that we are talking about this! Can I tell you how I think about these things? I think that most people would feel a great sadness and grief, as you do, after watching their child die after suffering through a long illness.

ALEX: So, you are not saying it is all in my head.

THERAPIST: Absolutely not! And, at the same time, isn't it interesting how you and your daughter both read the same book and had such different reactions?

ALEX: Yeah, I guess we did.

THERAPIST: So, the situation—reading the book—was the same, right? But your reactions were different. One of the key ideas in cognitive therapy is that the kinds of thoughts we have in response to a situation will influence how we feel. Can you summarize the thoughts that you had when you were reading the book?

ALEX: Well, I thought it was saying that I was overreacting to my son dying.

THERAPIST: And when you thought that, you felt sad or discouraged?

ALEX: Yeah, I thought, "what's the point of going back there?"

THERAPIST: And what about your daughter? What do you think her thoughts were?

ALEX: I think she thought it was interesting and a new perspective on things, and she was excited about it. I guess that is a little different take on it, huh? (laughing)

THERAPIST: Yes! So the point is really that it's possible to see the same situation in different ways, and that the way you see a situation can have a big impact on how you feel. When you thought I was saying "It's all in your head," you felt sad and hopeless. When your daughter thought, "Wow, here is some new valuable information," she felt excited.

ALEX: Yes, that is true.

THERAPIST: I wonder, when you think about your depression these last couple years, do you think it is possible that some of how you have been feeling is related to how you are thinking about David's death or perhaps the situations you have faced since then?

ALEX: Oh, yes. Well, I know I failed him in a lot of ways, and I do feel much worse when I dwell on those thoughts. And I guess I feel worse, too, when I think about how I have nothing left to give or do that is worthwhile anymore—when I think, "What is the point of any of it?"

THERAPIST: Yes, my guess is that those sorts of thoughts are closely connected to your feelings of depression. And those are just the kinds of thoughts we can look at together, maybe get curious about them together. We can explore those thoughts and perhaps see whether there may be some other perspectives to bring to the table. Would you be open to doing that?

ALEX: Yes, I think so.

THERAPIST: Great!

Openly and genuinely discussing the treatment model and Alex's concerns allowed the therapist and Alex to establish a foundation of collaboration for therapy. Based on this foundation, they moved on to focus on behavioral activation strategies. The therapist introduced the activity schedule as a way to track both feelings and the links between feelings and activities. The therapist asked Alex to complete the activity schedule each day until their next session, which was 3 days later. She specifically suggested that Alex record the activity in which she engaged and a corresponding depression rating (from 1 to 10) for each hour of the day.

When assigning the activity schedule, it is important to inquire about the patient's thoughts and feelings about completing the assignment. More severely depressed patients may think that the assignment is overwhelming or impossible, but they may be reluctant to disclose this to the therapist. It is important for therapists to elicit such information and to be open to modifying the assignment to maximize the patient's experience of success (e.g., keeping the schedule for a briefer period of time).

In the third session, Alex and the therapist reviewed the activity schedule. Alex commented on how much she had learned about herself, although the assignment had taken some time and effort. She reported that she could see certain patterns emerging as she recorded day-to-day activities. Alex recorded having no social contact for 2 days, and accompanying feelings of sadness. On the third day, however, when she received a phone call from a friend, she found that her mood improved. The therapist inquired about Alex's beliefs about her depression and lack of social contact. Alex reported that she avoided social contact because she "didn't want to bring people down." Although she took great pleasure in helping others and acknowledged that her isolation decreased her self-worth, Alex was convinced that her presence had a negative impact on others. The therapist asked Alex whether she was willing to do an experiment before the next session, to explore what happened when she spent time with others. Alex was amenable to this and made a commitment to call her friend back to schedule a visit. The therapist and Alex also identified possible thoughts and situations that might interfere with Alex's commitment. Alex reported that if she felt down in the morning, she might be tempted to stay in bed instead of going for the visit. Together, Alex and the therapist decided that she could experiment with telling herself, "Even though I want to stay in bed, staying in bed usually makes me feel worse. Getting up, showering, eating breakfast, and calling my friend is more likely to help improve my mood." Alex wrote this statement down on a card to take home with her. She also suggested and recorded the following thought: "I'm not giving myself any more reasons to get down on myself for being lazy. That thinking gets me nowhere."

Review of the activity schedule also illustrated the relationship between Alex's depression, and her eating and physical activity routines. Alex had recorded several episodes of overeating, followed by exacerbation of her mood. In reviewing these times, Alex reported feeling very discouraged about her recent weight gain and lack of physical activity. The therapist asked Alex what she thought her activity routines would be if she were not depressed. Alex talked about taking her dog for long walks twice a day before David became seriously ill. Based on this, the therapist introduced the principle of graded task assignment. They agreed that Alex would first walk for 5 minutes total. The next day she could walk for 5–7 minutes, adding 2 minutes each day (or at least maintaining the previous day's total as a minimum) for 5 days a week. A homework assignment of walking the dog once a day, with gradual increases in distance or time, was planned as an experiment.

At the following session Alex reported that she had in fact spent time with several friends, which helped her mood, although she reported still believed that they were visiting with her out of pity. Similarly, she had walked the dog on 4 of the days since the last session. Moreover, she had taken the bus and walked a short distance to the therapy session (as opposed to being dropped off by her daughter). The therapist highlighted these walks as significant increases in Alex's activity and inquired about their impact on her mood. Alex reported feeling better but dismissed her increased activity as something anyone ought to be able to do, thereby disregarding her own progress.

The subsequent six therapy sessions focused heavily on activity scheduling and monitoring. Over time, Alex increased her social contact, physical activity, and skill at monitoring her activities and feelings. She responded well to small behavioral steps, especially those that targeted avoidance, improved her physical activity, and increased social interaction. Alex began to attend her eating self-help group again and found it rewarding; she brought her "healthy eating charts" to discuss in session.

As Alex's depressive severity improved, the therapist began to target some of Alex's negative thinking patterns more explicitly. Alex understood and accepted the cognitive model of depression and could discuss with her therapist examples of thoughts influencing feelings. On this basis, the therapist introduced in the session and assigned for homework a Daily Thought Record. Alex returned the following session, stating that it was impossible to do thought records on her own, although she found that her mood improved when she and the therapist completed the log together in sessions. The therapist experimented with different versions of the thought log, and found that Alex preferred the Testing Your Thoughts form (J. S. Beck). She identified the thought, "I don't have a reason to go on. There's no purpose in my life," which made her feel "very tired." As in standard CT, the therapist used Socratic questioning to help Alex explore and examine these key thoughts. The following dialogue illustrates these discussions:

ALEX: My purpose was to be a parent. I guess I did good work at my job, too, but when David got sick, the most important thing I could do was to take good care of him. And I failed at that. He suffered a lot at the end. And now my daughter is suffering, too. I am such a burden on her, and I know her life would be easier without me.

THERAPIST: What do you feel and think when you picture your last days with David?

ALEX: I really want David to be alive (crying). It's just so hard to imagine what my purpose is now. I wish I could have cured him or kept him alive. I miss him all the time, just seeing him and hearing his voice.

THERAPIST: I know this is so hard. There is so much sadness and grief now when you think about how much you wanted to help him and how powerless you were to cure his illness.

ALEX: Yes, I do think that if I couldn't do something so important, what is the point now? What is my purpose at all?

THERAPIST: I wonder, Alex, if you had a friend who had cared for her child like you, and experienced such a sad loss and was feeling she had no purpose in life, what might you tell her?

ALEX: Oh, I do have a friend like that. And I know what I say when I see her, which is "You can still do something good with your life." My friend Mary feels at loose ends since her husband died, but I know she still has a lot to give, even though she doesn't think so.

THERAPIST: Do you think that there is any chance the same might be true for you?

ALEX: I guess there is. I know when I think that I can't help anyone and that I have nothing to contribute, I feel a lot worse. Sometimes it's just so hard to see what to do, but as I think about Mary, I'm realizing that it might be possible for me to help others again, like my daughter. I guess maybe I help Mary when I see her, too.

With Socratic questioning, Alex remembered that she had done an effective and important job raising her children, caring for David as best that she could, and that even the most loving and hardworking parents cannot protect their children from all sources of pain and suffering, particularly illness. Gradually, Alex came to the realization that she could work to develop another purpose in life. Although she could not bring David back, she could have an important influence on her daughter, reengage with her friendships, and enjoy the independence of this phase of her life.

The foundation of collaboration and positive regard was critical in exploring and evaluating Alex's thoughts about her care of David and her future. The therapist frequently expressed hope that Alex's mood would improve, particularly during times of acute sadness, grief, and hopelessness. The therapist consistently encouraged an experimental approach and also utilized aspects of the therapeutic relationship as a vehicle to address some of Alex's therapy goals. For instance, when the therapist expressed respect for Alex's many skills and talents, Alex would frequently minimize or dismiss this feedback. The therapist used humor to draw attention to Alex's tendency to dismiss her own progress and to take responsibility for all that ever went wrong, but never for success. The therapist gave examples of when this had transpired in therapy, calling attention to Alex's tendency to attribute all progress to the therapist, rather than to their collaboration and to her own hard work outside of sessions.

Together, Alex and the therapist built on these conversations with specific activity scheduling assignments to enhance Alex's sense of contribution and her competence in doing so. In addition, the therapist continued to use Socratic questioning to review Alex's history and to look for examples of competence and resilience in her life. For example, they identified that she had given birth to David in her late teens, then helped her husband build a house while raising their family. When the marriage was at its worst, Alex had asked her husband to leave, and she was proud of her "strength and stubbornness" in ensuring that her children did not grow up in a home characterized by a high level of conflict and alcoholism. After the divorce, Alex finished high school by attending night classes, then studied business at a technical college, so that she could earn money to send both of her children to college.

As Alex began to identify her sadness and grief about her son's death, she began to cry more in sessions—some of the first times she had cried openly since David's death. As Alex grieved, she also began to discuss her experience of David's death in a more comprehensive way. For instance, she reported that she had felt very controlled by David's illness. When he was very sick, he often asked her to sit with him for long periods of time, and the sedentary and consuming nature of much of her caretaking resulted in much of her weight gain and in losing her sense of purpose outside of her parenting and caretaking role.

Alex also found it very helpful to complete the cognitive conceptualization diagram (J. S. Beck, 1995). Use of this strategy undermined her negative core belief and enabled Alex to see her current life and her past more realistically and with a broader view. In particular, she saw how verbal and physical abuse by a rejecting stepfather had encouraged her early marriage and her belief in his opinion of her, summarized in the core belief "I'm not a good person." As a result of being self-reliant early, she had developed many skills but devalued them with the negative assumption, "I have some skills, but I'm really a fraud." At home, Alex had also learned, "If I build myself up or brag, I'll fall or be pushed back."

Compensatory strategies associated with this history and way of thinking were to suppress her talents, to hide her real self and never feel pride, to work hard, always to do for others, and never to take credit. For example, Alex enjoyed painting with watercolors and had won some awards, but she never told anyone about this. After describing this in therapy, Alex began again to paint and to give her small watercolors to others; she received many compliments, which she practiced describing with pride in therapy. She developed a new belief about herself—"I'm good at things I love"—that caused her to smile and to feel hopeful.

By the end of treatment, Alex reported feeling "fantastic" and being very busy. She was planning to do more watercolors and to go on a long outing with her eating support group. The therapist and Alex planned for the third anniversary of her son's death, about which she said, "I am so deeply sad that he died, but I know I gave him love and care to his last moment." She also found that looking at his picture brought her comfort:

"His memory is always with me." Alex acknowledged that she was a hard worker and discovered that she liked to learn new things.

At the final session, Alex was smiling and happy, having enjoyed a trip with her group. She reported that she had met many of her goals for therapy and felt understood, respected, and challenged. She stated that she found the activity logs extremely helpful and was continuing to use them on a regular basis to plan activities and occasionally monitor her mood. She disliked the repetitiveness of the thought logs, but found that the Core Belief Worksheet helped her change her self-perceptions (e.g., as someone who likes to learn new things). Alex made herself a folder of her paintings and her photographs of David, which she intended to use to prevent a relapse of depression. She planned to look at this folder to remember good times with David and her daughter, and her hard work caring for both of them. The paintings also reminded Alex that she was creative and that others appreciated this part of her. She was sad to end therapy and continued to mourn the loss of her son; however, she did not feel the weight of depression. She was now working on finding a new purpose in her new life, and she felt hopeful about this process.

REVIEW OF EFFICACY RESEARCH

In 1989, Elkin and colleagues published the first report from what would soon become one of the most influential and controversial treatment studies, the National Institute of Mental Health (NIMH) Treatment of Depression Collaborative Research Program (TDCRP). This multisite study was designed to test the efficacy of CT, interpersonal therapy, and pharmacotherapy in the context of a placebo-controlled, multisite trial (Elkin et al., 1989). Initial analyses found few significant differences between treatments across multiple outcomes; however, subsequent analyses, exploring the role of baseline severity, found that more severely depressed patients experienced significantly better outcomes in pharmacotherapy than in CT; moreover, there were no differences between CT and placebo (Elkin et al., 1995).

The lack of significant differences between CT and placebo among more severely depressed patients was extremely influential. Treatment guidelines stipulated a highly limited role for CT in the treatment of severely depressed patients (e.g., American Psychiatric Association, 2000), stating, for instance, "Antidepressant medications should be provided for moderate to severe major depressive disorder unless ECT [electroconvulsive therapy] is planned. . . . A specific, effective psychotherapy alone as an initial treatment modality may be considered for patients with mild to moderate major depressive disorder" (p. 2).

The findings of the TDCRP and their codification in treatment guidelines were not without controversy (e.g., Jacobson & Hollon, 1996). Critics questioned the implementation of CT based on both the pattern of site differences (sites with greater CT experience had better outcomes) and the comparison of TDCRP relapse rates with other published studies (TDCRP rates were notably higher). In addition, providing supervision relatively infrequently for TDCRP therapists (i.e., monthly), critics argued, was insufficient for newly trained cognitive therapists. Critics also noted that irrespective of CT's performance during acute treatment, there were no differences in longer-term outcomes, with CT performing as well as antidepressant medication (ADM) across the 18-month follow-up.

In addition, a subsequent mega-analysis compared CT and pharmacotherapy for more severely depressed patients across pooled data from four studies, including the TDCRP, and found no differences between CT and medication for such patients (DeRubeis, Gelfand, Tang, & Simons, 1999). The impact of these data, however, has been tempered by methodological problems of the studies included. Specifically, the quality of ADM implementation has been questioned, and the role of allegiance effects has been highlighted in the trials whose outcomes favored CT (Hollon et al., 2002). Moreover, of the studies included, only the TDCRP was placebo-controlled, thus compromising the ability of the other trials to demonstrate that the samples were pharmacologically responsive and that the ADM conditions were properly implemented (e.g., Klein, 2000).

Two recent studies have addressed specifically the role of severity in the treatment of depression. First, DeRubeis et al. (2005) compared CT to ADM (paroxetine) in a two-site, placebo-controlled design with moderate to severely depressed patients. Across the two sites (University of Pennsylvania and Vanderbilt University), 240 patients were enrolled. Results across sites suggested that CT was comparable to ADM, with overall response rates of approximately 58% in both treatment groups. However, there was a significant site × treatment interaction, with ADM significantly outperforming CT at the Vanderbilt site (and CT showing a nonsignificant advantage over ADM at the University of Pennsylvania site). This was accounted for by patient and treatment quality differences between sites. Patients with comorbid anxiety disorders showed better outcomes in ADM than in CT across sites; however, the greater number of comorbid patients enrolled at Vanderbilt contributed to the superior outcomes of ADM compared to CT at this site. Moreover, the therapists at the University of Pennsylvania site had greater expertise in CT, and their patients demonstrated better outcomes than ADM, in contrast to the less experienced therapists at Vanderbilt (who did better over the second half of the study once they had more training and experience).

Second, our group also recently completed a placebo-controlled trial comparing CT, ADM, and stand-alone BA therapy among depressed adults (Dimidjian et al., 2006). Randomization in this study was stratified, based on depressive severity. Results indicated no significant differences among treatments for the less severely depressed patients (consistent with the TDCRP findings). Among more severely depressed patients, BA and ADM demonstrated comparable outcomes, and both were superior to CT. In fact, approximately 25% of severely depressed patients who received CT demonstrated a pattern of "extreme nonresponse" to treatment, defined as ending treatment with scores above 30 on the BDI. In contrast to the other patients who received CT, this subgroup also showed greater functional impairment and more frequent problems with primary supports groups at intake (Coffman, Martell, Dimidjian, & Hollon, 2007). Across the 2-year follow-up, BA performance was comparable to that of CT in the prevention of relapse and recurrence (Dobson et al., in preparation).

In general, the findings from our recent study underscore the potential importance of severity in considering the provision of CT. Consistent with TDCRP findings, our results suggest that the selection of particular treatment strategies is not as critical among less severely depressed patients. The lack of significant differences among treatments for patients with less severe depression in both studies suggests an important role for psychosocial treatments, such as CT, among less severely depressed patients, particularly in light of the potential side effects associated with the use of antidepressants.

Among more severely depressed patients, however, the findings are equivocal. The results highlight the possibility that the behavioral strategies in CT may be not only necessary but also sufficient ingredients for change. Although the importance of replicating our recent work cannot be overstated, these findings highlight the promise of behavioral strategies in the treatment of depression. Additionally, the findings reported by DeRubeis and colleagues (2005) highlight the importance of ensuring high therapist competence in the delivery of CT when working with more severely depressed patients.

CONCLUSIONS

The preceding treatment guidelines and clinical illustration highlight areas of importance when implementing CT with more severely depressed patients. Frequently, patients with severe depression require longer use of activity monitoring and scheduling than is the case for less severely depressed patients. This sustained focus on behavioral activation is important in increasing activities associated with positive mood generally, and with experiences of pleasure and mastery specifically. As indicated in our review, recent data suggest the promise of purely behavioral approaches to depression and underscore the importance of emphasizing such strategies within the CT approach. This recommendation is consistent with the seminal formulation of CT (Beck et al., 1979), as well as recent work emphasizing the importance of behavioral experiments in CT (Bennett-Levy et al., 2004). Special attention to the therapeutic relationship is also important. Particularly for patients with interpersonal stressors, it may be important to inquire regularly about whether patients experience the exploration of their beliefs and behavior as critical or judgmental. Finally, current evidence suggests that discussion of possible concurrent pharmacotherapy is advised. The guidelines reviewed here are intended to help maximize clinical competence, and ongoing formal monitoring of competence in CT is highly recommended to ensure that more severely depressed patients receive the most efficacious treatment possible.

REFERENCES

American Psychiatric Association. (1994). *Diagnostic and statistical manual of mental disorders* (4th ed.). Washington, DC: Author.

American Psychiatric Association. (2000). Practice guidelines for the treatment of patients with major depressive disorder (revision). *American Journal of Psychiatry, 157,* 1–45.

Beck, A. T., Freeman, A., & Associates. (1990). *Cognitive therapy of personality disorders.* New York: Guilford Press.

Beck, A. T., Rush, A. J., Shaw, B. F., & Emery, G. (1979). *Cognitive therapy of depression.* New York: Guilford Press.

Beck, A. T., Steer, R. A., & Brown, G. K. (1996). *Manual for the BDI-II.* San Antonio, TX: Psychological Corporation.

Beck, J. S. (1995). *Cognitive therapy: Basics and beyond.* New York: Guilford Press.

Bennett-Levy, J., Butler, G., Fennell, M., Hackman, A., Mueller, M., & Westbrook, D. (2004). *Oxford guide to behavioural experiments in cognitive therapy.* Oxford, UK: Oxford University Press.

Coffman, S., Martell, C. R., Dimidjian, S., Gallop, R., & Hollon, S. D. (2007). Extreme non-response to cognitive therapy: Can behavioral activation succeed where cognitive therapy fails? *Journal of Consulting and Clinical Psychology, 75,* 531–541.

DeRubeis, R. J., Gelfand, L. A., Tang, T. Z., & Simons, A. D. (1999). Medications versus cognitive behavior therapy for severely depressed outpatients: Mega-analysis of four randomized comparisons. *American Journal of Psychiatry, 156,* 1007–1013.

DeRubeis, R. J., Hollon, S. D., Amsterdam, J. D., Shelton, R. C., Young, P. R., Salomon, R. M., et al. (2005). Cognitive therapy vs medications in the treatment of moderate to severe depression. *Archives of General Psychiatry, 62,* 409–416.

Dimidjian, S., Hollon, S. D., Dobson, K. S., Schmaling, K. B., Kohlenberg, R. J., Addis, M., et al. (2006). Randomized trial of behavioral activation, cognitive therapy, and antidepressant medication in the acute treatment of adults with major depression. *Journal of Consulting and Clinical Psychology, 74,* 658–670.

Dobson, K. S., Hollon, S. D., Dimidjian, S., Schmaling, K. B., Kohlenberg, R., Gallop, R., et al. (2005). *Behavioral activation therapy, cognitive therapy and pharmacotherapy for depression: Relapse prevention.* Manuscript in preparation.

Dobson, K. S., Shaw, B. F., & Vallis, T. M. (1985). Reliability of a measure of the quality of cognitive therapy. *British Journal of Clinical Psychology, 24,* 295–300.

Elkin, I., Gibbons, R. D., Shea, M. T., Sotsky, S. M., Watkins, J. T., Pilkonis, P. A., et al. (1995). Initial severity and differential treatment outcome in the National Institute of Mental Health Treatment of Depression Collaborative Research Program. *Journal of Consulting and Clinical Psychology, 63,* 841–847.

Elkin, I., Shea, M. T., Watkins, J. T., Imber, S. D., Sotsky, S. M., Collins, J. F., et al. (1989). National Institute of Mental Health Treatment of Depression Collaborative Research Program: General effectiveness of treatments. *Archives of General Psychiatry, 46,* 971–982.

Ferster, C. B. (1973). A functional analysis of depression. *American Psychologist, 28,* 857–870.

Hamilton, M. (1960). A rating scale for depression. *Journal of Neurology, Neurosurgery and Psychiatry, 23,* 56–61.

Hayes, A. M., Castonguay, L. G., & Goldfried, M. R. (1996). Effectiveness of targeting the vulnerability factors of depression in cognitive therapy. *Journal of Consulting and Clinical Psychology, 64,* 623–627.

Hollon, S. D., Thase, M. E., & Markowitz, J. C. (2002). Treatment and prevention of depression. *Psychological Science in the Public Interest, 3,* 39–77.

Jacobson, N. S., Dobson, K., Truax, P. A., Addis, M. E., Koerner, K., Gollan, J. K., et al. (1996). A component analysis of cognitive-behavioral treatment for depression. *Journal of Consulting and Clinical Psychology, 64,* 295–304.

Jacobson, N. S., & Hollon, S. D. (1996). Cognitive behavior therapy vs pharmacotherapy: Now that the jury's returned its verdict, its time to present the rest of the evidence. *Journal of Consulting and Clinical Psychology, 64,* 74–80.

Jacobson, N. S., Martell, C. R., & Dimidjian, S. (2001). Behavioral activation treatment for depression: Returning to contextual roots. *Clinical Psychology: Science and Practice, 8,* 255–270.

James, I. A., Blackburn, I. M., Milne, D. L., & Reichfelt, F. K. (2001). Moderators of trainee therapists' competence in cognitive therapy. *British Journal of Clinical Psychology, 40,* 131–141.

Klein, D. F. (2000). Flawed meta-analyses comparing psychotherapy with pharmaco-therapy. *American Journal of Psychiatry, 157,* 1204–1211.

Kohlenberg, R. J., & Tsai, M. (1994). Improving cognitive therapy for depression with functional analytic psychotherapy: Theory and case study. *Behavior Analyst, 17,* 305–319.

Lewinsohn, P. M. (1974). A behavioral approach to depression. In R. M. Friedman & M. M. Katz (Eds.), *The psychology of depression: Contemporary theory and research* (pp. 157–185). New York: Wiley.

Martell, C. R., Addis, M. E., & Jacobson, N. S. (2001). *Depression in context: Strategies for guided action.* New York: Norton.

Safran, J. D., & Segal, Z. V. (1990). *Interpersonal process in cognitive therapy.* New York: Basic Books.

Shapiro, D. A., Barkham, M., Rees, A., Hardy, G. E., Reynolds, S., & Startup, M. (1994). Effects of treatment duration and severity of depression on the effectiveness of cognitive-behavioral and psychodynamic–interpersonal psychotherapy. *Journal of Consulting and Clinical Psychotherapy, 62,* 522–534.

Sholomskas, D. E., Syracuse-Siewert, G., Rounsaville, B. J., Ball, S. A., Nuro, K. F., & Carroll, K. M. (2005). We don't train in vain: A dissemination trial of three strategies of training clinicians in cognitive-behavioral therapy. *Journal of Consulting and Clinical Psychology, 73,* 106–115.

Vallis, T. M., Shaw, B. F., & Dobson, K. S. (1986). The Cognitive Therapy Scale: Psychometric properties. *Journal of Consulting and Clinical Psychology, 54,* 381–385.

Young, J., & Beck, A. T. (1980). *Cognitive Therapy Scale: Rating manual.* Unpublished manuscript, University of Pennsylvania, Philadelphia.

┌─────┐
│ 4 │
└─────┘

CHRONIC DEPRESSION

Anne Garland
Jan Scott

Chronic depression is a disorder defined by its symptom severity and its course. There are several manifestations of this problem, but most classification systems differentiate these according to whether symptoms meet criteria for major depression or other forms of depression, and/or whether the symptoms persist at a syndromal or subsyndromal level. Using these parameters, there are four recognized subtypes: (1) chronic major depressive disorder, (2) dysthymic disorder, (3) dysthymic disorder with major depressive disorder ("double depression"), and (4) major depressive disorder with poor interepisodic recovery (i.e., incomplete remission). According to these definitions it is estimated that the prevalence of chronic depressions is 3–6% of the general population, but probably affects about 30% of depressed patients following acute treatment, suggesting that a significant number of patients do not fully respond to available treatments, and, in particular, to the most common treatment, namely, antidepressant medication (Cornwall & Scott, 1997; Paykel et al., 1995). In addition to increasing risk for future relapse (e.g., see Judd, 1997), persistent depressive symptoms are an important clinical target in their own right, because they produce substantial distress and suffering, are frequently drug refractory, are associated with a history of

loss
gradual
helplessness
hopeless

recurrent depression, and significantly impair work and social performance (Cornwall & Scott, 1997; Judd, 1997; Paykel et al., 1995).

In this chapter, we provide an overview of conceptualization, assessment, and cognitive therapy (CT) for chronic major depression, dysthymia, and their combination; CT for partially remitted depression is described by Fava and Fabric, Chapter 5, this volume.

CONCEPTUALIZATION OF CHRONIC DEPRESSION

Chronic depression is not a homogenous problem, and patient history, course of current episode, and presentation can vary widely. As in the standard CT model for acute depression (Beck, Rush, Shaw, & Emery, 1979), the theme of loss (actual and perceived) and the negative cognitive triad (negative view of self, world, and future) are helpful as an initial starting point for formulating the patient's problems. However, in the model of chronic depression, the losses are often more enduring and may arise as a consequence of the depression itself. Similarly, the negative thoughts that characterize a chronic presentation are more enduring in nature and have over time become interwoven with associated behavioral strategies, and their social and environmental consequences. On the basis of this observation we propose a chronic cognitive triad as follows: low self-esteem (negative view of self), helplessness (negative view of the world), and hopelessness (negative view of the future).

Furthermore, we propose that the chronicity of negative thinking in each domain is a direct product of three factors. First, extreme and rigidly held conditional and unconditional beliefs provide an enduring vulnerability to negative automatic thoughts in each domain. Second, cognitive, affective, and behavioral avoidance are used to manage distress that would otherwise be constantly present when these belief are activated. Finally, the implementation of avoidant coping strategies leads to the recurrence of negative situations and events, which then provides the individual with confirmatory evidence to support his/her conditional and unconditional beliefs. This in turn further entrenches those beliefs and provides fuel for further negative automatic thoughts. Thus, an especially pernicious maintenance cycle is established.

A further aspect of the proposed model is that, over time, the person with chronic depression integrates the illness into his/her sense of self. The resulting emergence of beliefs about depression itself forms an important aspect of the maintenance of the disorder.

THE ROLE OF AVOIDANCE IN CHRONIC DEPRESSION

Clinical experience tells us that one common factor unifies most patients' problems in this homogenous clinical presentation: avoidance. Avoidant coping manifests itself in a number of ways in chronic depression and takes three interrelated forms: behavioral avoidance of certain external situations; cognitive avoidance of certain mental ideas or images; and emotional avoidance, through the direct suppression of emotional experiences.

The successful execution of many CT interventions is predicated on the patient's ability to identify, label, experience, and tolerate negative affect and upsetting thoughts. Each of these forms of avoidance is utilized to mask distressing feelings and thoughts, therefore representing a significant obstacle to be overcome if CT is to be implemented successfully. Whereas most patients in acute depression concur that avoidance is wholly unhelpful, the picture is not so clear-cut for patients in chronic depression. Frequently, over the course of years of illness, avoidance becomes adaptive and helps patients to manage both their mood states and their social environment. The adaptive nature of avoidant coping strategies can often be traced back to early childhood and may be shared within families, subcultures, and communities (see Bedrosian & Bozicas, 1994). Formulating different forms of avoidance and how they work for the patient is a vital step to promoting lasting change, because avoidance is pivotal in blocking change.

ASSESSMENT OF CHRONIC DEPRESSION

When therapists work with patients with chronic depression, the assessment process can be challenging on a number of fronts. Generally speaking, a patient comes to therapy with a long history of the disorder, and there is a lot of ground for the therapist to cover in terms of gathering sufficient information to make sense of current problems, sharing a treatment rationale with the patient, and devising an initial formulation of the development and maintenance of the disorder. A further consideration is the fact that patients with chronic depression can be vague or evasive when giving information, as well as interpersonally sensitive, especially in novel social situations such as assessment. These two factors alone mean that the pacing of the interview needs to be slower, with more time and attention given to rapport building. This latter point is especially important given the interpersonal sensitivity that characterizes many patients' presentations can be disruptive to the process of systematic information gathering.

longer
more freq

The Format of Assessment

Bearing these issues in mind, the following format is recommended for conducting a CT assessment in which the patient's presenting complaint is chronic depression. The assessment consists of two to three sessions, the first of 90 minutes' duration and the following of 60 minutes each. Clear goals are established for each session, with relevant homework assignments in between; at the end of the process, therapist and patient should have collaboratively arrived at the following:

- A comprehensive assessment of current symptoms and problems.
- An assessment of current and past risk.
- A shared treatment rationale based on a cognitive formulation of the development and maintenance of current problems.
- A time-line history of illness episodes and their treatment, including inpatient admissions and periods of involuntary detention.
- Detailed account of prescribed medications, concordance with these and treatment response.
- Completion and interpretation of psychometric and idiographic measures
- Problem and target lists.
- A negotiated treatment contract.

Assessing Current Presenting Problems

In working with a patient with chronic depression, the assessment process is structured around three areas:

- The patient's current symptoms and problems.
- The development of the patient's problems and personal history, including early childhood experiences, and the social and environmental factors potentially contributing to depression.
- The patient's view of depression as an illness and its treatment.

Psychometric Measures

Although formal diagnosis is not a standard part of a CT assessment, diagnostic interview schedules such as the Structured Clinical Interview for DSM-IV (SCID; Spitzer, Williams, Gibbon, & First, 1992) can provide a useful template to cover the main symptoms of depression. It is helpful to focus on a specific, recent time period (e.g., the last week), but the therapist should ascertain whether the chosen time period is reasonably representative of the patient's usual experience of depressive symptoms.

It is also helpful to assess the severity of the patient's overall symptomatology; and standard measures such as the Beck Depression Inventory–II (BDI-II; Steer & Brown, 1996) have a useful role. However, we provide a note of caution. Given that a proportion of patients with chronic depression are reluctant to acknowledge and discuss depressive symptoms, they may underrate their symptoms when completing standard measures. Therefore, as a rule of thumb, such measures should always be supplemented by more detailed questioning about each symptom, with some subjective measure of frequency, intensity, and duration.

Idiographic Measures

Given the level of complexity in chronic depression, idiographic measures play a crucial role in assessing in detail the nature and extent of the patient's current difficulties. In this respect, idiographic measures should be introduced from the assessment stage onward. Typically the most useful tool to introduce at assessment is an activity schedule (Beck et al., 1979). This can be used in a standard way to monitor activity and to rate mastery and pleasure, or it can be used to gather baseline data regarding mood states, including depression, anxiety, or anger. It may also be useful if patients are using alcohol to manage mood or are consuming excessive amounts of caffeine. Such data can be vital in terms of making sense of patients' problems and in developing an initial problem list.

TREATMENT OF CHRONIC DEPRESSION

The application of the standard cognitive model in the treatment of chronic depression can result in confusion and frustration for both patient and therapist. For treatment to be effective, a number of adaptations need to be made in the application and delivery of standard interventions. Our starting point in approaching treatment of chronic depression is to retain the essential features of CT that have contributed to its established efficacy in treating acute depression. In particular, we endorse a highly structured and focused intervention, both in individual sessions and across the intervention. We advocate actively fostering a collaborative therapeutic relationship and explicitly sharing a formulation of the factors that maintain the patient's current difficulties. Realistic problem and target lists are used to guide treatment, and an explicit treatment contract (between 18 and 25 sessions) is negotiated with the patient. Initially we advocate twice-weekly sessions for 2–3 weeks. This disrupts avoidant coping strategies sufficiently to promote active engagement in treatment. This is followed by weekly sessions for 10 weeks and, subsequently, sessions every 2 weeks for 4 weeks. Finally there is a graded reduction in frequency 1-month and then 2-month intervals. Standard, session length is 60 minutes, although extending the session length to 75 minutes has in some cases proven to be clinically very productive with highly avoidant patients who take time to break through avoidant coping tactics.

In terms of standard interventions, equal weight is given to behavioral interventions, such as activity scheduling and graded task assignment (although these would be used within a cognitive treatment rationale), and standard cognitive interventions, such as identifying and modifying auto-matic thoughts with behavioral experiments. However, within this a great deal of emphasis, both within and outside of sessions, is placed on action-oriented behavioral experiments to test out predictions and to act against avoidant coping strategies. In addition, we advocate the following essential components:

- Each session is audiotaped, and the patient is encouraged to listen to this tape between sessions.
- The patient is encouraged to develop a personal therapy folder con-taining all written materials used in the course of therapy. This acts as a self-help folder once therapy is completed.
- Homework is an integral aspect of every therapy session.
- A written handout supports every intervention, with guidance on how to implement the intervention outside the session.
- Written summaries of learning are made from homework assign-ments and at the end of each session.

As a rule of thumb, patients with chronic depression may present three obstacles to successful therapy. First, patients with chronic depression may lack motivation to engage in a treatment they perceive as bound to fail. Sec-ond, their level of passivity and avoidant coping strategies may make therapy more difficult. Third, their negative thoughts may be more refractory to disconfirmatory evidence. We recommend the following adaptations as ways of dealing with these obstacles (for more details, see Moore & Garland, 2003).

Cultivating the Therapist's Mind-Set to Work Effectively with Chronic Depression

Most standard CT texts do not give a great deal of attention to the treating clinics contribution to therapy outcome. Expert opinion and research evidence suggests that experienced clinicians achieve better outcomes than novice therapists when working with patients with more chronic presentations (Burns & Nolen-Hoeksema, 1992). Indeed, with regard to acute depression, the application of the standard Beckian treatment protocol (Beck et al., 1979) is considered the bread and butter of CT. Often there is an assumption that this same protocol is easily and readily translated to the treatment of more chronic and refractory presentations. When protocols fail to yield their intended results, the source of the problem is often located with the limitations of the intervention itself or the complexity of the patient presentation. Rarely is attention given to therapist qualities and skills that are likely to contribute to a beneficial outcome. Let us look at each of these in turn.

Therapist Personal Qualities

McCullough (2000) observed that fundamentally, in therapy, chronically depressed patients need to have an experience of engaging with a "decent, caring, human being." This is a position we also endorse. Chronically depressed patients can present considerable obstacles to the therapist conveying warmth and care, and there is the potential for supposedly therapeutic encounters to be damaging, unless the therapist has some capacity to recognize and manage his/her own contribution to interpersonal encounters in therapy. The therapist also needs to be consistent and reliable, and have the tenacity to stick with the therapy process and structure, and remain proactive, often in the face of extreme hopelessness, helplessness, and negativity.

Importantly, the therapist needs to be motivated and have an internal sense of confidence and that he/she can help the patient. It is very easy for the therapist taking on a patient's hopelessness and negativity to reach the point that he/she dreads the next session and is rendered powerless by his/her own automatic thoughts about perceived inabilities as a therapist or the intractable difficulties that place the patient beyond help. To counter this and to work effectively with patients with chronic depression, the therapist needs to adopt a certain mind-set, which is perhaps summed up by the phrase "Everything is grist for the mill." What we mean by this is that the therapist is accepting of the territory he/she is in (no matter how difficult) and works with the patient to use the difficulties, so that they work to the patient's advantage to progress in therapy. From this position there are always opportunities to learn and understand. Thus, for example, even incomplete homework assignments are not a waste of time. Collaboration can be fostered and responsibility for change can be shared when the therapist and patient ask, "What can we learn from this?" and "How does this develop our formulation?" It is important to emphasize the need for an equitable balance between optimism and realism in taking this mindful position, so that the messages given to the patient induce sufficient hope to motivate the patient's engagement but are not so unrealistic that they raise impossible expectations in the patient regarding the therapist and the therapy.

Therapist Skills

Increasingly, the CT literature is turning its attention to issues related to the training and clinical supervision of cognitive therapists (Padesky, 1996). It is our view that clinical outcomes for patients with chronic depression will be enhanced if the treating clinician has undertaken robust CT training; has extensive clinical experience working with this patient group; and is backed up by an effective clinical supervisor who has undertaken specific CT training and who is experienced in working with chronic depression.

A standard feature of all CT is explicitly sharing with the patient a cogent treatment rationale. The aim is to help the patient to understand at an experiential level the connection between specific experiences in his/her daily life, his/her emotional responses to these experiences, and the thoughts and thought processes, biological/physiological symptoms, and behaviors that occur at these times. There is a specific emphasis on how these domains feed into each other to create a vicious circle maintenance cycle.

This socialization process is usually initiated at the end of the first assessment session. It is important that the model not be presented in purely generalized and abstract terms, because this only enhances the global, overgeneral processing of information that characterizes chronic depression. Traditionally, CT uses metaphors to illustrate the treatment rationale (e.g., "You are lying in bed at night and you hear a loud bang. What is your first thought?"). In our experience, such metaphors may be less useful in chronic depression. We strongly encourage use of a concrete, recent example (the last 2–3 days) from the patient's experience to illustrate the vicious circle. In addition recounting the event needs to be located in time, place, and person, and recalled in the first person, present tense. For CT to be effective, the patient needs to engage emotionally at an experiential level. Therefore, the treatment rationale needs to have a high degree of personal relevance and emotional meaning to the patient. This is more likely to be achieved with the use of recent, personally relevant material that contains some emotional resonance. Given the role that cognitive and affective avoidance play in the maintenance of chronic depression, the use of abstract metaphors is more likely to enable the patient to distance him- or herself from the socialization process and declare that the example in the metaphor is not relevant to his/her particular circumstances. There is, however, a need for a note of caution.

How the model is communicated to the patient is important. Given the cognitive deficits that characterize chronic depression, the patient may find it hard to remember what has been discussed. In addition, the patient's rigidly held beliefs might result in subsequent distortion of any conclusions. It is therefore advisable to diagram the vicious circle, with the patient example included, on a piece of paper for the patient to take home. Again this needs to be communicated sensitively. Many patients do not see words written on the paper. They see themselves, and this has potential to escalate feelings of humiliation and hopelessness. In addition, a supplementary handout that reiterates the treatment rationale is vital. An audiotape of the session containing the treatment rationale is also beneficial.

It may also be helpful with some patients to include cognitive processes within the treatment rationale, for example, negative, overgeneral, and black-and-white thinking; rumination; and depressive intrusive memories. This can be particularly effective when a patient cites an example of an incident that affected his/her mood over several hours. This enables the patient to incorporate the idea that the lower the mood, the more negative, black-and-white, and overgeneral the thinking, and the patient becomes less active and more internally focused. This can give rise to rumination and the intrusion of depressogenic memories from the past. The use of the metaphor that thinking becomes like ink on blotting paper can be very helpful in the beginning to engage the patient in a metacognitive perspective in which he/she observes not only the content of his/her thinking but also how he/she thinks when depressed (negative, over general, black-and-white, and ruminative thinking and accessing past unpleasant memories), and contrasting this with his/her thinking when in a less depressed mood.

One of the key goals in sharing the treatment rationale is to engender hope. One means of engendering hope is to strike an optimistic but realistic tone with the patient regarding what CT can achieve. Often, therefore, it is more helpful to sell the patient on the idea that CT may not cure the depression, but it may have an impact in terms of improving function and symptom management as part of a treatment package that may include medication and social inclusion initiatives.

Adaptations to Standard CT When Working with Chronic Depression

Many aspects of how chronically depressed patients present indicate that unless there is active management of a structured process, therapy can disintegrate into a diffuse entity that lacks focus and direction. This can lead to hopelessness and despondence in both patient and therapist. It is in this area that, if the therapist can accept the idea that "everything is grist for the mill" and not become exasperated at him/herself or the patient, therapy can be its most productive and rewarding.

Separating the patient from the depression can be very liberating in terms of increasing the therapist's level of empathy, care, and motivation toward the patient. The cognitive deficits that characterize chronic depression include poor recall, poor problem-solving skills, over general autobiographical memory, and rumination. All of these have a real and vivid impact in terms of how the patient functions in the session and go a long way to account for the paralyzing negativity, passivity, and seeming intransigence that manifests itself during treatment sessions. It is all too easy when confronted with a chronically depressed patient to attribute these factors to personality. We encourage the therapist to be mindful in considering what part of the patient's presentation is personality and what part of the patient's depression and the very real cognitive deficits that result from it. How the therapist attributes these factors impacts the level of hope the therapist is likely to bring to the therapy.

The Therapeutic Relationship

CT is predicated on the ability of the therapist and patient being able to establish a sound therapeutic relationship. However, patients with chronic depression can present considerable obstacles to conveying the warmth, genuineness, and empathy that are considered the foundation stones of the therapeutic alliance.

Given that cognitive, emotional, and behavioral avoidance are so central in chronic depression, many patients react to the therapist's display of warmth and empathy in an aloof or hostile manner. The patient's beliefs about him/herself and others also influence his/her interactions with the therapist. A patient may find it hard to accept expressions of warmth and care and may greet them with suspicion and distrust. A highly autonomous patient, or one who sees emotionality as weakness, may interpret signs of care and concern as confirmation of his/her own perceived inadequacy and become more hopeless and passive, as well as hostile toward the therapist. These processes are best managed by adopting the therapeutic stance that takes into consideration the impact of the patient's belief system has on the therapist's interpersonal style.

Session Structure

The "style of therapy" refers to the role the therapist takes in shaping the nature of the interaction with the patient. In chronic depression, structure is vital. The hallmark of CT is its proactive, goal-orientated intervention in which the therapist is active and collaborative and uses primarily a questioning format to facilitate guided discovery. There are several ways in which different facets of chronic depression impact on therapy style. These include passivity in behavior and social interaction, rigidity of thinking, and avoidance of emotion. The style of therapy thus needs to be adapted in order to gain a balance between the activity level of the patient and that of the therapist as well as to maximize the chances of cognitive and behavioral change and evoke emotion within the session. Using standard CT interventions is painstaking and their implementation requires a good deal of patience and persistence on both sides before yielding results. This can be frustrating for both patient and therapist. Being explicit about this and articulating the nature of the ballpark the therapy is occupying can be beneficial in terms of establishing expectations that it usual for progress to be slow but systematic.

As a guiding principle, each session needs to be structured and action orientated with a clear goal in mind. Ideally the aim of both patient and therapist is to tackle a problem actively in session and generate a homework assignment that builds on that session's work.

Homework

Homework is a central mechanism of change in CT (Burns & Spangle, 2000; Garland & Scott, 2000), and there is some evidence that the extent to which patients engage in homework predicts outcome in CT (Kazantzis, Dean, & Roman, 2000). In chronically depressed patients, a number of factors are likely to interfere with the completion of homework assignments. Behavioral and cognitive avoidance work directly against the patient's engagement with any task that has the potential to require effort or to generate distress or negative automatic thoughts. Emotional avoidance and suppression can lead to the patient's passivity and result in a deficit in the motivation to execute new tasks. The following strategies maximize the likelihood of the patient engaging in homework assignments:

- Establish assigning and reviewing homework as a routine part of the structure of each session.
- Establish homework assignments collaboratively to increase patient ownership of the works.
- Use the work of the session to generate homework tasks and assign these as the session progresses rather than at the end.
- Make the task realistic and achievable from the patient's perspective and set a maximum of two tasks.
- When asking the patient to monitor or modify automatic thoughts, ask him/her to work with a maximum of two examples. This minimizes the chance that the task will feel overwhelming to the patient.
- Be clear regarding what the task is, and use a written plan, with the audiotape to support it.
- Anticipate obstacles to non completion and try and minimize their impact by having alternate plans.
- Always review homework and reinforce verbally and in a written summary what the patient has learned, even when (which is the most common scenario) it has not gone according to plan.

Questioning Style

Given the level of passivity in chronic depression, the therapist is left with no option in the early stages of therapy other than to be more active than usual. Because there is a danger that such a stance will reinforce patients' passivity and lack of engagement, the therapist maintains a questioning style. However, one of the greatest challenges in chronic depression is that patients often respond to the therapist's questions with caution, anxiety, or even hostility. This response may be governed by a number of factors. For example patients who have high standards and perceive themselves as failures may become anxious in the face of questions. They may experience automatic thoughts about appearing stupid, not knowing the answer, and failing. Other, more interpersonally sensitive patients may experience the questioning style as undermining and perceive that the therapist is trying to catch them out in some way. It is therefore par for the course that standard CT techniques are likely to trigger patients' conditional and unconditional beliefs. The therapist needs to articulate and formulate these concerns with the patient to manage them effectively.

Experience tells us that when introducing interventions, therapists need to explain them carefully and provide written guidelines. It is also helpful to prepare the patient for how he/she might react to the intervention and seek permission to proceed. Furthermore, once the patient's foibles are known, the therapist can preempt possible activation of beliefs with statements such as "I need to ask a difficult question that may be upsetting, but if you can consider it, we may be able to understand the problem more clearly." This often gives the patient sufficient time to approach the question and to have a sense of control within the interaction. It also may help to create a path toward a productive dialogue about how a patient's perceptions about him-/herself and others influence everything he/she does, including therapy. This is often a very useful lever for promoting effective change. However, it is difficult to convey in text the style of this kind of therapy. It is frequently painstakingly slow, often with silences and long pauses, and requires a lot of proactive engagement from the therapist to see an intervention to the end. A reasonable summary would be that it is more akin to taking the long and winding road than to taking the route the crow flies.

Regulating Affect

Given the different kinds of avoidance described in the chronic depression model, the therapist has to adapt the style of therapy to regulate the intensity of affect in the session. In therapy for patients with acute depression, therapist regulation of the intensity of emotion occurs through engagement in different tasks of therapy. Thus, the distress evoked by focusing on problems or painful thoughts and feelings can be ameliorated by identifying coping strategies. In chronic depression, inappropriate levels of affect can interfere with many of the tasks of therapy. This interference may result from the suppression of affect or from the overwhelmingly high levels of emotion that result when cognitive and emotional avoidance break down.

When there is insufficient emotional arousal, it is difficult to identify problems, and any negative automatic thoughts that are elicited possess little emotional immediacy or resonance: They are "cold" rather than "hot" thoughts. Attempts at questioning these "cold" thoughts are more likely to lead to rationalization or rumination than to genuine evaluation. Thus, the therapist needs to gear therapy in a way that provokes a degree of affect, and this is achieved by playing dumb and adopting an inquisitive style. In doing so, the therapist creates the impression that he/she makes no assumptions about what the patient is doing, thinking, or feeling. This puts the onus on the patient to go into detail to inform the therapist. Using this method over time, the patient gradually increases the emotional relevance of the discussion and subtle signs of emotional arousal, such as fidgeting or increase in speed of speech, may occur. This opens the way for the therapist to use standard interventions to optimum effectiveness.

In contrast, with patients who have little control over seemingly overwhelming emotional reactions, the use of standard interventions may be experienced as aversive, and the therapist can feel like he/she is walking on eggshells. A useful tactic here is for the therapist to be a step ahead of the patient, to guide him/her over what might seem to the patient like rugged and dangerous terrain. In working to contain excessive emotion, the therapist needs to be directive rather than to probe. When a patient is clearly struggling to contain strong emotion, asking more questions may further escalate the intensity of emotion, leading the patient to feel very out of control. This can be experienced by the patient as potentially catastrophic. To maintain collaboration, the therapist needs to indicate that although the patient feels very out of control, some control remains in the therapeutic situation. The therapist can facilitate a degree of control over the emotional intensity in the session by offering an explanation for the patient's emotional state (e.g., activation of a core conditional or unconditional belief), and suggesting and trying out ways of dealing with it and managing it in the session. It is also useful, as discussed previously, to help the patient anticipate an increase in distress by warning him/her that this is likely to occur and is indeed necessary to promote change. The therapist can explain how these emotions in a therapy session can be experienced more safely than in the outside world, with less likelihood of additional ramifications based on the patient's reactions. This is tempered as the therapist overtly displays in both verbal and nonverbal communication a level of confidence that he/she can and will guide the patient through this painful process in a way that is beneficial.

CASE ILLUSTRATION

Background Information

Alan is a 55-year-old married man with two adult children. His depression emerged 6 years ago, when a local company for whom he worked was taken over by a multinational. This led to redundancies in a close-knit community, which Alan had to implement. Alan not only found the idea of redundancies unbearable but he also became the subject of criticism and hostility from work colleagues. Born and raised in Scotland, Alan described a typical working-class upbringing with an emphasis on hard work. He left school at 15 and commenced an apprenticeship in a local firm where he remained for 30 years, working his way up from the shop floor to a middle-management position.

Current Problems

At intake, Alan scored a 35 on the BDI-II. The main problems he identified at assessment were as follows:

- Poor sleep, reduced concentration and memory, and excessive tiredness
- Feelings of shame regarding the fact he had become depressed
- Loss of purpose and meaning in daily life since retiring from work on grounds of ill health
- Avoidance of social activities to keep from meeting work colleagues and friends
- Unpleasant memories of events at work that intruded on his mind daily, giving rise to feelings of guilt and anger

From Alan's perspective, his main problem was the loss of his work role. He believed that if he could return to work his depression would resolve itself. Alan blamed himself for not having handled the circumstances leading up to his illness. Alan tried hard not to think about events at work, but experienced frequent intrusive memories and thoughts about particular incidents that occurred in the months before he commenced sick leave. He interpreted how he had handled the situation at work, the intrusive memories that he experienced, and the distress that these caused as a sign that he was not in control of himself or his life.

Initial Formulation

On the basis of information gleaned at assessment, the treating therapist hypothesized the following mechanisms as being central to the maintenance of Alan's depression:

- *A perceived loss of control over events at work and a perception he had made mistakes in how he conducted himself.* This had compromised Alan's self-esteem, which was based entirely on work and the sense of role, purpose, and status that this inferred. Prior to the onset of his illness, Alan perceived himself as capable, competent, and master of his own domain.

- *His view that becoming depressed was a sign of weakness.* Alan viewed the persistence of his illness as further evidence of his weakness. This further undermined his self-esteem.
- *His sense of shame at becoming depressed.* Although Alan admitted feeling ashamed regarding his depression, he did not readily articulate the concomitant sense of himself as weak that was hypothesized by the therapist but rather, he expressed a strong view that his depression was biological in origin.

Alan expressed reservations regarding the utility of CT as a treatment. This, in conjunction with his sense of shame, led the therapist to exercise caution in terms of sharing the formulation with Alan. The therapist was concerned that being too explicit with Alan regarding his sense of himself as weak might lead him to disengage. Therefore, the initial formulation was presented tentatively, with ample opportunity for Alan to contribute and to disagree. The initial formulation drew on the Beck et al.'s (1979). model by considering the practical (actual) losses that Alan was confronting. The therapist then developed this further by looking at the personal (perceived) losses that arose from them. This was presented in written form as follows:

Practical losses I have suffered as a result of becoming depressed:
- Loss of job
- Loss of ability to be as active as I used to be
- Loss of financial security
- Loss of retirement plan

Personal losses I have suffered since becoming depressed and losing my job:
- Loss of a sense of security
- Loss of a role in life
- Loss of purpose and meaning in life
- Loss of status
- Loss of respect for self and in the eyes of others

Alan responded favorably to the formulation and was able to make a connection with the idea that certain practical external losses had also triggered internal change and losses.

A number of important conditional beliefs were hypothesized and subsequently endorsed by Alan: *If you are not in control, it is a sign of weakness.* The theme of control was central to the onset and maintenance of his illness. Alan perceived that he had not taken control of events in a climate of change at work. He also invested a great deal of mental and emotional effort into trying to control his depression. *If you show your emotions, you will be ridiculed and humiliated.* This belief to a large extent reflected a cultural norm. The environment in which Alan was raised and currently lived endorsed men who were strong and did not show their feelings. *If you work hard, you will be rewarded.* Alan saw working hard as a virtue in itself that also conferred a sense of self-worth. Hence, his self-esteem was predicated on work. This belief was a contributory factor in the onset of Alan's depression, because he always believed that if he worked hard (which he did), he would gain not only material reward (which he would deserve for working hard) but also self-respect and respect in the eyes of others.

Formulating Alan's unconditional beliefs presented more of a dilemma. Since becoming depressed, he interpreted much of what went on in his life in terms of his own weakness. In contrast, prior to becoming depressed Alan had viewed himself, and had perceived that others viewed him, as strong, capable, and in control of his life. On this basis within the formulation, Alan and the therapist made sense of his problems in terms of his positive view of himself as strong, capable, and in control as having been shattered by an inability to control events at work and by his resultant depressive illness. Alan's view of himself as weak related only to having become depressed, not as a pre morbid, global negative view of self. In terms of his view of the world, Alan believed it should be a fair place was closely linked to his belief that if he worked hard, he would be rewarded. Prior to the changes at work, Alan believed life had treated him fairly, and it had done so because he had worked hard.

The extremity (all or nothing nature) and rigidity with which Alan held his beliefs was formulated as being an important contributor to his distress and fundamental to his vulnerability.

Manifestations of Beliefs

The beliefs hypothesized in the formulation manifested themselves in a number of ways. Alan's beliefs about the importance of control accounted for his self-blaming automatic thoughts and feelings of guilt regarding events at work. They also explained his persistent attempts to control his symptoms and memories, and his interpretation of his difficulties in doing so as evidence of weakness. His belief that lack of emotional control would lead to humiliation accounted for his complete social avoidance since becoming depressed and his high levels of anxiety when in the company of others. These beliefs also fed his marked cognitive avoidance, as shown in his efforts to suppress distressing intrusive thoughts and memories, and behavioral avoidance, as shown in his general inactivity.

Treatment

Alan found the development of the formulation to be one of the most help-ful aspects of therapy. It enabled him to make sense of his experiences and, despite his biological view of depression, to consider the role his own per-ceptions and beliefs might play in maintaining his difficulties. The formula-tion also provided Alan with a cogent rationale for engaging in interven-tions that were difficult and distressing for him. Examples of how standard interventions were adapted to tackle Alan's problems were described earlier.

REVIEW OF EFFICACY RESEARCH

One of the strengths of CT is its strong empirical base, and this is well estab-lished in relation to acute depression. Much of the research evidence that addresses the effectiveness of CT on persistent symptoms comes from small-scale studies that have not been rigorously controlled. The earliest studies (e.g., Fennell & Teasdale, 1982) sounded a note of caution due to the low response rate. Response rates in subsequent studies (Harping, Letterman, Marks, Stern, & Johann, 1982; Gonzales, Levin, & Clarke, 1985; Stravynski, Shah, & Verreault, 1991; Fava, Rafanelli, Grandi, Canestrari, & Morphy, 1998; Fava, Savron, Grandi, & Rafanelli, 1997) have varied widely between 20 and 75%. The small sample sizes mean that such studies are highly sus-ceptible to biases. In addition, only two of these studies (Harpin et al., 1982; Moore & Blackburn, 1997) included any kind of control condition. There were however, signs of promise that CT might be of benefit in some cases of chronic depression (Teasdale, Scott, Moore, Hayhurst, Pope, & Paykel, 2001).

The approach to CT for chronic depression described briefly here (and elaborated in Moore & Garland, 2003) was first developed for use in a rigor-ous, randomized controlled trial of CT for chronic depression, known as the Cambridge–Newcastle Depression Study (Paykel et al., 1999; Scott et al., 2000). This study (the results of which are described in detail in Moore & Garland, 2003) indicated that CT, as outlined here, produced a significant but modest additional improvement in remission rates, overall symptom functioning, and social functioning when added to good clinical manage-ment and medication. CT also resulted in significant improvement in the key symptoms of hopelessness and low self-esteem. Most importantly, it achieved a worthwhile reduction in the rate of relapse into full major depression, over and above the effects of continued medication. Analysis of the mechanism of change by which CT prevented relapse found little evi-dence to support the idea that this occurs by changing the content of cognition. In contrast, substantial evidence indicated that CT may prevent relapse by enabling patients to influence the way they process depression-related material rather than thought content. CT also demonstrated a reduction in the extremity of emotionally relevant thinking and an increase in patients' ability to experience upsetting cognitions as thoughts rather than facts. Both of these types of change were associated with reduced relapse.

CONCLUSIONS

The primary goal of this chapter is to provide an overview of the clinical adaptations to CT for depression that may make it more effective for individuals with persistent depressive symptoms. The evidence from research studies is that a combination of CT and antidepressants can help to resolve or ameliorate the symptoms and social problems associated with this debilitating condition. In day-to-day practice, CT alone or in combination with medication appears to be a highly acceptable intervention for individuals with chronic depression and may produce durable benefits for 50–70% patients. However, it would be wrong to assume that we have gone as far as we can in conceptualizing and treating chronic depression with CT. A number of exciting cognitive theory and therapy developments are being explored. For example, research on rumination (which may play a crucial role in the maintenance of depressive symptoms) suggests that it may be useful to conceptualize rumination in terms of processing styles rather than simply as recurrent negative thought content. To date, psychological treatments for chronic depression have not explicitly focused on shifting processing modes during focus on negative self-experience. The work on mindfulness-based CT (MBCT) has only been used for patients with fully remitted, rather than partially remitted, depression (Teasdale et al., 2000), so we do not yet know if this approach is suitable for chronic depression. However, the success of MBCT in preventing relapse is consistent with the argument that a shift processing style when faced with negative self-experience may be of therapeutic benefit. It is therefore timely to consider exploring how CT might be varied to explicitly shift the mode of processing negative self-experience in residual depression, without requiring a background in mindfulness meditation (Watkins, 2004). Such work is now underway and will perhaps offer another useful advance on our current CT models that may then allow us to understand further the causes of chronic depression, as well as to offer a range of CT approaches to tackle this problem.

REFERENCES

Beck, A. T., Rush, A. J., Shaw, B. F., & Emery, G. (1979). *Cognitive therapy of depression*. New York: Guilford Press.

Bedrosian, R. C., & Bozicas, G. D. (1994). *Treating family of origin problems: A cognitive approach*. New York: Guilford Press.

Burns, D. D., & Nolan, S. N. (1992). Therapeutic empathy and recovery form depression in cognitive behavioral therapy: A structural equation model. *Journal of Consulting and Clinical Psychology, 60,* 441–449.

Burns, D. D., & Spangler, D. L. (2000). Does psychotherapy homework lead to improvement in depression in cognitive behavioural psychotherapy or does improvement lead to increased homework compliance? *Journal of Consulting and Clinical Psychology, 68,* 46–56.

Cornwall, P. L., & Scott, J. (1997). Partial remission in depressive disorders. *Acta Psychiatrica Scandinavica, 95,* 265–271.

Cornwall, P. L., Scott, J., Garland, A., & Pollinger, B. R. (2005). Beliefs about depression and their partners. *Behavioural and Cognitive Psychotherapy, 33,* 131–138.

Fava, G. A., Rafanelli, C., Grandi, S., Canestrari, M. D., & Morphy, M. A. (1998). Six year outcome for cognitive behavioural treatment of residual symptoms in major depression. *American Journal of Psychiatry, 155,* 1443–1445.

Fava, G. A., Savron, G., Grandi, S., & Rafanelli, C. (1997). Cognitive behavioural management of drug resistant major depressive disorder. *Journal of Clinical Psychiatry, 58,* 278–282.

Fennell, M. J. V., & Teasdale, J. D. (1982). Cognitive therapy with chronic drug refractory depressed outpatients: A note of caution. *Cognitive Therapy and Research, 6,* 455–460.

Fennell, M. J. V., & Teasdale, J. (1987). Cognitive therapy for depression: Individual differences and process of change. *Cognitive Therapy and Research, 11,* 253–271.

Garland, A., & Scott, J. (2000). Using homework in therapy for depression. *Journal of Clinical Psychology, 58*(5), 489–498.

Gonzales, L. R., Lewinsohn, P. M., & Clarke, G. N. (1985). Longitudinal follow-up of unipolar depressives: An investigation of predictors of relapse. *Journal of Consulting and Clinical Psychology, 53,* 461–420.

Harpin, E., Lieberman, R. T. P., Marks, I., Stern, R., & Bohannon, W. E. (1982). Cognitive-behaviour therapy from chronically depressed patients: A controlled pilot study. *Journal of Nervous and Mental Disease, 170,* 295–301.

Judd, L. L. (1997). The clinical course of unipolar major depressive disorders. *Archives of General Psychiatry, 54,* 989–991.

Kazantzis, N., Deane, F. P., & Ronan, K. R. (2000). Homework assignments in cognitive and behavioural therapy: A meta-analysis. *Clinical Psychology, Science and Practice, 2,* 189–202.

McCullough, J. P. (2000). *Treatment of chronic depression: Cognitive behavioural analysis system of psychotherapy approach*. New York: Guilford Press.

Mercier, M. A., Stewart, J. W., & Quitkin, F. M. (1992). A pilot sequential study of cognitive therapy and pharmacotherapy of atypical depression. *Journal of Clinical Psychiatry, 53,* 166–170.

Moore, R. G., & Blackburn, I. M. (1997). Cognitive therapy in the treatment of non-responders to antidepressant medication"controlled pilot study. *Behavioural and Cognitive Psychotherapy,* 25, 251–259.

Moore, R. G., & Garland, A. (2003). *Cognitive therapy for chronic and persistent depression.* Chichester, England: Wiley.

Padesky, C. A. (1996). Developing cognitive therapist competency: Teaching and supervision models. In P. M. Salkovskis (Ed.), *Frontiers of cognitive therapy.* London: Guilford Press.

Paykel, E.S., Jonhson, A.L., Abott, R., Hayhurst, H., et al. (2000). Effects of cognitive therapy on psychological symptoms and social functioning in residual depression. *British Journal of Psychiatry, 177,* 440–446.

Paykel, E. S., Scott, J., Cornwall, P. L., Abbott, R., Crane, C., Pope, M., et al. (2005). Duration of relapse prevention after cognitive therapy in residual depression: Follow-up of controlled trial. *Psychological Medicine, 35,* 59–68.

Paykel, E. S., Ramana, R., Cooper, Z., Hayhurst, H., Kerr, J., & Barocka, A. (1995). Residual symptoms after partial remission: An important outcome in depression. *Psychological Medicine, 25,* 1171–1180.

Paykel, E. S., Scott, J., Teasdale, J. D., Johnson, A. L., Garland, A., Moore, R., et al. (1999). Prevention for relapse in residual depression by cognitive therapy. *Archives of General Psychiatry, 56,* 829–835.

Schatzberg, A. F., Rush, A. J., Arnow, B. A., Banks, P. L., Blalock, J. A., Borian, F. E., et al. (2005). Chronic depression: medication (nefazodone) or psychotherapy (CBASP) is effective when the other is not. *Archives of General Psychiatry, 62,* 513–520.

Scott, J. (2000). Treatment of chronic depression. *New England Journal of Medicine.* 342, 518–520.

Shaw, B. F., Elkin, I., Yamaguchi, J., Olmstead, M., Vallis, T. M., Dobson, K.S., et al. (1999). Therapist competence ratings in relation to clinical outcome in cognitive therapy for depression. *Journal of Consulting and Clinical Psychology, 67,* 837–846.

Spitzer, R. L., Williams, J. B. W., Gibbon, M., & First, M. B. (1992). The structured clinical interview for DSM-IIIR (SCID): I. History, rationale and description. *Archives of General Psychiatry, 49,* 624–629.

Steer, A. T., & Brown, R. A. (1996). *Manual for the Beck Depression Inventory–II.* San Antonio, TX: Harcourt Assessment, Inc.

Stravynski, A., Shahar, A., & Verreault, R. (1991). A pilot study of the cognitive treatment of dysthymic disorder. *Behavioural Psychotherapy, 19,* 369–372.

Teasdale, J. D., Scott, J., Moorell, R. G., Hayhurst, H., Pope, M., & Paykel, E. S.(2001). How does cognitive therapy prevent relapse in residual depression? Evidence from a controlled trial. *Journal of Consulting and Clinical Psychology, 69,* 347–357.

Teasdale, J. D., Segal, Z. V., Williams, J. M. G., Ridgeway, V. A., Soulsby, J. M., & Lau, M. A. (2000). Prevention of relapse/recurrence in major depression by mindfulness-based cognitive therapy. *Journal of Consulting and Clinical Psychology, 68,* 615–623.

Watkins, E. (2004). Adaptive and maladaptive ruminative self-focus during emotional processing. *Behaviour Research and Therapy, 42,* 1037–1052.

Wegner, D. M., Schneider, D. J., Carter, S., III, & White, T. (1987). Paradoxical effects of thought suppression. *Journal of Personality and Social Psychology, 53,* 5–13.

5

DRUG-RESISTANT AND PARTIALLY REMITTED DEPRESSION

Giovanni A. Fava
Stefania Fabbri

There is increasing awareness that the majority of depressed patients fails to respond to an appropriate trial of antidepressant drug of adequate dose and duration (less then 25% symptom reduction from baseline) or shows a partial response (25–49% symptom reduction from baseline), or achieves a response without remission (50% or greater symptom reduction from baseline but presence of residual symptomatology) (Fava, 2003). Several pharmacological strategies have been developed for depressed patients who fail to respond to standard drug treatment (Fava, 2003; Fava & Rush, 2006; Thase & Rush, 1995) but limited research has been done on nonpharmacological approaches despite the logical appeal of treating patients who do not respond to antidepressant medication with psychotherapy (McPherson et al., 2005). There has been an upsurge of research, however, on cognitive strategies in prevention of relapse of mood disorders (Fava, Ruini, & Rafanelli, 2005). In this chapter, we discuss the role of cognitive therapy (CT) in drug-resistant depression and when remission is partial and associated with substantial residual symptomatology.

110

DRUG-RESISTANT DEPRESSION

There is no accepted definition of "drug-resistant depression" (Fava, 2003; Sackeim, 2001). The most common definition is failure to achieve a satisfactory response to at least one antidepressant trial of adequate dose and duration. A more conservative definition is a poor response to two appropriate trials of different classes of antidepressants (Fava, 2003).

We report here an abridged account of our cognitive protocol developed from standard cognitive strategies. Unfortunately, because large-scale, randomized controlled trials of CT in the treatment of resistant depression have not been published yet, our suggestions are purely tentative, based only on an open trial and on our experience in our Affective Disorder Program.

Assessment

A first issue that is important when assessing a case of drug-resistant depression is that of "pseudoresistance." Nierenberg and Amsterdam (1990) used this expression in reference to nonresponse to inadequate treatment, in terms of duration or dose of the antidepressant used. Certain pharmacokinetic factors, such as concomitant use of metabolic inducers (e.g., drugs that may increase the metabolism and elimination rate of coadministered agents) may also contribute to the phenomenon of pseudoresistance. In the Affective Disorder Program, our very conservative definition of "treatment-resistant depression" (TRD) is the persistence of major depression despite at least two courses of adequate drug treatment. "Appropriate drug treatment" is defined as use of standard doses of antidepressant drugs administered continuously for a minimum duration of 6 weeks. Furthermore, as suggested by Simpson and Kessel (1991), one trial should include the use of a high-dose (200–300 mg) tricyclic, such as imipramine, for a minimum of 6 weeks.

Another aspect of pseudoresistance concerns patients who are misdiagnosed as having unipolar depressive disorder (Nierenberg & Amsterdam, 1990) when they have suffering from diseases such as bipolar illness, vascular dementia, or anxiety disorders. But even when unipolar depression disorder is confirmed by a careful assessment, the issue of comorbidity needs to be explored (Fava et al., 2005).

The majority of depressed patients qualify not for one, but for several Axis I and Axis II disorders, which is exemplified by the occurrence of comorbidity in major depression (van Praag, 2000). Very seldom do these different diagnoses undergo hierarchical organization or is attention paid to the longitudinal development of disorders (Fava & Kellner, 1991; e.g., the primary–secondary distinction in depression; Feighner et al., 1972). There is comorbidity that wanes upon successful treatment of one disorder (e.g., recovery from major depression may result in remission from co-occurring hypochondriasis), without any specific treatment for the latter (Kellner, Fava, Lisansky, Perini, & Zielezny, 1986). Other times, treatment of one disorder does not result in the disappearance of comorbidity. For instance, successful treatment of depression may not affect preexisting anxiety disturbances (Fava, Rafanelli, Grandi, Conti, & Belluardo, 1998). As a result, longitudinal development of disorders may not always provide a hierarchical link, and the response to treatment should be evaluated.

Emmelkamp, Bouman, and Scholing (1992) distinguish two levels of functional analysis in psychological assessment: "macroanalysis" (a relationship between co-occurring syndromes is established on the basis of where treatment should commence) and "microanalysis" (a detailed analysis of symptoms). For instance, a patient may present with a major depressive disorder, obsessive–compulsive disorder, and hypochondriasis. In terms of macroanalysis, the clinician may give priority to the pharmacological treatment of depression, leaving to posttherapy assessment the determination of the relationship of depression to obsessive–compulsive disorder and hypochondriasis. Will they wane as depressive epiphenomena, or will they persist, despite some degree of improvement? In this latter case, should further treatment be necessary? What type of relationship do obsessive–compulsive symptoms and hypochondriasis entertain? On the basis of the type and longitudinal development of hypochondriacal fears and beliefs (Savron et al., 1996), the clinician may decide to tackle the obsessive–compulsive disorder, regarding hypochondriasis as an ensuing phenomenon, or he/she may consider them as independent syndromes. Thus, macroanalysis allows disentangling of the complexity of comorbid disorders by establishing treatment priorities. The clinician may in fact decide not to consider drug-resistant depression as the primary target of treatment but to concentrate his/her efforts on a co-occurring syndrome.

A final aspect that needs to be explored in assessing the patient is the presence of medical comorbidity: Several disorders (e.g., Cushing's syndrome, hyperprolactinemia) in their acute phase hinder satisfactory response to antidepressant drugs (Fava & Sonino, 1996).

Cognitive Treatment

It has been frequently reported that management of refractory depression requires modifications from standard CT (Beck, Rush, Shaw, & Emery, 1979). Cole, Brittlebank, and Scott (1994) emphasized the importance of brief but frequent (20 minutes, three times a week) initial sessions, as well as incorporating techniques developed in CT of personality disorders. Thase and Howland (1994) suggested the need for frequent sessions to enhance learning and retention of homework assignments and in-session rehearsal, and of involvement of the spouse or significant others to provide psychoeducation.

Treatment of drug-resistant major depressive disorder may consist of 10–20 sessions, once every week. Treatment is articulated in three phases.

First Phase

The first phase of treatment is characterized by refraining from use of cognitive techniques, which are deferred to a later stage, and extensive use of behavioral strategies. Patients are asked to make a list of situations, rated on a 0- to 100-point scale, that cause distress and/or induce avoidance. Anxiety is regarded as much a target for treatment as is depression. Exposure therapy (assignment of homework activities in a structured diary) is implemented when avoidance is identified (e.g., phobia disturbances). *In vivo* situational exposure exercises should be specific for each day and well defined in terms of duration, situation, and what the patient must do or not do.

It is important that patients understand that exposure must induce discomfort: Patients should be informed that the increase of anxiety during exposure exercises is a sign that what they are doing is working.

In general, patients' disturbances are conceptualized in terms of inhibited central pleasure–reward mechanisms (e.g., low self-esteem, pessimism), central pain disturbances (e.g., sadness, anxiety, excessive regard for potentially adverse consequences of action), and psychomotor regulation (e.g., exhaustion, slowing of thoughts), according to the model advanced by Carroll (1991). This first phase of treatment is mainly involved with behavioral techniques for inhibited psychomotor regulation and anxiety in central pain disturbances.

We feel that treatment of anxiety is often insufficiently emphasized during CT for depression, probably since anxiety is regarded as a by-product of depression. However, as discussed in detail elsewhere (Fava, 1999), at least in certain types of depression, anxiety and irritability are prominent in the prodromal phase of depression, may be concealed by mood disturbances in the acute phase, and are again a prominent feature of the residual phase. Behavioral techniques are implemented also to increase general activities by writing simple tasks in a diary, which may counteract loss of activities related to fatigue and anhedonia.

This initial phase extends over four to six sessions. During this part of treatment, the antidepressant drug that the patient was taking on intake is kept at the same dosage. Attitudes of the patient toward pharmacotherapy are explored. Often patients conceive treatment of depression in purely pharmacological (external) terms and need to be educated about the importance of self-therapy. An example we frequently use has to do with lowering cholesterol levels. Drugs may be important, but they achieve insufficient results if the patient does not attempt in his/her diet to lower the intake of food high in saturated fats. Other patients perceive their lack of response to drug treatment as personal failure and confirmation of their inadequacies. We tell these patients that because drugs are effective only for two out of three patients, and no drug is effective for everybody, other strategies frequently need to be involved.

Middle Phase

When a certain degree of psychomotor activation and cooperation has been achieved, use of the diary for monitoring automatic thoughts and cognitive restructuring, according to standard CT protocols, is introduced (Beck et al., 1979). During this second phase, cognitive strategies are mainly targeted to change mood and to inhibit central pleasure–reward mechanisms.

Patients are at first asked to identify situations that evoke discomfort and rate them on a scale from 0 to 100. Gradually patients should be encouraged to label their discomfort more specifically, using appropriate terms that better describe their emotions. Once they become familiar with identifying the situations and recognizing their emotions, we bring in the concept of automatic thoughts and ask subjects to start monitoring them and writing them down in the diary. Thinking errors are addressed as they arise in patients' reports. Finally, patients are asked to counteract their automatic thoughts with a more objective and rational point of view, and to add this last part to their diary. When discussing automatic thoughts and dysfunctional beliefs in session, it is important to start working with the most weakly held beliefs, which are less likely to induce resistance from patients and are therefore more amenable to change. Automatic thoughts are introduced only at a later stage, when patients have satisfactorily monitored their episodes of distress. Thus, patients are gradually exposed to the need for and cognitive restructuring with a self-disclosing strategy.

Behavioral homework is continued throughout this phase, and medication tapering is also initiated at the lowest possible rate (e.g., 25 mg of tricyclic antidepressant every other week). This phase may extend over 4–10 sessions until clinical improvement in mood occurs.

Final Phase

In the final phase of treatment, the antidepressant drug is finally discontinued. We are reluctant to decrease antidepressant drugs in the initial phase of treatment, because this may be a source of further distress. At the same time, we do not intend to keep a patient indefinitely on a medication that has yielded limited benefit. Patients are monitored closely for signs of relapse. In this phase, attention is given to the transformation of cognitive insights into behavioral changes, with particular reference to lifestyle modification. For instance, a patient may become aware of his/her cognitive errors in an interpersonal situation but be unable to endorse alternative modalities of interaction. This phase of psychotherapy extends over two to four sessions. Furthermore, we place emphasis on continuation of self-therapy once the psychotherapy sessions are over and on education recognizing prodromal symptoms of relapse.

Review of Efficacy Research

There is little literature on CT approaches to drug-resistant depression. Fennell and Teasdale (1982) failed to detect a significant effect of CT in five chronic, drug-refractory, depressed outpatients. Antonuccio et al. (1984) applied a psychoeducational group treatment (including relaxation, increasing pleasant activities, cognitive strategies, and social skills) to 10 outpatients with unipolar depression who had not responded to antidepressant medication. All patients continued drug treatment. One patient dropped out of group treatment, four were no longer depressed, two showed some improvement, and three patients were still depressed after psychoeducational group treatment. Improvements were maintained at 9-month follow-up. Miller, Bishop, Norman, and Keitner (1985) examined the effectiveness of a treatment program comprising CT, pharmacotherapy, and short-term hospitalization in six chronic, drug-resistant, depressed females. The approach produced a substantial improvement in the majority of patients. De Jong, Treiber, and Henrich (1988) studied a group of 30 chronically depressed patients who failed to respond to antidepressant drugs. Patients were randomly assigned to an intensive inpatient cognitive-behavioral program, to an inpatient low-intensity milieu therapy, and to a waiting-list control group. Patients treated with the intense cognitive-behavioral program had the better outcome. Cole et al. (1994) treated 16 inpatients who had refractory major depression with CT and found a remission rate of 69%, with a significant decrease in depression ratings. Thase and Howland (1994) reported that after participation in an inpatient cognitive-behavioral program, 17 patients with major depression who were resistant to antidepressant treatment had a 47% remission. In one of our studies (Fava, Savron, Grandi, & Rafanelli, 1997), 19 patients who failed to respond to at least two trials of antidepressant drugs of adequate dosage and duration (minimum of 6 weeks) were treated by cognitive-behavioral methods in an open trial. Three patients dropped out of treatment. The remaining 16 subjects displayed a significant decrease in scores on the Clinical Interview of Depression (Paykel, 1985) after therapy. Twelve patients were judged to be in remission at the end of the trial; only one of these patients was found to have relapsed at a 2-year follow-up. Antidepressant drugs were discontinued in 8 of the 12 patients who responded to CT.

PARTIALLY REMITTED DEPRESSION

The notion that the majority of depressed patients experience mild but chronic residual symptoms or recurrence of symptoms after complete remission, a perspective that was well delineated in the 1970s (Weissman, Kasl, & Klerman, 1976), did not receive the attention it deserved in subsequent years. Moreover, the presence of residual symptoms after completion of drug treatment (Fava, 1999; Fava, Fabbri, & Sonino, 2002) or CT (Simons, Murphy, Levine, & Wetzel, 1986; Thase et al., 1992) for depression has been correlated with poor long-term outcome.

The awareness on the one hand that pharmacotherapy is the most cost-effective therapeutic strategy for treatment of the acute phase of a major depression, and on the other hand that cognitive-behavioral approaches are the most valuable intervention for the treatment of residual symptoms and relapse prevention (so that the residual symptomatology does not turn into the prodromal phase of a new depressive episode) is the basis for the sequential administration of pharmacotherapy (as the first ingredient) and psychotherapy (as the second one) according to the stages of the disorder. This sequential approach allows us to use what has been found to be the most effective therapeutic ingredient for each specific phase of the disorder.

The results of several randomized controlled trials, reviewed in detail elsewhere (Fava et al., 2002, 2005) support to the use of a sequential treatment model (pharmacotherapy followed by psychotherapy) to prevent relapse in unipolar depression.

This approach appears to be particularly important in recurrent depression. However, because incomplete recovery from the first lifetime major depressive episode was found to predict a chronic course of illness during a

12-year prospective naturalistic follow-up (Judd et al., 2000), this sequential approach may be indicated whenever substantial residual symptomatology is present.

Suitability and Motivation for Treatment

Before undergoing sequential treatment, patients should already have displayed a satisfactory response to antidepressant drug treatment. They should have been treated for at least 3 months with drug treatment and no longer present with depressed mood. During pharmacological treatment and clinical management, however, it is essential to introduce the subsequent part of treatment.

A helpful way to introduce the sequential approach (Fava et al., 1998) follows:

> "When we first saw you, you were very depressed. You went off the road. We gave you antidepressant drugs, and these put you back on the road. Things are much better now. However, if you keep on driving the way you did, sooner or later, you will go off the road again."

This example highlights the need for lifestyle modification and introduces a sense of control in the patient relative to his/her depressive illness. This psychological preparation paves the way for subsequent psychotherapeutic approaches.

Standard Format

Psychotherapeutic intervention extends over 10 sessions, 30–45 minutes each session every other week. The first session is mainly concerned with assessment and introduction of the psychotherapeutic treatment by the therapist, rehearsing the example provided before formal initiation of treatment. Sessions 2 through 6 are concerned with cognitive treatment of residual symptoms and lifestyle modification. The last four sessions involve well-being therapy. Because this technique is rather new, we describe it in greater detail.

Assessment

It is of considerable importance to reassess the remitted patient after pharmacological treatment as if he/she were a new patient. This means reviewing carefully the patient's symptoms in the most recent weeks. Exploration should concern not only symptoms that characterize the diagnosis of major depressive disorder but also those that characterize anxiety disturbances (including phobic and obsessive–compulsive symptoms) and irritability. In the original studies (Fava, Grandi, Zielezny, Canestrari, & Morphy, 1994; Fava et al., 1998) a modified version of Paykel's (1985) Clinical Interview for Depression was employed, but other semistructured interviews may be used as long as they are sufficiently comprehensive to measure anxiety and irritability. This is the first step in recognizing residual symptomatology.

The second method of assessment deals with the patient's self-observation. He/she is instructed to report in a diary all episodes of distress that ensue in the following 2 weeks. It is important to emphasize that the distress (which is left unspecified) does not need to be prolonged; it may also be short-lived. The patient is also instructed to build a list of situations that elicit distress and/or tend to induce avoidance. Each situation is rated on a 0- to 100-point scale (0, *No distress at all*; 100, *Extreme discomfort*). The patient is instructed to bring the diary to the following visit.

CT for Residual Symptoms

After completing the assessment of the patient, including reading his/her self-observation diary, the therapist formulates a cognitive package. This may encompass both exposure and cognitive restructuring. Exposure consists of homework exposure only. An exposure strategy is planned with the patient, based on the list of situations outlined in his/her diary. The therapist writes an assignment per day in the diary, following an *in vivo* graded exposure (Marks, 1987). The patient is asked to rate the discomfort caused by the assigned task on a scale from 0 to 100. At the following visit, the therapist reassesses the homework done, and discusses the next steps and/or problems in compliance that may have ensued.

Cognitive restructuring follows the classic format of Beck et al. (1979; Beck & Emery, 1985) and is based on introduction of the concept of automatic thoughts (Session 2) and of observer's interpretation (Session 3 and subsequent sessions). The problems that may be the object of cognitive restructuring strictly depend on the material offered by the patient. They may encompass insomnia (sleep hygiene instructions are added), hypersomnia, diminished energy and concentration, residual hopelessness, reentry problems (diminished functioning at work, avoidance and procrastination), lack of assertiveness and self-care, perfectionism, and unrealistic self-expectations.

Well-Being Therapy

At the seventh session well–being therapy is introduced (WBT; Fava & Ruini, 2003). WBT is a short-term psychotherapeutic strategy, with sessions taking place weekly or every other week. The duration of each session may range from 30 to 50 minutes. The technique emphasizes self-observation (Emmelkamp, 1974), with the use of a structured diary, and interaction between patient and therapist. WBT is based on Ryff's (1989) cognitive model of psychological well-being. This model was selected on the basis of its easy applicability to clinical populations (Fava et al., 2001; Rafanelli et al., 2000). WBT is structured, directive, problem-oriented, and based on an educational model.

In this phase of treatment, the target for intervention shifts from symptom reduction to the attainment of well-being. Underlying this treatment is the idea that the absence of well-being is a risk factor for future difficulties. WBT utilizes many of the traditional CT tools presented during the first phase of treatment (see Sessions 1–6). However, emphasis is shifted to patient monitoring of periods of well-being rather than periods of distress. The overall task of the patient is to attend to and enjoy periods of well-being, and to attend to cognitions or other events that may interfere with ongoing enjoyment. The therapist's role is to intervene with cognitive restructuring, activity assignments, and skills training to help the patient better maximize periods of well-being. The therapist uses a conceptual framework that defines domains in which well-being can be enhanced.

Seventh Session

The session focuses on introducing the concept of psychological well-being as a new target of treatment. The therapist, however, refrains from providing a description of Ryff's model and leaves the meaning to the patient. The therapist praises the patient for the successful completion of the first segment of therapy and encourages him/her to increase gains by working on psychological well-being. The session marks the first homework concerned with monitoring psychological well-being.

GOALS

Review of Homework. As before, the therapist asks whether the patient encountered any difficulty in completing the homework. If so, troubleshooting is done to identify obstacles to completion. The patient should be praised for efforts in employing CT techniques on his/her own. The therapist should emphasize the long-term importance of being able to employ such techniques to eliminate residual symptoms and reduce the risk for relapse. Therapist and patient note what types of situations/activities are associated with high mastery and pleasure ratings.

Introduction of a Well-Being Approach. The therapist uses an introduction such as the following:

> "During the last six sessions you have learned and practiced cognitive techniques to help you feel better during times of distress. In our work so far we have focused on *your major problem areas.* In addition to this we will now spend four sessions examining feelings of well-being and how to increase such feelings. Increasing your psychological well-being is important for making you less vulnerable to future life situations and stressors."

This introduction can be modified, as necessary, but the essential message should remain: The patient is now engaged in important work that is complementary to the first phase of treatment.

Ryff's (1989) Psychological Well-Being Scales, a self-rating scale for measuring autonomy, environmental mastery, personal growth, purpose in life, self-acceptance and positive relations with others, may also be given to patients to fill out at home. Completion of this scale takes approximately 10–20 minutes and provides additional information as to attitudes of well-being.

HOMEWORK ASSIGNMENT

The patient is asked to use the assessment diary to record circumstances surrounding episodes of well-being. As with recording episodes of distress, the patient is asked to rate the intensity of feelings of well-being on a 0- to 100-point scale (0 indicates the complete absence of well-being, whereas 100 indicates the most intense well-being that the patient could possibly experience). It is important to emphasize to the patient that moments of well-being will likely vary in length. However, the patient is instructed to record even the most brief moments of well-being. At this juncture it is important to anticipate with the patient any difficulties he/she might experience in completing the above assignment.

Meehl (1975, p. 305) described "how people with low hedonic capacity should pay greater attention to the 'hedonic book keeping' of their activities than would be necessary for people located midway or high on the hedonic capacity continuum. That is, it matters more to someone cursed with an inborn hedonic defect whether he is efficient and sagacious in selecting friends, jobs, cities, tasks, hobbies, and activities in general."

Session 8

This session focuses on enhancing the patient's ability to self-monitor periods of well-being, primarily by review of homework, but it can also occur through observing the patient's well-being during the session. If the therapist notices a positive change in affect, the patient is asked to describe what is happening cognitively. This session also marks the beginning of the process of identifying thoughts and beliefs that lead to premature interruption of well-being.

GOALS

Review of the Patient's Well-Being through the Assessment Diary. The patient presents data collected in his/her Well-Being Diary. Any difficulty the patient reports in completing this homework is discussed. As we mentioned earlier, some patients may report difficulty in identifying any periods of well-being. For such patients, strong emphasis must be placed on continuing to use the diary. These patients are typically described as having low hedonic capacity and need additional practice in identifying feelings of well-being. When working with such patients it is again helpful to look for the patient's moments of well-being that occur in session. The therapist may choose to evoke such feelings using praise, reviewing times of past success, or similar techniques. When a moment of well-being occurs in the session, it is critical to highlight this for the patient and encourage him/her to do the same outside of session using the Well-Being Diary. Some attention is paid to the ratings assigned by the patient to moments of well-being. If the ratings are consistently low (e.g., 30), the therapist asks the patient to describe what would potentially represent a rating of 70 or 80. This is done to avoid having the patient focus exclusively on lower levels of hedonia. The therapist comments on how the well-being instances reported in the assessment diary relate to Ryff's psychological dimensions of well-being (Ryff & Singer, 1996). These six dimensions of psychological well-being are summarized in Table 5.1.

Review of the Psychological Well-Being Scales. The therapist reviews with the patient the Psychological Well-Being Scales in case these have been administered in the previous session.

TABLE 5.1. Modification of the Six Dimensions of Psychological Well-Being

Dimensions	Impaired level	Optimal level
Environmental mastery	The patient has difficulties in managing everyday affairs; feels unable to change or improve surrounding context; is unaware of surrounding opportunities; lacks sense of control over external world.	The patient has a sense of mastery and competence in managing the environment; controls external activities; makes effective use of surrounding opportunities; is able to create or choose contexts suitable to personal needs and values.
Personal growth	The patient has a sense of personal stagnation; lacks sense of improvement or expansion over time; feels bored and uninterested with life; feels unable to develop new attitudes or behaviors.	The patient has a feeling of continued development; sees self as growing and expanding; is open to new experiences; has sense of realizing own potential; sees improvement in self and behavior over time.
Purpose in life	The patient lacks a sense of meaning in life; has few goals or aims, lacks sense of direction, does not see purpose in past life; has no outlooks or beliefs that give life meaning.	The patient has goals in life and a sense of directedness; feels there is meaning to present and past life; holds beliefs that give life purpose; has aims and objectives for living.
Autonomy	The patient is overconcerned with the expectations and evaluation of others; relies on judgment of others to make important decisions; conforms to social pressures to think or act in certain ways.	The patient is self-determining and independent; is able to resist social pressures; regulates behavior from within; evaluates self by personal standards.
Self-acceptance	The patient feels dissatisfied with self; is disappointed with what has occurred in past life; is troubled about certain personal qualities; wishes to be different than what he/she is.	The patient has a positive attitude toward the self; accepts his/her good and bad qualities; feels positive about past life.
Positive relations with others	The patient has few close, trusting relationships with others; finds it difficult to be open, and is isolated and frustrated in interpersonal relationships; is not willing to make compromises to sustain important ties with others.	The patient has warm and trusting relationships with others; is concerned about the welfare of others; is capable of strong empathy, affection, and intimacy; understands give and take of human relationships.

Note. Data from Ryff (1989).

Interruption of Well-Being. A critical step in WBT is to uncover thoughts and beliefs that lead to premature interruption of positive feelings. This can be accomplished by extending the use of the Well-Being Diary and by having the patient focus on the duration of feelings of well-being and the cognitions associated with an interruption in these feelings. An example would be receiving praise from a work supervisor and experiencing subsequent feelings of well-being, only to be interrupted by the thought, "He gives praise to everybody" or "He only wants me to stay late tonight." This is a perfect opportunity for the therapist to use the aforementioned CT techniques to intervene. At this point in therapy, the patient will have practiced these techniques on his/her own; thus, the therapist need supply only simple reinforcement and/or refinement of an existing skill set.

Homework Assignment. The patient is asked to continue use of the well-being assessment diary, with the additional instruction to look for interruptions of well-being. When a patient notices such an interruption as it occurs, he/she is encouraged to use previously learned CT techniques. The therapist also encourages the patient to engage in pleasurable activities on a regular basis (i.e., schedule a daily time to engage in a specific pleasurable activity). This increases the amount of time the patient spends in a well-being state, while offering more opportunities to self-monitor the interruption of well-being.

The similarities with the search for irrational, tension-evoking thoughts in Ellis and Becker's (1982) rational–emotive therapy and automatic thoughts in CT (Beck et al., 1979) are obvious. The trigger for self-observation is, however, different; it is based on well-being rather than distress.

Session 9

During this session, the therapist reviews the patient's efforts to monitor interruption of his/her well-being. Techniques to intervene with such interruptions are reviewed and reinforced with the patient. Therapist and patient also review the six key areas of well-being—environmental mastery, personal growth, purpose in life, autonomy, self-acceptance, and positive relations with others. They focus on the areas that are most relevant to the patient's current issues. Once the most relevant areas are selected, time is spent in session identifying and practicing techniques that facilitate the patient moving toward the optimal level of functioning in each of these areas. Because this is the next to last session, therapist and patient spend some time discussing progress achieved thus far in treatment and strategies to prevent relapse.

GOALS

Well-Being Therapy Techniques. The therapist reviews patient entries in the Well-Being Diary. At this point in treatment, the patient is expected to be able to identify readily moments of well-being (regardless of length), to be aware of interruptions in feelings of well-being (cognitions), and to utilize CT techniques to address these interruptions. If the patient completes this entire process with particular ease, only a brief review of examples from the patient's diary is necessary. However, if the patient seems to be struggling with one or more phases of this process, then the therapist reviews several examples—both fictitious and from the patient's life. It is important to emphasize to the patient that these skills help to prevent relapse and enhance feelings of well-being.

Review of Six Areas of Well-Being and Identification of Dimensions Relevant to Patient's Life. The therapist reviews the six dimensions of well-being and the corresponding impaired and optimal levels of functioning for each. The patient is asked to review each dimension consecutively and to indicate where it falls on the impaired–optimal continuum. This insession review, along with information gleaned from previous reviews of the patient's Well-Being Diary, greatly inform the therapist of the patient's most relevant dimensions. Strategies (used in session and at home) to move the patient toward optimal functioning in relevant dimensions encompass previously reviewed CT techniques. Examples are behavioral techniques (e.g., increasing assertive behavior and scheduling pleasant activities) and cognitive ones (e.g., use of the Dysfunctional Thought Record and the assessment diary, and the therapist challenging the patient's automatic negative thoughts in session). The overall goal here is to identify clearly those well-being dimensions that need work and to reinforce techniques that effectively increase the likelihood of optimal functioning.

Review of Progress and Preparation for Termination. It is important for the therapist to review progress the patient has made up to this point in therapy, and to remind the patient that the next session is the last of this treatment. Points to review include CT techniques utilized by the patient in and out of session that produced relief from distress, dimensions of well-being and how to prevent interruptions of these feelings, and the importance of the patient's ability to conduct "self-therapy."

Homework Assignment. The patient is asked to write a review of what he/she have learned in therapy. The therapist provides some guidance for this assignment by asking that the patient focus on the key elements to coping with distress, his/her particular problem areas, and the tactics he/she can use to enhance well-being. In addition, the patient is asked again to keep a Well-Being Diary for the 2-week interim period, adding a column of observer's interpretations.

Session 10

This represents the last session of this course of psychotherapy. As such, it is important for the therapist to praise the patient's efforts during the course of therapy, to reinforce techniques that have been helpful to the patient, and to facilitate the patient's planning of a self-therapy session.

GOALS

Review of Homework. The therapist reviews both the patient's summary of what he/she has been learned in therapy and the Well-Being Diary covering the last 2 weeks. Although it is expected that patients will be able to identify specific tools they have acquired in the course of therapy, some patients provide only a global description of progress they have made (e.g., "I'm feeling better" or "I can cope better now"). In this case, the therapist needs to ask the patient for the specifics supporting such general statements. A review of the Well-Being Diary indicates whether a patient has reached the point of understanding the details of the interactions among his/her feelings, cognitions, and behavior. The therapist should, in any case, remind the patient of the depressed person's tendency to discount the positive and make internal, negative, global attributions. These should serve as signs to the patient that he/she is engaging in unhealthy thought processes. Another important message to reinforce with the patient is that continued self-monitoring and practice of techniques learned in therapy serve a vital role in protecting against relapse/recurrence.

Planning a Self-Therapy Session. In many ways, the patient has learned to be his/her own therapist through this 10-session course of psychotherapy. However, some patients may attribute much or all of their progress to the therapist's efforts and/or expertise. In such cases it is critical to remind the patient that he/she has done the majority of work in session and, of course, outside of session. If it seems necessary, the therapist can review the original problem list, the gains achieved, and the techniques used by the patient to make this progress. Particular emphasis is placed on highlighting specific situations in which the patient used these techniques in his/her life. The patient is asked to schedule a self-therapy session at the normal meeting time in 2 weeks. The therapist suggests that the patient follow the same format used in previous sessions. The patient can use imagery to help remind him/her of what it was like to participate in a therapy session. As in medication therapy, the therapist introduces the idea that "booster" therapy sessions are available in the future, while emphasizing that a period of going without psychotherapy is a positive sign and a step forward.

Lifestyle Modification

One of the aims of therapy is also to make the patient aware of allostatic loads (i.e., chronic and often subtle life stresses that exert harmful consequences on the individual over a certain amount of time). Examples may be excessive work loads, lack of awareness of the longer time that increasing age requires for recovering from demanding days, inability to protect oneself from requests that exceed one's potential, and inappropriate sleeping habits. Such awareness (and the resulting lifestyle implementation) is pursued in all phases of psychotherapy, but particularly with WBT. Patients are given instructions in the diary as to this implementation. For instance, patients are encouraged to modify their work overcommitments, to refuse inappropriate requests from relatives and colleagues, and to dedicate more time to pleasurable activities.

Drug Tapering and Discontinuation

Sequential treatment offers a unique opportunity for antidepressant drug tapering and discontinuation. In fact, it offers the opportunity to monitor the patient in one of the most delicate aspects of treatment. In the original studies (Fava et al., 1994, 1998) antidepressant drugs, mainly tricyclics, were decreased at the rate of 25 mg of amitriptyline or its equivalent every other week. When selective serotonin reuptake inhibitors (SSRIs) are involved, more gradual tapering is the better.

It is important to warn the patient that he/she should not perceive "steps" (as one patient defined them) in this tapering (i.e., patients should not perceive substantial differences in their sleep, energy, mood, and appetite in going from 200 mg to 175 mg of amitriptyline per day). If they do, the appropriateness of tapering the antidepressant drug should be questioned. Indeed, in the original studies, drug discontinuation did not take place in a few patients.

The sequential format offers an ideal opportunity to support the patient psychologically when withdrawal syndromes (despite slow tapering, particularly with SSRI) do occur. At times when patients are fearful of drug discontinuation, it is helpful to emphasize that a drug-free status is a step forward in therapy and may be associated with increased quality of life. Thus, it is a sign of progress. Antidepressant drugs may be prescribed again, if needed, in the event of prodromal symptoms of mood deterioration, and patients should be reassured that this option is always available.

Review of Efficacy Research

There is now extensive research evidence, based on five randomized controlled trials reviewed in detail elsewhere (Fava et al., 2005), on the long-term benefits, including a lowered relapse rate, of increasing the level of remission with cognitive-behavioral strategies. In one trial, Fava et al. (1998) used the combination of CT and WBT described in this chapter and yielded dramatic differences in relapse rate compared to clinical management. In two trials, follow-up was up to 6 years (Fava et al., 2004; Paykel et al., 2005).

CASE ILLUSTRATION

The patient, a 44-year-old man who works as a county clerk, has a major depressive disorder of recent onset. He had two previous episodes 1 and 3 years earlier that were treated by his primary care physician with fluvoxamine (100 mg per day) for 4 months each time. Although in this case his physician has prescribed fluvoxamine (100 mg per day), he wonders whether a different treatment may be justified. Careful assessment discloses only partial remission after each episode. The psychiatrist confirms treatment with fluvoxamine, but introduces the need of a sequential approach. After 3 months of drug treatment, the patient is given the combined treatment, CT + WBT. The CT part of treatment yields important insights and modification of some of his maladaptive attitudes. WBT allows him to realize how his lack of autonomy leads his workmates consistently to take advantage of him. This results in workloads that, because of their diverse nature, undermine the patient's environmental mastery, constitute a significant stress, and increase his work hours. The patient accepts the situation by virtue of his low degree of self-acceptance: He claims that this is the way he is, but at the same time he is dissatisfied with himself and chronically irritable. When he learns to say "no" to his colleagues (assertiveness training) and to endorse this attitude consistently, a significant degree of distress ensues, linked to perceived disapproval by others. However, as time goes by, his tolerance to disapproval gradually increases, and in the last session he is able to make the following remark: "Now my workmates say that I have changed and that I have become a bastard. In a way I am sorry, since I have always tried to be helpful and kind to people. But in another way I am happy, because this means that—for the first time in my life—I have been able to protect myself." Fluvoxamine was tapered and discontinued during psychotherapy. The patient had no further relapse at an 8-year follow-up, while being drug-free. This clinical picture illustrates how an initial feeling of well-being (being helpful to others) identified in the patient's diary was likely to lead to overwhelming distress. Its appraisal and the resulting change in behavior initially led to more distress, then yielded a lasting remission.

CONCLUSIONS

Isaac Marks (1999) suggested that the prevailing therapeutic mechanisms for explaining therapeutic effectiveness in psychotherapy are about to change. Foa and Kozak (1997) wondered whether the slowing advance of CT might be the result of an alienation from psychopathology. The sequential model introduces a conceptual shift in psychotherapy research and practice. The target of psychotherapeutic efforts is not predetermined and therapy-driven (e.g., cognitive triad) but depends on the type and intensity of residual symptomatology (Fava et al., 1994, 1998) or the specific impairments in psychological well-being (Fava et al., 1998; Fava & Ruini, 2003). Therefore, the cognitive approach in the sequential model is pragmatic and realistic instead of idealistic, based on a strictly evidence-based appraisal of its components (Fava, 2000). There is limited awareness that current techniques of treating affective disorders are geared more toward acute situations than toward residual phases of illness, and that they neglect psychological well-being (Fava, 1999). The model may be frustrating to the purist because of its blurring of clear-cut interpretive instruments. However, it is more in keeping with the complexity of the balance of positive and negative affects (Ryff & Singer, 1998) in health and disease, and the clinical needs of patients with affective disorders.

REFERENCES

Antonuccio, D. O., Akins, W. T., Chathan, P. M., Monagin, J. A., Tearnan, B. H., & Ziegler, B. L. (1984). An exploratory study: The psychoeducational group treatment of drug-refractory unipolar depression. *Journal of Behavior Therapy and Experimental Psychiatry, 15*, 309–313.

Beck, A. T., & Emery, G. (1985). *Anxiety disorders and phobias.* New York: Basic Books.

Beck, A. T., Rush, A. J., Shaw, B. F., & Emery, G. (1979). *Cognitive therapy of depression.* New York: Guilford Press.

Carroll, B. J. (1991). Psychopathology and neurobiology of manic depressive disorders. In B. J. Carroll & J. E. Barrett (Eds.), *Psychopathology and the brain* (pp. 265–285). New York: Raven Press.

Cole, A. J., Brittlebank, A. D., & Scott, J. (1994). The role of cognitive therapy in refractory depression. In W. A., Nolen, J. Zohar, S. P. Roose, & J. D. Amsterdam (Eds.), *Refractory depression* (pp. 117–120). Chichester, UK: Wiley.

De Jong, R., Treiber, R., & Henrich, G. (1988). Effectiveness of two psychological treatments for inpatients with severe and chronic depression. *Cognitive Therapy and Research, 10,* 645–663.

Ellis, A., & Becker, I. (1982). *A guide to personal happiness.* Hollywood, CA: Wilshire.

Emmelkamp, P. M. G. (1974). Self-observation versus flooding in the treatment of agoraphobia. *Behaviour Research and Therapy, 12,* 229–237.

Emmelkamp, P. M. G., Bouman, T. K., & Scholing, A. (1992). *Anxiety disorders. A practitioner's guide.* Chichester, UK: Wiley.

Fava, G. A. (1999). Subclinical symptoms in mood disorders. *Psychological Medicine, 29,* 49–61.

Fava, G. A. (2000). Cognitive behavioral therapy. In M. Fink (Eds.), *Encyclopedia of stress* (pp. 484–487). San Diego: Academic Press.

Fava, G. A., Fabbri, S., & Sonino, N. (2002). Residual symptoms in depression: An emerging therapeutic target. *Progress in Neuro-Psychopharmacology and Biological Psychiatry, 26,* 1019–1027.

Fava, G. A., Grandi, S., Zielezny, M., Canestrari, R., & Morphy, M. A. (1994). Cognitive behavioral treatment of residual symptoms in primary major depressive disorder. *American Journal of Psychiatry, 151,* 1295–1299.

Fava, G. A., & Kellner R. (1991). Prodromal symptoms in affective disorders. *American Journal of Psychiatry, 148,* 823–830.

Fava, G. A., Rafanelli, C., Grandi, S., Conti, S., & Belluardo, P. (1998). Prevention of recurrent depression with cognitive–behavioral therapy. *Archives of General Psychiatry 55,* 816–820.

Fava, G. A., Rafanelli, C., Ottolini, F., Ruini, C., Cazzaro, M., & Grandi, S. (2001). Psychological well-being and residual symptoms in remitted patients with panic disorder and agoraphobia. *Journal of Affective Disorders, 65,* 185–190.

Fava, G. A., & Ruini, C. (2003). Development and characteristics of a well-being enhancing psychotherapeutic strategy: Well-being therapy. *Journal of Behavior Therapy and Experimental Psychiatry, 34,* 45–63.

Fava, G. A., Ruini, C., & Rafanelli, C. (2005). Sequential treatment of mood and anxiety disorders. *Journal of Clinical Psychiatry, 66,* 1392–1400.

Fava, G. A., Ruini, C., Rafanelli, C., Finos, L., Conti, S., & Grandi, S. (2004). Six year outcome of cognitive behavior therapy for prevention of recurrent depression. *American Journal of Psychiatry, 161,* 1872–1876.

Fava, G. A., Savron, G., Grandi, S., & Rafanelli, C. (1997). Cognitive-behavioral management of drug resistant major depressive disorder. *Journal of Clinical Psychiatry, 58*(6), 278–282.

Fava, G. A., & Sonino, N. (1996). Depression associated with medical illness. *CNS Drugs, 5,* 175–189.

Fava, M. (2003). Diagnosis and definition of treatment-resistant depression. *Biological Psychiatry, 53,* 639–659.

Fava, M., & Rush, A. J. (2006). Current status of augmentation and combination treatments for major depressive disorder. *Psychotherapy and Psychosomatics, 75,* 139–153.

Feighner, J. P., Robins, E., Guze, S. B., Woodruff, R. A., Winokur, R. A., Winokur, G., et al. (1972). Diagnostic criteria for use in psychiatric research. *Archives of General Psychiatry, 26,* 57–63.

Fennell, M. J. V., & Teasdale, J. D. (1982). Cognitive therapy with chronic, drug-refractory depressed outpatients: A note of caution. *Cognitive Therapy and Research, 6,* 455–460.

Foa, E. B., & Kozak, M. J. (1997). Beyond the efficacy ceiling?: Cognitive behavior therapy in search of theory. *Behavior Therapy, 28,* 601–611.

Judd, L. J., Paulus, M. J., Schettler, P. J., Akiskal, H. S., Endicott, J., Leon, A. C., et al. (2000). Does incomplete recovery from first lifetime major depressive episode herald a chronic course of illness? *American Journal of Psychiatry, 157,* 1501–1504.

Kellner, R., Fava, G. A., Lisansky, J., Perini, G. I., & Zielezny, M. (1986). Hypochondriacal fears and beliefs in DSM-III melancholia: Changes with amitriptyline. *Journal of Affective Disorders, 10,* 21–26.

Marks, I. M. (1987). *Fears, phobias, and rituals: Panic, anxiety and their disorders.* New York: Oxford University Press.

Marks, I. M. (1999). Is a paradigm shift occurring in brief psychological treatments? *Psychotherapy and Psychosomatics, 68,* 169–170.

McPherson, S., Cairns, P., Carlyle, J., Shapiro, D. A., Richardson, P., & Taylor, D. (2005). The effectiveness of psychological treatments for treatment-resistant depression: A systematic review. *Acta Psychiatrica Scandinavica, 111,* 331–340.

Meehl, P. E. (1975). Hedonic capacity: Some conjectures. *Bulletin of the Menninger Clinic, 39,* 295–307.

Miller, I. W., Bishop, S. B., Norman, W. H., & Keitner, G. I. (1985). Cognitive-behavioral therapy and pharmacotherapy with chronic, drug refractory depressed inpatients: A note of optimism. *Behavioural Psychotherapy, 13,* 320–327.

Nierenberg, A. A., & Amsterdam, J. D. (1990). Treatment-resistant depression. *Journal of Clinical Psychiatry, 51*(Suppl.), 39–47.

Paykel, E. S. (1985). The Clinical Interview for Depression. *Journal of Affective Disorders, 9,* 85–96.

Paykel, E. S., Scott, J., Teasdale, J. D., Johnson, A. L., Garland, A., Moore, R., et al. (2005). Duration of relapse prevention after cognitive therapy in residual depression. *Psychological Medicine, 35,* 59–68.

Rafanelli, C., Park, S. K., Ruini, C., Ottolini, F., Cazzaro, M., & Fava, G. A. (2000). Rating well-being and distress. *Stress Medicine, 16*, 55–61.

Ryff, C. D. (1989). Happiness is everything, or is it?: Explorations on the meaning of psychological well-being. *Journal of Personality and Social Psychology, 57*, 1069–1081.

Ryff, C. D., & Singer, B. (1996). Psychological well-being: Meaning, measurement, and implications for psychotherapy research. *Psychotherapy and Psychosomatics, 65*, 14–23.

Ryff, C. D., & Singer, B. (1998). The contours of positive human health. *Psychological Inquiry, 9*, 1–28.

Sackeim, H. (2001). The definition and meaning of treatment-resistant depression. *Journal of Clinical Psychiatry, 62*(Suppl. 16), 10–17.

Savron, G., Fava, G. A., Grandi, S., Rafanelli, C., Raffi, A. R., & Belluardo, P. (1996). Hypochondriacal fears and beliefs in obsessive–compulsive disorder. *Acta Psychiatrica Scandinavica, 93*, 345–348.

Simons, A. D., Murphy, G. E., Levine, J. L., & Wetzel, R. D. (1986). Cognitive therapy and pharmacotherapy of depression. *Archives of General Psychiatry, 43*, 43–50.

Simpson, G. M., & Kessel, J. B. (1991). Treatment-resistant depression. *British Journal of Psychiatry, 159*, 162–163.

Thase, M. E., & Howland, R. H. (1994). Refractory depression: Relevance of psychosocial factors and therapies. *Psychiatric Annals, 24*, 232–240.

Thase, M. E., & Rush, A. J. (1995). Treatment-resistant depression. In F. E. Bloom & D. J. Kupfer (Eds.), *Psychopharmacology: The fourth generation of progress* (pp. 1081–1097). New York: Raven Press.

Thase, M. E., Simons, A. D., McGeary, J., Cahalane, J. F., Hughes, C., Harden, T., et al. (1992). Relapse after cognitive behavior therapy of depression. *American Journal of Psychiatry, 149*, 1046–1052.

van Praag, H. M. (2000). Nosologomania: A disorder of psychiatry. *World Journal of Biological Psychiatry, 1*, 151–158.

Weissman, M. M., Kasl, S. V., & Klerman, G. L. (1976). Follow-up of depressed women after maintenance treatment. *American Journal of Psychiatry, 133*, 757–760.

6

PREVENTING RECURRENT DEPRESSION

Robin B. Jarrett
Jeffrey R. Vittengl
Lee Anna Clark

Relapse and recurrence prevention are essential to improving treatments for depressed individuals. In this chapter, we describe how to reduce the likelihood of relapse by using "continuation-phase cognitive therapy" (C-CT) for adults with recurrent major depressive disorder (Jarrett, 1989; Jarrett & Kraft, 1997), and we present an overview of the conceptual and empirical foundations of C-CT. We show why many patients may benefit from C-CT; how to begin implementing this treatment to reduce relapse, and to promote remission and recovery; and why diagnostic evaluation is central in caring for patients with recurrent major depressive disorder across their lifespan.

MULTIFACTORIAL MODEL OF RISK AND PREVENTION OF MOOD DISORDERS

While developing C-CT, Jarrett (1989) constructed an integrative, multifactorial, model of vulnerability for—and prevention of—mood disorders.

a. Risk Factors

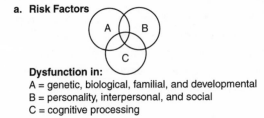

Dysfunction in:
A = genetic, biological, familial, and developmental
B = personality, interpersonal, and social
C = cognitive processing

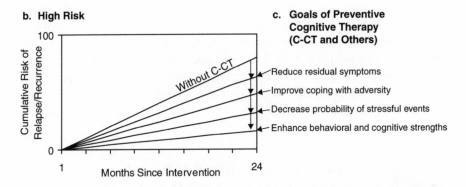

b. High Risk

c. Goals of Preventive Cognitive Therapy (C-CT and Others)

Reduce residual symptoms

Improve coping with adversity

Decrease probability of stressful events

Enhance behavioral and cognitive strengths

Cumulative Risk of Relapse/Recurrence

Without C-CT

Months Since Intervention

FIGURE 6.1. Multifactorial model of depression onset and prevention.

This biopsychosocial model is organized into three overlapping domains of risk factors that identify the conditions that increase the chance of an initial major depressive episode (MDE), of relapse (MDE prior to recovery from the index episode), and of recurrence (MDE after recovery from the index episode), and specify the key goals of preventive intervention. Vulnerability for first onset, relapse, and recurrence of depression is associated with dysfunction in (1) genetic, biological, familial, and developmental functioning; (2) personality, interpersonal, and social functioning; and (3) cognitive functioning. In this model, risk for developing depressive episodes is highest when dysfunction overlaps across domains (Figure 6.1a) and preventive intervention is not used (Figure 6.1b). In short, relapse and recurrence are probable when the patient (1) has untreated or unresolved genetic, biological, or developmental dysfunction; (2) continues to experience residual depressive symptoms and/or impairment in cognitive processing or in personality, interpersonal, or social functioning; (3) experiences a "challenge" (e.g., stressful life event), or set of challenges, that exceed coping skills, thus activating previous ideas and behaviors associated with distress or unhealthy outcomes; and/or (4) either did not learn or no longer practices the coping skills taught during CT (Figure 6.1b). The goals of preventive interventions, including C-CT and other therapies, are to reduce residual symptoms across risk domains, to improve coping with adversity, to decrease the probability of stressful events, and to enhance behavioral and cognitive strengths (Figure 1.6c). An underlying premise of this model is that vulnerability for and prevention of mood disorders are influenced by risk, and by what people learn and experience.

The preventive model of C-CT focuses on lowering the strength of—and possibly eliminating—dynamic, changeable risk factors (e.g., negative cognitions) and reducing the impact of static, unchangeable ones (e.g., basic temperament). In C-CT, learning centers on recognizing when to activate new coping or compensatory skills. The more the patient understands the interrelations of risk factors, recognizes that challenges such as stressful life events (e.g., familial conflict) or symptoms (e.g., transient insomnia) increase risk, and uses compensatory skills when these occur, the lower the chance of relapse and recurrence (Figure 6.1b).

The Central Role of Evaluation and Follow-Up in Relapse Prevention: Prerequisites to Learning and to Providing C-CT

A therapist with a firm foundation in cognitive theory *and diagnostic and behavioral assessment* has the background to learn to provide C-CT to promote remission and recovery, and to reduce relapse. Cognitive theory guides therapists in identifying patients' emotional vulnerabilities, and learning theory guides them in teaching patients new behaviors to cope with the inherent vulnerabilities of suffering from a recurrent, often chronic illness, to cope with coming to painful conclusions about the self, world, and future. Behavioral assessment aids the therapist in knowing when to modify the therapy content, homework, or schedule.

Specific prerequisite skills that therapists need to produce preventive effects with C-CT include (1) mastery of CT (as described by Beck, Rush, Shaw, & Emery, 1979), defined as scores above 39 on the Cognitive Therapy Scale (Young & Beck, 1980); and (2) competence in diagnosing psychiatric syndromes and symptoms both at initial presentation and longitudinally. Therapists who are competent in C-CT know how (1) to use collaborative empiricism (Beck et al., 1979) and case conceptualization (J. S. Beck, 1995; Persons, 1989; see Whisman & Weinstock, Chapter 2, this volume) to develop a multifactorial model for an at-risk patient; (2) to identify and to teach the patient "key" skills to promote recovery and reduce risk; and (3) to structure and monitor the patient's acquisition and generalization of key skills.

Assessment of Recurrent Depression Is Initial, Psychoeducational, and Longitudinal

Why Assess?

Prior to beginning acute-phase cognitive therapy (A-CT; the treatment phase focused on symptom reduction and skills acquisition), an initial diagnostic evaluation is essential (for an overview see Jarrett, 1995). During this evaluation the clinician determines whether a mood disorder is present and characterizes its severity, current subtype (e.g., single vs. recurrent episodes), and lifetime course, as well as its association with other concurrent or past psychiatric disorders. Eliciting information regarding temporal associations with developmental hurdles, psychosocial stressors (e.g., past physical and/or emotional trauma or maltreatment), and functioning, and past response to treatment is key. Evaluating the history of family members' psychiatric illnesses and treatment history is also important. Patients (or, when available, the family members themselves) are given referrals for currently ill but untreated family members.

The evaluator shares the diagnoses, treatment alternatives, and prognoses with patients (and, when appropriate, with significant others) using the medical model as detailed by Klerman, Weissman, Rounsaville, and Cheveron (1984) and Jarrett (1995). Patients and their significant other(s) learn that recurrent depression is a disorder (rather than a character flaw) that carries risks requiring symptom detection, lifetime assessment, and follow-up. Psychoeducation about mood disorders and how depressions can be treated effectively is an important component of obtaining informed consent for treatment from patients and their significant others. Over the course of evaluation and treatment, continuous review of the definition of the syndrome and symptoms of major depressive disorder (MDD) helps to prepare patients to recognize the signs and symptoms of recurrent depression over the lifespan. They learn that early detection facilitates effective treatment for depression. Videotapes, pamphlets, handouts, books, and selected websites (e.g., the home page of the NIMH [National Institute of Mental Health]) aid busy clinicians in providing this information to patients and their families.

Single-Case Design

A key to providing C-CT to patients with recurrent MDD is the single-case design (Hayes, Barlow, & Nelson-Gray, 1999). One of the most practical single-case designs is the A (baseline)–B (single-treatment) design. The absence of a control condition limits inference in the A–B design, but clinicians can extend the reversal design to include all treatment phases when monitoring the depressive episode and symptoms during A1 (initial evaluation)–B (A–CT)–C (C–CT) and A2 (treatment-free longitudinal evaluation or follow-up).

After diagnoses are established, one of the initial steps is for clinicians and patients to select and use a measure of syndromal status and severity. Ideally, charting or graphing scores at each visit result in a longitudinal snapshot of the course of disorder—a prospective extension of the retrospective lifeline developed during the initial evaluation. Along the way, they can mark when the criteria for MDD (and other psychiatric disorders) are and are not met, when treatment changes, when key psychosocial events or stressors occur, when critical CT skills are learned and used, and when therapeutic goals have been accomplished.

Teaching patients to monitor depressive symptoms and their own functioning (e.g., as family members, workers, or friends) is key to helping them to recognize when treatment may need to be reinitiated or changed, and to helping therapists decide which areas to target in sessions and as homework. Improvements in psychosocial functioning may be tied to the A–CT targets or goals that a patient has set in the areas of "love, work, and play." In addition, patients learn which psychosocial factors or stressors tend to increase the chance that depressive symptoms will progress into a full depressive syndrome, and which symptoms or type of functional impairment may be predictive of the entire syndrome recurring. Finally, patients learn which cognitive-behavioral strategies work best to promote return to full functioning and euthymia.

These single-case data that allow clinicians and patients to distinguish the phases and stages of treatment thereby determine whether treatment and homework need to be based on (1) engaging the patient in a treatment that reduces symptoms (acute phase); (2) achieving full remission and preventing relapse of the index episode (continuation phase); (3) preventing relapse and maintaining remission or achieving recovery (continuation phase); or (4) maintaining recovery and preventing recurrence or a new depressive episode (maintenance phase). Throughout the process, patients and therapists monitor levels of symptoms and functioning, and remain vigilant for increases in risk factors (i.e., predictors).

Selecting Measurements: What's Available?

At intake, differential diagnosis of MDD is necessary to identify appropriate alternative acute-phase treatment options, and throughout A-CT, symptom assessment is key in structuring therapy sessions, gauging acute-phase treatment response, and identifying which patients need C-CT. Instruments that clinicians may use to measure the syndrome and severity of depressive symptoms are described below.

To assess the syndrome of depression, to rule out other disorders, and to diagnose concurrent psychiatric disorders, the Structured Clinical Interview for DSM (SCID; First, Spitzer, Gibbon, & Williams, 1996; Spitzer, Williams, Gibbon, & First, 1992) is a benchmark instrument. With appropriately trained clinicians, SCID diagnoses for MDD have demonstrated strong psychometric properties (Zanarini et al., 2000; Miller, Dasher, Collins, Griffiths, & Brown, 2001), although administering the full interview can be relatively time-consuming (typically 1–2 hours).

Clinicians who do not have the time to use the SCID may use screening measures such as the Primary Care Evaluation of Mental Disorders (PRIME-MD; Spitzer et al., 1994) or its patient-report version, the Patient Health Questionnaire (PHQ; Spitzer, Kroenke, & Williams, 1999), also available as a short form (PHQ-9; Kroenke, Spitzer, & Williams, 2001). The self-report measures have shown adequate agreement with interview-based diagnoses, and sufficient validity to be used to track progress during treatment (Kroenke & Spitzer, 2002). Because differentiating patients with bipolar disorders who require pharmacotherapy is especially important, we recommend that clinicians include a screen for a history of mania, such as the Mood Disorder Questionnaire (MDQ; Hirschfeld et al., 2000), a brief patient-report measure.

After making a primary diagnosis of MDD and beginning A-CT, clinicians need to assess depressive symptom severity frequently to structure therapy sessions, to gauge patients' progress over time, to identify treatment response, and to make an informed and collaborative decision about continuing or discontinuing treatment. Depressive symptoms may be assessed equally well with both self- and clinician reports (Vittengl, Clark, Kraft, & Jarrett, 2005), so time-pressured clinicians may prefer to use shorter patient reports. Measures of depressive symptom severity with acceptable psychometric properties include the Hamilton Rating Scale for Depression (HRSD; Hamilton, 1960), the Beck Depression Inventory (BDI; Beck, Ward, Mendelson, Mock, & Erbaugh, 1961) or the BDI-II (Beck, Steer, & Brown, 1996), and the Inventory for Depressive Symptomatology (IDS; Rush et al., 1986; Rush, Gullion, Basco, Jarrett, & Trivedi, 1996; Trivedi, Rush, Ibrahim, Carmody, Biggs, et al., 2004), which is available in parallel Self-Report (IDS-SR) and Clinician (IDS-C) versions.

Vittengl et al. (2005) found that total scores on these four measures demonstrated high convergence in their pattern and degree of change during A-CT. Moreover, the 16-item Quick IDS (Q-IDS; Rush et al., 2003), available in both Self-Report (Q-IDS-SR) and Clinician (Q-IDS-C) versions, correlates highly (r's = .94) with these measures. Using conversions of scores among the four measures (derived from their common factor; Vittengl et al., 2005; Jarrett, Vittengl, & Clark, 2005), clinicians can compare their patients' progress during CT to the modal or mean progress of patients treated in research studies. When CT fails to produce typical results, clinicians should consider an alternative approach (e.g., pharmacotherapy as an alternative or adjunct).

DECIDING WHEN TO CONTINUE AND WHEN TO STOP CT

What Risk Factors Have Been Documented?

For patients who no longer meet DSM-IV criteria for MDD after an A-CT trial, a critical decision is whether to continue or discontinue CT. Whereas some patients who respond to A-CT have fewer risk factors for relapse and recurrence and may discontinue treatment safely and proceed to periodic, longitudinal evaluation, other responders to A-CT have a high risk for relapse and are strong candidates for C-CT. Although there are numerous risk factors for relapse and recurrence (e.g., unstable remission and early onset), residual symptoms at the end of acute-phase treatment are a robust predictor (e.g., Jarrett et al., 2001; Thase et al., 1992), and their assessment is practical, so we expand on this finding below. Specifically, we describe a method that enables clinicians to use any of several of these popular symptom measures to identify patients who likely require C-CT to avoid relapse and recurrence.

Stopping or Continuing CT: Using Levels of Residual Symptoms to Decide

To demonstrate the ability of depressive symptoms at the *last A-CT session* (residual symptoms) to predict relapse/recurrence among responders to A-CT (Jarrett et al., 2005), we operationalized depressive symptoms as the common factor score we mentioned earlier and examined the data in two different ways. First, we examined 8 points on the survival function (the probability of remaining well over time), and found that higher depressive symptom factor scores at the last A-CT session predicted quicker relapse/ recurrence as a main effect and also interacted with assignment to C-CT versus assessment only. Specifically, C-CT does not reduce the probability of relapse/recurrence for patients with no or low residual symptoms, but patients with progressively higher residual symptoms relapse less in C-CT compared to assessment-only controls. Thus, the practical value of these results is that patients' scores on any one of a number of readily available symptom severity measures after 20 sessions of CT can aid clinicians and patients in assessing risk for relapse/recurrence and using predicted risk to decide whether to provide C-CT.

As a further illustration, we then divided these same patients (from the clinical trial reported by Jarrett et al., 2001) into lower versus higher residual symptoms, assignment to C-CT or to assessment only, and relapse/recurrence within 24 months. Residual symptoms at the end of A-CT were dichotomized as lower versus higher (approximate cutoffs on individual scale: HRSD $\leq$ 4 vs. $\geq$ 5, BDI $\leq$ 6 vs. $\geq$ 7, IDS-C $\leq$ 9 vs. $\geq$ 10, IDS-SR $\leq$ 11 vs. $\geq$ 12, QIDS-C $\leq$ 3 vs. $\geq$ 4, and QIDS-SR $\leq$ 4 vs. $\geq$ 5) based on the level of depressive symptoms that consistently differentiated C-CT from the control group in relapse/recurrence probabilities. Residual symptom level did not predict relapse/recurrence for patients in C-CT (Fisher's exact test $p =$ .41), but high residual symptoms predicted more relapses/recurrences for patients who did not receive C-CT (Fisher's exact test $p < .01$). Among patients with lower residual symptoms at the end of A-CT, 30% relapsed or experienced recurrence within 24 months in both the C-CT and assessment-only groups. In contrast, among patients with higher residual symptoms, 90% relapsed or experienced recurrence in assessment-only compared to 50% in C-CT. Moreover, relapses or recurrences tended to come earlier (in the experimental phase) for the assessment-only control, and later (during the follow-up phase) for the C-CT group. Although C-CT does not prevent *all* relapses or recurrences in high-risk patients, the clinical conclusion is clear: Patients with higher residual symptoms after A-CT experience relapse and recurrence less and later with C-CT. In contrast, patients with lower residual symptoms, who do not have other risk factors, may not require C-CT.

THE STRUCTURE, GOALS, AND STAGES OF C-CT

Preparation for Therapy Termination: Start at the Initial Session and Revisit Repeatedly

Therapists begin the process of CT termination at the first A-CT session by focusing on the fact that effective CT results from learning and practicing new skills, and learning when and how to apply these skills in different situations. Therapists describe themselves as teachers, collaborators, and coaches, who in the process, transfer to patients more of the intervention planning and problem solving as patients' mastery grows over time. They emphasize the concept of using affect shifts and depressive symptoms to trigger the use of skills to reduce both symptoms and relapse. Therapists reinforce these concepts repeatedly throughout C-CT.

Transitioning from A-CT to C-CT: Avoid the Discontinuation Effect

Based on the operant conditioning literature, Jarrett (1989) used fading the schedule of therapy sessions as a tool for reducing relapse and recurrence. It appears that patients with depression are exquisitely sensitive to abrupt changes in the schedule of treatment and may develop symptoms when the schedule is thinned or stopped abruptly, regardless of the type of treatment. This so-called "discontinuation effect" has been observed not only with CT (Jarrett et al., 1998), but also pharmacotherapy (e.g., Baldessarini et al., 1996). To reduce the impact of this effect, it is important to provide the patient with an expectation and rationale for the change, and to thin the frequency of sessions gradually, thus avoiding abrupt and/or unexpected discontinuation of sessions and/or rapid shifts in the time between sessions.

The 8-month, 10-session "formulation" of C-CT (Jarrett, 1989) respected this principle of thinning in the following manner. The continuation phase followed a 3- to 4-month, 20-session A-CT aimed at reducing symptoms, facilitating basic skills, and increasing adaptive functioning. During A-CT, the first 16 sessions were provided twice a week and the last four sessions were thinned to once weekly. During C-CT, the first four sessions occurred every other week, then the remaining six sessions occurred monthly. If a crisis arose, or if relapse appeared eminent, one of the 10 sessions could be scheduled as needed. When rescheduling sessions, therapists attempted to approximate the original plan, gradually thinning the schedule of sessions across the 10 months to minimize discontinuation effects.

A comparable process also occurs in the therapy itself. During A-CT, the therapist emphasizes the importance of mastering and using the crucial skills of CT independently, proactively, and when negative affect occurs. As the therapy advances, the therapist encourages patients to take more "control" of the therapy and to apply the critical skills to new problems and situations independently. Therapists "fade" direct guidance of the session, and patients assume greater responsibility. For example, therapists can promote such independence by asking patients to set and prioritize the agenda, to identify what coping strategies helped previously to reduce similar symptoms, to design homework assignments, and to conduct their own "therapy sessions" at home between sessions and on a regular basis. The therapist's goal is for the patient to attribute

gains in adaptive changes in thinking and other behaviors to using understandable and easily accessible compensatory skills. The assumption is that mastering these tools is the first step to being able to use them in times of high need,
and to making their use automatic and habitual.

THE GOAL OF C-CT

The goal of C-CT is to teach, generalize, and maintain critical skills that
prevent relapse and promote remission and recovery (Jarrett & Kraft, 1997).
In short, cognitive therapists not only treat depressive symptoms but also
teach new coping strategies. As in A-CT, therapists work to decrease, eliminate, and prevent the symptoms and syndrome of depression by teaching
patients compensatory skills that include (1) understanding relations between cognition and other behavior, (2) self-monitoring emotions and cognition, (3) restructuring automatic thoughts via logical analysis, (4) restructuring automatic thoughts through hypothesis testing, (5) identifying
schemas, (6) restructuring schema through logical analysis, and (7) testing
alternative schemas through experimentation. During C-CT, hypothesis
testing draws heavily on contingency-based strategies described as "behavioral activation" (Martell, Addis, & Jacobson, 2001) and emphasizes pairing
cognitive changes with practical, daily behavioral changes (e.g., What does a
future that looks more promising mean about one's job search this week?
What goals has the patient set for homework? How does homework [i.e.,
cognitions, behaviors] relate to overall and weekly goals for therapy?). It is
assumed that for cognitive changes to have a prophylactic effect (i.e., result
in relapse prevention after sessions are discontinued) behavioral changes are
required. Ideally, each patient will have mastered all these skills during A-
CT; realistically however, not all patients, even those who respond to A-CT,
accomplish this. When therapists must decide which skills to eliminate (or
to teach last), skills 1–3 and/or 4 represent the "basics" (and homework
assignments focus throughout on associated behavioral changes). Table 6.1
provides a sample of available CT compensatory skills used to teach patients
and assess their mastery throughout the course of treatment.

Stages of Learning: Acquisition, Generalization, and Maintenance of New Skills

C-CT draws liberally from learning theory and emphasizes strategies to
promote acquiring, generalizing, and maintaining new responses (Ferster,
1973). Social learning theory (e.g., Bandura, 1977) emphasizes the impor-

TABLE 6.1. Sample Compensatory Skills Learned during Cognitive Therapy

Cognitive model	Behavioral targets	Restructuring via logical analysis	Restructuring via hypothesis testing	Restructuring schemas
Understands that thoughts, feelings, and behaviors can contribute to depression.	Schedules and participates in activities that improve mood.	Identifies automatic negative thoughts and completes thought records.	Identifies automatic negative thoughts and completes thought records.	Examines underlying assumptions (or schemas) and how they contribute to his/her depression.
Notices how view of self, world, and future influences behavior.	Applies CT tools to problems in family.	Identifies thinking or logical errors.[a]	Tests automatic thoughts or beliefs by setting up experiments.	Identifies automatic negative thoughts and completed thought records.
Recognizes and records thoughts, feelings, and other behaviors with a mood shift.	Applies CT tools to problems with feelings.	Notices a change in mood after analyzing automatic thoughts.	Looks at how negative thinking affects his/her predictions about the future.	Identifies underlying assumptions (or schemas) that increase depressive assumptions.
Identifies automatic negative thoughts and completes thought records.	Applies CT tools to problems with relationships.	Examines automatic negative thoughts logically and/or rationally.	States thoughts in ways that could be tested.	Uses CT skills (e.g., logical analysis or hypothesis testing) to challenge depressive assumptions.
Uses CT skills when a mood shift occurs on a typical day.	Applies CT tools to depressive symptoms.	Looks for alternative explanations when he/she has negative thoughts.	Identifies ways to test thoughts.	Tests alternatives to depressive schemas or assumptions by testing what it would be like to have different beliefs.
	Applies CT tools to problems at work.	Weighs the evidence for and against negative thoughts.	Decides how to evaluate the results of his/her test.	Uses CT skills when a mood shift occurs on a typical day.
		Is able to separate facts from beliefs.	Compares the results of experiment to thoughts or predictions.	
		Sees the difference between thinking styles when feeling depressed versus not.	Asks whether additional tests are necessary to evaluate beliefs.	
		Looks at the consequences or advantages/disadvantages of holding certain beliefs.	Results of the tests influence thinking.	
		Changes thinking when it was illogical.		
		Argues with automatic thoughts.		

Note. From Jarrett and Kraft (1998). Reprinted by permission of the authors.

[a]For example: overgeneralization, negative filtering of information, discounting the positive personalization, jumping to conclusions, mind readings, fortune-telling, catastrophizing, all-or-none thinking, emotional reasoning, excessive use of "should" statements, labeling, minimization, and magnification.

tance of modeling and vicarious learning, guided practice, and attitudes about learning and mastery (i.e., self-efficacy) that help to facilitate these processes in therapy. As such, role plays, homework, and insession responding can aid therapists in assessing where patients' skills fall in the stages of learning.

Specifically, during each session the therapist not only assesses the signs and symptoms of depression and sets goals for the therapy based on symptoms and functioning level, but he/she also evaluates how far the patient has progressed in learning compensatory skills by asking him/herself, whether, the patient learning has reached the acquisition stage. Is more practice needed to grasp the basics? What specific skills have been learned? Can the patient name the skill? Can the patient describe aloud when and how to use the skill or demonstrate its use in session? Can the patient teach a peer to use the skill, proving a rationale for when and how to use it? If the patient has acquired basic skills (based on homework and in-session usage), then how well can he/she generalize the skills to new environments or new problems? How likely is it that the patient will be able to maintain these skills over time? Has he/she learned a sufficient number of skills to be prepared for psychosocial stressors in multiple risk domains? How many "psychosocial challenges" has the patient encountered and successfully used coping skills? How confident and comfortable is the patient in his/her ability to use the skills?

Therapists decide how many skills to teach depending on which interventions their patients learn and use most easily, which interventions and life changes have occurred with symptom reductions during A-CT, and which interventions may promote and enhance "stress inoculation." Therapists help patients identify and name these so-called "critical or key skills" that can be used most effectively and frequently. They design in-session role plays and homework assignments in which critical skills can be practiced (repetitively) in highly probable, high-risk situations occurring *in vivo*, in session, and in imagination.

Individualizing the Multifactorial Model of Risk and Prevention

Therapists use the results of the diagnostic and behavioral assessment to personalize the model of risk and prevention (described earlier) for each patient. Patient and therapist collaboratively address the following questions: (1) What risk factors have been involved in the initial and recurrent pattern of the patient's depression, and (2) which compensatory skills, and changes in behavior and outlook, have been associated with a decrease in depressive symptoms and improved functioning and life satisfaction? Depending on how the patient's skills building has progressed, his/her use of the concept of depressive assumptions, or schemas, as "shorthand" for recurrent ideas about the self, the world, and the future may increase or decrease risk of future depressions. Then the patient attempts to alter the vulnerabilities or to minimize their impact on the course of his/her illness. To promote remission and recovery, the therapist teaches the patient how to monitor the syndrome, symptoms, characteristic risk factors, and use of skills.

The model we described earlier specifies that the more a patient repeatedly and successfully uses the compensatory strategies, the higher the probability (1) that a fundamental shift will occur in his/her perception of the self, the world, and the future, resulting in a view that is more congruent with natural environmental contingencies; and (2) that his/her vulnerability will decrease accordingly.

A "Road Map" within C-CT

Patients start and progress through C-CT with different levels of skills development, durations of symptom remission, and composites of risks. Behavioral assessment of patients' skills aids therapists in knowing when to modify the focus or content of the therapy, its homework, or its schedule. To determine where to focus C-CT, therapists consider (1) syndromal status (i.e., the presence or absence of a mood and other psychiatric disorder, noting that all patients begin C-CT without MDD); (2) severity of residual depressive symptoms; (3) the degree to which patients have mastered, are using, and can generalize compensatory skills; and (4) the continuation or emergence of risk factors that might necessitate a change in the treatment schedule or homework recommended. Below we describe some typical combinations and describe the associated therapeutic focus or goal.

Residual Symptoms and/or Low Skills Acquisition: Goal—Complete Remission and Promotion of Basic Skills Mastery

At times C-CT can look a lot like A-CT continued! This occurs when patients' symptoms no longer meet criteria for MDD, yet they have not achieved full and sustained remission and/or have not completely mastered the use of efficacious compensatory strategies, in which case C-CT and A-CT are very similar. Therapists then help patients identify cognitive, emotional, and environmental obstacles that support and impede their use of critical skills. For example, consider a patient who no longer meets criteria for MDD, yet whose HRSD score is above 5. The patient does not consistently note a reduction in negative affect when he/she attempts a thought record and continues to blame him/herself solely for chronic relationship discord. Then the C–CT focus may be finding the skills deficit in the application of the thought record or determining whether a different compensatory skill (see Table 6.1; problem solving regarding conflictual issues) might be useful in lowering and maintaining an HRSD score consistently below 5.

Fewer Symptoms and Skills Acquired: Goal—Prevent Relapse and Generalize Gains over Time and Environments; Promote Resilience

When the HRSD has often been below 5 and patients know how to use one or more skills to produce symptomatic relief, the focus of C–CT moves to relapse prevention, stress inoculation, and promotion of sustained remission and a full recovery. "Stress inoculation" comprises constructing an individualized model of depression onsets, offsets, and prevention. Patient and therapist work together to make the model of depression and prevention practical and usable in daily life. They examine common themes associated with prior onsets of depression or with increases in negative affect. They examine the cognitive and behavioral patterns associated with offsets in prior depressions or negative affect. For example, if onsets of prior depressions were associated with the end of romantic relationships and offsets were correlated with starting a new romantic relationship, the therapist would attempt to elicit an underlying belief, such as "I am only worthwhile and happy if I have a partner." Patient and therapist consider the effect of this belief across the life cycle and hypothetical adverse events (e.g., the patient never bonds with a partner, experiences a breakup, loses a partner to death). In session and through homework, they work through the alternative beliefs and behaviors that allow the patient to experience these difficulties without developing another depressive episode.

The patient is encouraged to keep a notebook through therapy and in between sessions. The patient brings thought records to C–CT sessions and identifies the most important entries for review. If the patient does not bring these materials, thought records can be completed retrospectively in session and obstacles to completing these can be identified in session. Recurrent or new symptoms and targets are placed on the agenda and prioritized. The therapist encourages independence by asking the patient to generate solutions and skills that may have helped before (e.g., "What has helped in the past? Are you using these strategies now? What is getting in the way? What is helping you stay on track?").

What Happens When There Is a "Lapse" (vs. a Relapse) during C-CT?

It is important to teach patients to discriminate a full "relapse" (a syndrome with impairment that lasts 2 weeks or more) from a "blip" or "lapse" (transient symptoms that may resolve with intensified use of critical skills). Attention to the temporal aspects of the diagnosis and the effect of symptoms on functioning helps with this discrimination. Furthermore, it can be helpful to teach patients to use self-rating scales (e.g., BDI or IDS-SR) to detect depressive symptoms and to learn when to intensify the use of critical skills, to call the therapist for extra help, or to request an appointment.

A "lapse" can cue therapist and patient to design specialized homework over the telephone to address the symptoms and to determine whether a session should be scheduled soon or "out of sequence." The therapist's aim is to promote a sense of mastery and self-efficacy and to help the patient learn that he/she can use compensatory strategies successfully and independently to reduce depressive symptoms. If a patient relapses during C-CT, the frequency of sessions can be increased until the symptoms of MDD have remitted and functioning is restored. If the relapse is detected immediately rather than later, we predict that fewer sessions of C-CT will be necessary to restore remission.

Asymptomatic, Recovered, with Skills: Goal—Maintain Gains (Initiate M-CT)

When patients' symptoms have not met criteria for major depression, the HRSD (or other symptom severity measure) score has been below 5 (or the measure's equivalent) more weeks than not during the past 8 or more consecutive *months*, and psychosocial functioning is fully restored, then patients can be declared "recovered" from an episode of MDD. When patients also have acquired the basic CT compensatory skills and have learned to generalize the so-called "critical skills" to new target problems and situations, they are ready to "graduate" from C-CT to maintenance-phase CT (M-CT). The aims of M-CT are to maintain recovery and to prevent recurrence or new depressive episodes. During M-CT some patients move from habitually using compensatory skills to achieving a *fundamental and meaningful* change in their lifestyle and perceptions of the world, self, and future. The few data that exist on M-CT suggest that (1) the preventive effects of C-CT are finite for most patients (Jarrett et al., 2001), (2) M-CT may have a preventive effect (Blackburn & Moore, 1997), and (3) M-CT my be necessary to help at-risk patients stay well. At this time, it is unknown how many sessions of M-CT are necessary and/or sufficient to prevent recurrence and to sustain

recovery, the optimal time between sessions, or the duration of the maintenance phase needed to accomplish these goals. This area is ripe for research.

CASE ILLUSTRATION

Presenting Problem/Client Description

The following case illustration was adapted from Jarrett and Kraft (1997).
Mr. Turner, a 50-year-old European American, widowed father of two
daughters and Protestant choir director, met DSM-IV criteria for moderately severe, recurrent MDE, with good recovery between episodes. At the
beginning of treatment, he had been depressed for 5 months following the
terminal illness of a family member. He could not complete basic requirements of his job and had difficulty caring for his daughters. Mr. Turner
described his relationships with congregation members as severely discor-
dant, and he resented many interactions. He reported that he frequently
thought about death and suicide, but said he would not commit suicide
because it would be too painful to his family. His stated his main complaint
as "self-doubt about my job, my family."

Mr. Turner described his nondepressed self as confident, successful, and
competent; he thought of himself as a loving father, loyal son, kind and gen-
erous friend with concern for others and, most importantly, respected choir
director. He experienced his first episode of depression at age 21; the current episode was his fifth, and each had lasted approximately 6 months to 1
year. His self-view had become increasingly negative with each successive
episode. Mr. Turner considered his depression to indicate personal weakness,
so he experienced recurring episodes as threatening to his sense of self, his
vocation, and his life itself. He began to feel like an imposter to his friends
and congregants, his family, and even to God.

Case Formulation

Mr. Turner held himself to unrealistically high standards for serving the congregation, his family, and God, and he was extremely harsh on himself when
he inevitably failed to meet them. He also held his daughters and church
members to these same excessively high standards. He believed that because
of his position as choir director, his family was always being scrutinized by
church members, so that any imperfection indicated that he and his family
were poor role models. Similarly, he blamed himself when church members
did not meet his unrealistically high standards, because it indicated he had
failed to motivate them sufficiently. Furthermore, he interpreted any criti-

cism from choir members to mean that he was a "bad person." Therefore, to please others and avoid criticism, Mr. Turner was unassertive—even with his daughters and choir members.

Course of Treatment

Over the course of 20 A-CT sessions, Mr. Turner was taught the cognitive model. His forte was identifying and reevaluating logical errors in cognition, such as all-or-none thinking, overuse of *should* statements, perfectionism, and personalization. Because he was able to distance himself from his depression, he viewed himself as having a recurrent illness that could be treated rather than as weak and incompetent. The therapist used role plays and homework assignments to help Mr. Turner increase his assertive behavior and respond effectively when choir members criticized him. He also learned to prioritize and schedule his major responsibilities, to have time for himself and his family.

When he began therapy, Mr. Turner was uncertain about his value as a choir director, so he was ambivalent about his occupation. The therapist hypothesized that this stemmed in part from the anxiety and dissatisfaction with being a choir director as a result of his excessively high standards. As he was able to lower his unrealistic expectations, Mr. Turner came to experience being a choir director as a choice rather than an obligation.

When Mr. Turner began C-CT after completing the 20 A-CT sessions, he had been depression-free for 9 weeks. During C-CT, he continued working on the way he viewed himself. He came to see his depression as a medical disorder rather than a sign of weakness and to change his belief that "people with a strong faith don't ask for help." He also continued to reevaluate how he interpreted his mood shifts. Mr. Turner came to view shifts in his mood as triggers to use the skills he had acquired in A-CT, rather than as signs of inevitable depression. Furthermore, he applied the social skills he had acquired to speaking with religious colleagues, parishioners, and family about his stressors and pressures, and asked for their help. He even began to encourage others to seek help for problems they experienced.

During the fourth session of C-CT, Mr. Turner was distressed about his relationship with his oldest daughter. On the one hand, he feared that she would not comply with any limits he tried to place on her behavior, so their difficulties would intensify. On the other hand, he was upset with himself for being passive rather than assertive. With the therapist, he generated alternative explanations for his unassertiveness and determined the minimal changes he wanted to see in his daughter's behavior. When he discussed these changes with his daughter, she surprised him by agreeing to try to change. She also requested changes, for example, that he be less critical of her. As a result, he became more hopeful that their relationship could improve and more confident about asserting himself.

In C–CT, Mr. Turner became very active and "took charge" of the sessions. He first reported on his successful use of coping skills, complete with specific examples. By reviewing successful experiences with these skills, the therapist encouraged Mr. Turner to take credit for the changes he was making in his life. As C–CT was nearing an end, the therapist had Mr. Turner review the major changes he had made over the course of treatment. Mr. Turner stated that over the course of therapy he had come to see that he could be "proud to be average," that he had "permission to be imperfect," and that he had multiple important roles (father, choir director, friend), in contrast to his former self-view as someone who must please everyone and always achieve perfection. He also recognized the importance of using the social support of members of his church, of prioritizing family time, and of taking care of himself.

In the final C–CT sessions, therapy focused on termination and relapse prevention. Mr. Turner was encouraged to view treatment outcome not in terms of success or failure (i.e., being or not being depressed), but as an ongoing collaboration to examine evidence that the interepisode interval had increased. He also was encouraged to use skills such as logical analysis and cognitive restructuring to shorten any episodes of depression, should they recur. The therapist worked with Mr. Turner in identifying and handling future stressors. Together, they predicted that either job or relationship stressors could be associated with depression recurrence, for example, if the church failed to meet its budget (resulting in a salary cut), or if he received repeated negative feedback from the choir. They spent session time rehearsing ways to cope with excessive responsibility, such as practicing ways to delegate responsibility. In addition to identifying future stressors, the therapist worked to change Mr. Turner's views of future sad mood and hopelessness, to think of them as signals for treatment seeking rather than for planning suicide. Finally, the therapist made sure that Mr. Turner knew when and where to seek help.

REVIEW OF EFFICACY RESEARCH

Outcomes with Formulations of C-CT for Adults

The problem of relapse and recurrence after acute-phase treatments, including A–CT, has been recognized for decades and underscores the need for preventive treatment (e.g., Elkin et al., 1989; Klerman, DiMascio, Weissman,

Prusoff, & Paykel, 1974; Thase et al., 1992). Below we review research test-ing relapse/recurrence prevention with C-CT, including the "formulations" that Jarrett and other developers have tested. A meta-analysis of this litera-ture is available (Vittengl, Clark, Dunn, & Jarrett, 2007). Empirical support for CT for medication-resistant and partially remitted depression is reviewed by Fava and Fabbri, Chapter 5, this volume.

C-CT Reduces Relapse after Response to A-CT

Jarrett et al. (1998) compared sequential cohorts of patients responding to A-CT. The first cohort discontinued treatment after A-CT and experienced relapse/recurrence (met MDE criteria at any time during longitudinal follow-up) more frequently (45% over 8 months, 74% over 24 months) than the second cohort that received 8 months of C-CT, followed by 16 months of treatment-free assessment (20% over 8 months, 36% over 24 months). Jarrett et al. (2001) conducted a full-scale randomized clinical trial of C-CT for responders to A-CT, including independent assessment of treatment outcomes. Patients were randomized to 8 months of C-CT or assessment only, followed by 16 months of treatment-free assessment. C-CT reduced relapse (met MDE criteria by Longitudinal Interval Follow-up Evaluation [LIFE; Keller, Lavori, Friedman, Nielsen, Endicott, et al., 1987] depression scores 5 for 2 consecutive weeks) over 8 months (10 vs. 31%), and reduced relapse for patients with unstable remission (37 vs. 62%) and with early-onset MDD (16 vs. 67%) over 24 months compared to controls. As described earlier, those with residual symptoms are most in need of C-CT for prevention of relapse/recurrence.

Group CT May Reduce Relapse and Recurrence

For example, Teasdale et al. (2000) randomized patients with recurrent MDD who were in recovery/remission (i.e., who did not meet MDE crite-ria) for 12 or more weeks after discontinuing antidepressant medication, to treatment as usual (TAU; i.e., patients sought help on their own, as needed) or to TAU plus mindfulness-based cognitive therapy (MBCT). CT included eight weekly group sessions followed by four monthly group sessions lasting 2 hours. Over 60 weeks, for 105 patients with a history of more than three depressive episodes, CT reduced relapse (40%; defined as meeting MDE cri-teria) compared to TAU (67%) alone. For a smaller subset of 32 patients with two depressive episodes, relapse/recurrence rates did not differ signifi-cantly (56% CT, 31% TAU). Very similar results were found in a replication study (Ma & Teasdale, 2004). Over 60 weeks, MBCT reduced relapse (defined as meeting MDE criteria) compared to TAU for patients with more than three episodes (36 vs. 78%; $N = 55$), but the effect was not significant for patients with two depressive episodes (50 vs. 20%; $N = 18$). However, the null results for the latter may be due to low power and replication in a larger sample is needed.

Benefits of M-CT Have Been Identified

Fewer data are available for M–CT than for C–CT. Blackburn and Moore (1997) found that 2-year relapse/recurrence rates (HRSD ≥ 15) did not differ significantly among depressed patients randomized to acute-phase followed by maintenance-phase pharmacotherapy (31%), A–CT followed by M–CT (24%), and acute-phase pharmacotherapy followed by M–CT (36%). This study suggested that M–CT is as effective as maintenance-phase pharmacotherapy but lacked a no- or minimal-treatment condition to establish firmly the benefits of M-phase CT. Helping to fill this gap, Klein et al. (2004) randomized patients with chronic depression who responded (reduction in baseline 24-item HRSD score by ≥ 50% to a total score ≤ 15) to *cognitive-behavioral analysis system of psychotherapy* (CBASP) as an acute-phase treatment (either alone or after failed pharmacotherapy), and who maintained response for 16 weeks with continuation CBASP, to monthly maintenance CBASP or assessment only. After 1 year, maintenance CBASP reduced relapse (meeting MDE criteria by interview checklist or retrospective clinical consensus, plus 24-item HRSD scores ≥ 16 for 2 consecutive weeks) compared to assessment only, 11 versus 32%.

Outcomes with C-CT for Adolescents

In contrast to the research on adults we reviewed earlier, two studies have provided mixed support for postacute CT with adolescents. In a pilot study (Kroll, Harrington, Jayson, Fraser, & Gowers, 1996), adolescents who responded to A–CT and received continuation sessions every 2–4 weeks relapsed (met MDE criteria) less frequently over 6 months (20%) than did a historical control group that received no treatment beyond A–CT (50%). However, a larger randomized clinical trial (Clarke, Rohde, Lewinsohn, Hops, & Seeley, 1999) yielded less favorable results. Adolescents completing A–CT were assigned randomly to 24 months of assessments every 4 months plus CT booster sessions (including self-monitoring, lifestyle change interventions to cope with stress, and social support interventions) assessments only every 4 months, or assessments only every 12 months. Among A–CT responders, recurrence (meeting MDE criteria) did not differ significantly among booster session, frequent assessment, and annual assessment groups at 12 monthly (27, 0, and 14, respectively) or 24 months (36, 0, and 23%, respectively). Additional research is needed to develop and evaluate C–CT and M–CT for adolescents and for children.

Future and Additional Uses of Psychosocial Interventions to Prevent Relapse

In an ongoing, two-site randomized trial conducted by the team of Jarrett and Thase (Jarrett et al., 2003), patients who presented with recurrent MDD and showed incomplete remission after A–CT were randomized to receive continuation-phase pharmacotherapy. Preliminary experience with this sequential treatment of A–CT followed by continuation-phase pharmacotherapy (i.e., fluoxetine/Prozac) suggests that a group of responders to a *psychosocial* intervention will accept pharmacotherapy as a reasonable method to promote remission and reduce the risk of relapse. Psychoeducation regarding the risks of recurrent depression is important in promoting patient acceptability, engagement, and compliance relative to this sequence.

As the work from the teams of Fava, Grandi, Zielezny, Rafinelli, and Canestrari (1996), Blackburn and Moore (1997), Paykel et al. (1999), Teasdale et al. (2000), and Bockting et al. (2005) shows, psychosocial relapse prevention strategies similar to C–CT (by Jarrett, 1989) are efficacious after some level of remission has been achieved with pharmacotherapy. We look forward to learning what "ingredients," mechanisms, and moderators produce these comparable, preventive effects. We are curious about what similarities and differences in these "functionally related" psychosocial continuation-phase treatments are responsible for their important preventive effects.

CONCLUSIONS

In this chapter, we have described how to reduce the likelihood of relapse using C–CT for adults with recurrent MDD. We have outlined the theoretical model that serves as the foundation of C–CT and discussed assessment for and implementation of C–CT. Finally, we have provided a review of the empirical support for C–CT in preventing relapse.

Although we have no data on the concurrent use of C–CT plus pharmacotherapy, we think it is a reasonable treatment option for patients who do not achieve complete remission and/or recovery with C–CT alone. We look forward to promoting opportunities to apply and adapt what we have learned in working with adults with recurrent depression to preventing relapse and recurrence effectively and to promoting remission and recovery in other at-risk groups, including adolescents and children (see Kennard, Stewart, Hughes, Jarrett, & Emslie, in press, for initial efforts).

ACKNOWLEDGMENTS

We are grateful to Robin Jarrett's patients and team at The University of Texas Southwestern Medical Center (Psychosocial Research and Depression Clinic in the Department of Psychiatry), where the data we detail were collected. Our thanks to Amy McSpadden, BS, for her careful manuscript preparation. We appreciate the support provided by the National Institute of Mental Health that made this work and writing possible (Grant Nos. R01-MH-38238, R01-MH-58397, and K24-01571 [to Robin B. Jarrett, PhD]).

REFERENCES

Baldessarini, R. J., Tondo, L., Faedda, G. L., Suppes, T. R., Floris, G., & Rudis, N. (1996). Effects of the rate of discontinuing lithium maintenance treatment in bipolar disorders. *Journal of Clinical Psychiatry, 57*, 441–448.

Bandura, A. (1977). Self-efficacy: Toward a unifying theory of behavioral change. *Psychological Review, 2*, 191–215.

Beck, A. T., Rush, A. J., Shaw, B. F., & Emery, G. (1979). *Cognitive therapy of depression.* New York: Guilford Press.

Beck, A. T., Steer, R. A., & Brown, G. K. (1996). *Manual for the BDI-II.* San Antonio, TX: Psychological Corporation.

Beck, A. T., Ward, C. H., Mendelson, M., Mock, J., & Erbaugh, J. (1961). An inventory for measuring depression. *Archives of General Psychiatry, 4*, 561–571.

Beck, J. S. (1995). *Cognitive therapy: Basics and beyond.* New York: Guilford Press.

Blackburn, I. M., & Moore, R. G. (1997). Controlled acute and follow-up trial of cognitive therapy and pharmacotherapy in outpatients with recurrent depression. *British Journal of Psychiatry, 171*, 328–334.

Bockting, C. L., Schene, A. H., Spinhoven, P., Koeter, M. W., Wouters, L. F., Huyser, J., et al. (2005). Preventing relapse/recurrence in recurrent depression with cognitive therapy: A randomized controlled trial. *Journal of Consulting and Clinical Psychology, 73*, 647–657.

Clarke, G. N., Rohde, P., Lewinsohn, P. M., Hops, H., & Seeley, J. R. (1999). Cognitive-behavioral treatment of adolescent depression: Efficacy of acute treatment and booster sessions. *Journal of the American Academy of Child and Adolescent Psychiatry, 38*, 272–279.

Elkin, I., Shea, M. T., Watkins, J. T., Imber S. D., Sotsky, S. M., Collins, J. F., et al. (1989). National Institute of Mental Health Treatment of Depression Collaborative Research Program: General effectiveness of treatments. *Archives of General Psychiatry, 46,* 971–982.

Fava, G. A., Grandi, S., Zielezny, M., Rafanelli, C., & Canestrari, R. (1996). Four-year outcome for cognitive behavioral treatment of residual symptoms in major depression. *American Journal of Psychiatry, 153,* 945–947.

Ferster, C. B. (1973). A functional analysis of depression. *American Psychologist, 28,* 856–870.

First, M. B., Spitzer, R. L., Gibbon, M., & Williams, J. B. W. (1996). *Structured Clinical Interview for DSM-IV Axis I Disorders, Clinician Version (SCID-CV).* Washington, DC: American Psychiatric Press.

Hamilton, M. (1960). A rating scale for depression. *Journal of Neurology, Neurosurgery, and Psychiatry, 23,* 56–61.

Hayes, S. C., Barlow, D. H., & Nelson-Gray, R. O. (1999). *The scientist practitioner: Research and accountability in the age of managed care.* Boston: Allyn & Bacon.

Hirschfeld, R. M. A., Williams, J. B. W., Spitzer, R. L., Calabrese, J. R., Flynn, L., Keck, P. E., Jr., et al. (2000). Development and validation of a screening instrument for bipolar spectrum disorder: The Mood Disorder Questionnaire. *American Journal of Psychiatry, 157,* 1873–1875.

Jarrett, R. B. (1989). *Cognitive therapy for recurrent unipolar major depressive disorder: The continuation/maintenance phase.* Unpublished treatment manual, University of Texas Southwestern Medical Center at Dallas.

Jarrett, R. B. (1995). Comparing and combining short-term psychotherapy and pharmacotherapy for depression. In E. E. Beckham & W. R. Leber (Eds.), *Handbook of depression: Treatment, assessment, and research.* New York: Guilford Press.

Jarrett, R. B., Basco, M. R., Risser, R., Ramanan, J., Marwill, M., Kraft, D., et al. (1998). Is there a role for continuation-phase cognitive therapy for depressed outpatients? *Journal of Consulting and Clinical Psychology, 66,* 1036–1040.

Jarrett, R. B., Gershenfeld, H. K., Borman, P. D., Williams, M. J., Friedman, E. S., & Thase, M. E. (2003, November). *Cognitive reactivity and depressive relapse: Early signals from a randomized clinical trial.* Paper presented at the meeting of the Association for Advancement of Behavioral Therapy, Boston, MA.

Jarrett, R. B., & Kraft, D. (1997). Prophylactic cognitive therapy for major depressive disorder. *In Session, 3,* 65–79.

Jarrett, R. B., & Kraft, D. (1998). *Cognitive Therapy Skills Rating Scale—Patient and Observer Version.* Unpublished instruments, The University of Texas Southwestern Medical Center at Dallas.

Jarrett, R. B., Kraft, D., Doyle, J., Foster, B. M., Eaves, G. G., & Silver, P. C. (2001). Preventing recurrent depression using cognitive therapy with and without a continuation phase: A randomized clinical trial. *Archives of General Psychiatry, 58,* 381–388.

Jarrett, R. B., Vittengl, J. R., & Clark, L. A. (2005, November). *Which patients require continuation-phase cognitive therapy for depression?: Levels of residual symptoms pro-*

mote empirical practice and informed consent. Paper presented at the meeting of the Association for Behavioral and Cognitive Therapies, Washington, DC.

Keller, M. B., Lavori, P. W., Friedman, B., Nielsen, E., Endicott, J., et al. (1987). The Longitudinal Interval Follow-Up Evaluation: A comprehensive method for assessing outcome in prospective longitudinal studies. *Archives of General Psychiatry, 44,* 540–548.

Kennard, B., Stewart, S. M., Hughes, J. L., Jarrett, R. B., & Emslie, G. S. (in press). Developing cognitive behavioral therapy to prevent depressive relapse in youth. *Cognitive and Behavioral Practice.*

Klein, D. N., Santiago, N. J., Vivian, D., Arnow, B. A., Blalock, J. A., Dunner, D. L., et al. (2004). Cognitive-behavioral analysis system of psychotherapy as a maintenance treatment for chronic depression. *Journal of Consulting and Clinical Psychology, 72,* 681–688.

Klerman, G. L., DiMascio, A., Weissman, M., Prusoff, B., & Paykel, E. S. (1974). Treatment of depression by drugs and psychotherapy. *American Journal of Psychiatry, 131,* 186–191.

Klerman, G. L., Weissman, M. M., Rounsaville, B. J., & Chevron, E. S. (1984). *Interpersonal psychotherapy of depression.* New York: Basic Books.

Kroenke, K., & Spitzer, R. L. (2002). The PHQ-9: A new depression diagnostic and severity measure. *Psychiatric Annals, 32,* 509–515.

Kroenke, K., Spitzer, R. L., & Williams, J. B. (2001). The PHQ-9: Validity of a brief depression severity measure. *Journal of General Internal Medicine, 16,* 606–613.

Kroll, L., Harrington, R., Jayson, D., Fraser, J., & Gowers, S. (1996). Pilot study of continuation cognitive-behavioral therapy for major depression in adolescent psychiatric patients. *Journal of the American Academy of Child and Adolescent Psychiatry, 35,* 1156–1161.

Ma, S. H., & Teasdale, J. D. (2004). Mindfulness-based cognitive therapy for depression: Replication and exploration of differential relapse prevention effects. *Journal of Consulting and Clinical Psychology, 72,* 31–40.

Martell, C. R., Addis, M., & Jacobson, N. (2001). *Depression in context: Strategies for guided action.* New York: Norton.

Miller, P. R., Dasher, R., Collins, R., Griffiths, P., & Brown, F. (2001). Inpatient diagnostic assessments: 1. Accuracy of structured vs. unstructured interviews. *Psychiatry Research, 105,* 255–264.

Paykel, E. S., Scott, J., Teasdale, J. D., Johnson, A. L., Garland, A., Moore, R., et al. (1999). Prevention of relapse in residual depression by cognitive therapy: A controlled trial. *Archives of General Psychiatry, 56,* 829–835.

Persons, J. B. (1989). *Cognitive therapy in practice: A case formulation approach.* New York: Norton.

Rush, A. J., Giles, D. E., Schlesser, M. A., Fulton, C. L., Weissenburger, J. E., & Burns, C. T. (1986). The Inventory for Depressive Symptomatology (IDS): Preliminary findings. *Psychiatry Research, 18,* 65–87.

Rush, A. J., Gullion, C. M., Basco, M. R., Jarrett, R. B., & Trivedi, M. H. (1996), The

Inventory of Depressive Symptomatology (IDS): Psychometric properties. *Psychological Medicine, 26,* 477–486.

Rush, A. J., Trivedi, M. H., Ibrahim, H. M., Carmody, T. J., Arnow, B., Klein, D. N., et al. (2003). The 16-item Quick Inventory of Depressive Symptomatology (QIDS), Clinician Rating (QIDS-C), and Self-Report (QIDS-SR): A psychometric evaluation in patients with chronic major depression. *Biological Psychiatry, 54,* 573–583.

Spitzer, R. L., Kroenke, K., & Williams, J. B. W. (1999). Validation and utility of a self-report version of PRIME-MD: The PHQ Primary Care Study. *Journal of the American Medical Association, 282,* 1737–1744.

Spitzer, R. L., Williams, J. B., Gibbon, M., & First, M. B. (1992). The Structured Clinical Interview for DSM-III-R (SCID): I. History, rationale, and description. *Archives of General Psychiatry, 49,* 624–629.

Spitzer, R. L., Williams, J. B. W., Kroenke, K., Linzer, M., deGruy, F. V., Hahn, S. R., et al. (1994). Utility of a new procedure for diagnosing mental disorders in primary care: The PRIME-MD 1000 study. *Journal of the American Medical Association, 272,* 1749–1756.

Teasdale, J. D., Segal, Z. V., Williams, J. M. G., Ridgeway, V. A., Soulsby, J. M., & Lau, M. A. (2000). Prevention of relapse/recurrence in major depression by mindfulness-based cognitive therapy. *Journal of Consulting and Clinical Psychology, 68,* 615–623.

Thase, M. E., Simons, A. D., McGeary, J., Cahalane, J. F., Hughes, C., Harden, T., et al. (1992). Relapse after cognitive behavior therapy of depression: Potential implications for longer courses of treatment. *American Journal of Psychiatry, 149,* 1046–1052.

Trivedi, M. H., Rush, A. J., Ibrahim, H. M., Carmody, T. J., Biggs, M. M., Suppes, T., et al. (2004). The Inventory of Depressive Symptomatology, Clinician Rating (IDS-C) and Self-Report (IDS-SR), and the Quick Inventory of Depressive Symptomatology, Clinician Rating (QIDS-C) and Self-Report (QIDS-SR) in public sector patients with mood disorders: A psychometric evaluation. *Psychological Medicine, 34,* 73–82.

Vittengl, J. R., Clark, L. A., Dunn, T. W., & Jarrett, R. B. (2007). Reducing relapse and recurrence in unipolar depression: A comparative meta-analysis of cognitive therapy's effects. *Journal of Consulting and Clinical Psychology, 75,* 475–488.

Vittengl, J. R., Clark, L. A., Kraft, D., & Jarrett, R. B. (2005). Multiple measures, methods, and moments: A factor-analytic investigation of change in depressive symptoms during A-CT. *Psychological Medicine, 35,* 693–704.

Young, J., & Beck, A. T. (1980). *Cognitive Therapy Scale: Rating manual.* Philadelphia: Center for Cognitive Therapy.

Zanarini, M. C., Skodol, A. E., Bender, D., Dolan, R., Sanislow, C., Schaefer, E., et al. (2000). The Collaborative Longitudinal Personality Disorders Study: Reliability of Axis I and II disorders. *Journal of Personality Disorders, 14,* 291–299.

III

COGNITIVE THERAPY FOR COMORBID DEPRESSION

7

SUICIDE

Marjan Ghahramanlou-Holloway
Gregory K. Brown
Aaron T. Beck

Suicide is the 11th leading cause of death in the United States, with a rate of one completed suicide every 17 minutes (Hoyert, Kung, & Smith, 2005). Among individuals 15–24 years old, suicide is the third leading cause of death after accidents and homicide; among individuals 25–44 years old, suicide is the fourth leading cause of death after accidents, malignant tumors, and heart disease (Hoyert et al., 2005). Approximately 20% of all U.S. suicides occur in elderly persons; firearms account for up to 80% of these suicides (Oslin et al., 2004). Suicide ideation has been estimated in 2.3% of U.S. residents ages 18–54 within the past 12 months; within this group, 28.6% made a plan to kill themselves, and 32.8% of these individuals carried out a serious attempt to commit suicide (Cole & Glass, 2005).

Suicide among individuals with depression is a major public health problem. The lifetime risk of suicide for individuals with major depressive disorder (MDD) has been estimated to be 15% among psychiatric inpatients (Guze & Robins, 1970). Recent epidemiological data have suggested that the risk of suicide for individuals with MDD is approximately 3.4%, with males having a 7% risk and females having a 1% risk (Blair-West, Cantor, Mellsop, & Eyeson-Annan, 1999). An overall 6% risk of completed suicide for affective disorders has been reported in a recent meta-analysis (Inskip, Harris, & Barraclough, 1998). The National Comorbidity Survey indicates that individuals with MDD have odds ratios of 11.0 for suicide ideation and 9.6 for suicide planning (Kessler, Borges, & Walters, 1999). Yet few individuals with MDD receive adequate treatment for depression before and after a suicide attempt.

Most individuals with MDD are at the highest risk for suicide during the early years within the course of illness (Vieta, Nieto, Gasto, & Cirera, 1992); those who attempt suicide often do so in the first 3 months of a depressive episode and within 5 years of the onset of their depression (Malone, Haas, Sweeney, & Mann, 1995). Anxiety increases the risk of early suicide in the course of major depression, whereas stable levels of hopelessness increase long-term risk (Placidi et al., 2000). Together, these findings suggest that depressed individuals, especially those with suicide ideation or suicide attempts, constitute a high-risk group for suicide.

The *National Strategy for Suicide Prevention* identifies suicide as a "public health problem that is preventable," and one of its goals is the development and implementation of suicide prevention programs (U.S. Public Health Service, 2001, p. 46). Consequently, adequate training of mental health providers in assessment and treatment of depressed patients with suicide behavior is an important step in reducing subsequent suicide attempts. Interventions that target suicide attempters and achieve a 25% reduction in suicide attempts have been estimated to lead to a 2.6 reduction in the population rate of suicide (Lewis, Hawton, & Jones, 1997). Using national annual rates of suicide, approximately 1,000 deaths can be prevented each year.

Our primary objective in this chapter is to educate clinicians in empirically based strategies for the assessment and treatment of depressed individuals with suicide behavior. The first section addresses the relation between suicide behavior and psychotherapy outcome. The second section familiarizes the reader with assessment procedures to be utilized for depressed individuals with suicide behavior. The third section outlines the major components of an empirically based cognitive treatment protocol for adult depressed patients with recent suicide behavior.

SUICIDE BEHAVIOR AND PSYCHOTHERAPY OUTCOME

Few studies have examined the relation between treatment response and completed suicide. In general, individuals who have committed suicide are expected to demonstrate a history of poorer treatment outcomes compared to individuals who have not committed suicide. For instance, Motto,

Heilbron, and Juster (1985) found that in a sample of 2,753 inpatients, negative or variable results of previous efforts to obtain help predicted suicide risk. Modestin, Schwarzenbach, and Wurmle (1992) found that therapist experience was the most significant psychotherapy factor contributing to different outcome in a sample of suicide completers compared to matched controls. Goldstein, Black, Nasrallah, and Winokur (1991) found that a favorable outcome at discharge was a protective factor for suicide in a prospective study of 1,906 inpatients with affective disorders. Additionally, Borg and Stahl (1982) reported that patient dropout from treatment was a risk factor for suicide.

There is a paucity of studies that have examined patient response to cognitive therapy (CT) and completed suicide. Dahlsgaard, Beck, and Brown (1998) investigated response to CT as a predictor of suicide completion in a group of psychiatric outpatients. In this matched cohort study, suicide completers attended significantly fewer psychotherapy sessions and had a significantly higher rate of premature termination of therapy, as well as significantly higher hopelessness scores as compared to controls. Overall, the study suggested that nonresponsiveness to psychotherapy, as measured by the number of sessions attended; level of hopelessness; and premature termination serves as an important risk factor for suicide.

ASSESSMENT OF SUICIDE IDEATION AND BEHAVIOR

Comprehensive evaluations of past and current suicide behavior prior to and during treatment are needed for risk management and treatment planning. The ongoing assessment of a patient's risk for suicide cannot, at any time, rely solely on a single indicator. All available information should be used collectively by the clinician to identify potential risk factors, to address immediate safety concerns, and to consider appropriate approaches to ongoing risk management.

Comprehensive Assessment of Suicide

Clinical Interview

The first component of a comprehensive evaluation is a thorough clinical interview with the patient that covers the following domains: current mental status; sociodemographic factors; recent and chronic life stressors; coping style and resources; psychiatric, medical, and substance use history; family history of mental illness and suicide; past treatment history and compliance level; individual strengths and vulnerabilities; and general presentation of suicidality (for a comprehensive review on suicide risk assessment, see American Psychiatric Association, 2003; Jacobs, 1999). If the patient provides written permission, corroborating data from family members, other mental health professionals, and medical records may be obtained. However, in cases where the immediate safety of the patient or others is threatened, clinicians are permitted and highly encouraged to seek such information regardless of patient consent.

During the clinical interview, clinicians should directly assess suicide ideation, intent, and planning by asking the following three questions:

1. Are you currently having any *thoughts* of killing yourself?
2. Do you currently have any *desire* to kill yourself?
3. Do you have a specific *plan* to kill yourself?

To learn more about the nature of the patient's suicidal thinking, the clinician poses further questions about the frequency, timing, persistence, and the current severity of suicide ideation. If a patient describes a specific plan for suicide, his/her expectation about the lethality of such a plan should be examined directly. Overall, patients who report a detailed plan involving violent and/or irreversible methods are likely to be at significantly higher risk (Rudd, Joiner, & Rajab, 2001).

Because the clinical interview is an essential element of a comprehensive suicide evaluation, clinicians may benefit from the following recommendations (Ellis & Newman, 1996). Be attentive, remain calm, and provide the patient with a private, nonthreatening, and supportive environment to discuss experienced difficulties. Do not express anger, exasperation, or hostile passivity. Be forthright and confident in manner and speech to provide the patient with a stable source of support at a time of crisis. Stress a team approach to the problem(s) presented; for instance, freely use the collaborative pronoun "we" when discussing suicidal behavior. Model hopefulness, but make sure to acknowledge the patient's distress and perspective on the problem. Do not avoid using the word "suicide," because this gives the impression that you stigmatize the concept. Most importantly, do not immediately suggest hospitalization. In our experience, patients are most agreeable if the therapist carefully explores various safety options, then plans for the most appropriate clinical response to an acute suicidal episode.

Suicide Measures

The second component of a comprehensive evaluation involves the administration of suicide measures. We briefly review three clinically useful measures for the assessment of suicide ideation and hopelessness. For a comprehensive review of suicide assessment measures for adults and older adults, see Brown (2002).

Suicide ideation at the time of evaluation has been considered a potential predictor of suicide. Two commonly used interviewer-administered rating instruments for suicide ideation include the Scale for Suicide Ideation (SSI; Beck, Kovacs, & Weissman, 1979) and the Scale for Suicide Ideation—Worst (SSI-W; Beck, Brown, Steer, Dahlsgaard, & Grisham, 1999). The SSI assesses the severity of a patient's current suicidal ideation, intent, and plan, whereas the SSI-W assesses suicide ideation at the worst point in the patient's life. Evidence of the predictive validity of the SSI and the SSI-W for suicide has been found; however, the assessment of suicide ideation at its most severe point has been found to be a stronger risk factor for suicide than the assessment of current ideation (Beck et al., 1999).

In addition, hopelessness is one of the most commonly recognized and validated risk factors for suicide behavior. A recent study on patients with treatment-resistant depression indicated that more than half reported significant hopelessness or despair (Papakostas et al., 2003). The Beck Hopelessness Scale (BHS; Beck & Steer, 1988), a self-report instrument, comprises 20 true–false statements designed to assess the level of positive and negative beliefs about the future. Patients with scores of 9 and above on the BHS are approximately 11 times more likely to commit suicide than patients with scores of 8 or below (Beck et al., 1990).

Dahlsgaard et al. (1998) reported hopelessness to be significantly higher and more stable for suicide completers than for a control group. Empirical literature supports the notion that hopelessness should be assessed over time. Young et al. (1996) reported that stable levels of hopelessness in patients with remitted depression are more predictive of future suicide attempts than high levels at any one point. Similar findings have been reported for older adult patients whose high levels of persistent hopelessness after the remission of depression were related to suicide behavior (Szanto, Reynolds, Conwell, Begley, & Houck, 1998).

The three assessment instruments briefly reviewed here provide clinicians with cost-effective methods of identifying depressed patients at high risk for suicide. We know that nonresponsiveness to treatment and high scores on suicide ideation measures (e.g., SSI-W), in combination with consistently elevated BHS scores, are strong predictors of eventual suicide in psychiatric outpatients. Clinicians are cautioned that all suicide-screening measures are subject to response bias. Whereas some patients may conceal their suicide ideation and demonstrate low scores, others may report more chronic or elevated levels of ideation than what is experienced in actuality.

Although these assessment tools serve a function, they should never be used exclusively to determine a patient's level of risk.

Brief Ongoing Assessment of Suicide

Following a comprehensive evaluation, the clinician conducts brief ongoing assessments of suicide risk to monitor changes in the patient's overall status. Knowledge about established risk factors helps the clinician make informed judgments about potential risk. Table 7.1 provides a summary of several of these risk factors that are initially assessed during the comprehensive evaluation and subsequently monitored closely during the course of treatment.

During the therapy process, the clinician continues to collect information about the presence and severity of suicide ideation, intent, and planning. Clinicians may continue to administer measures of suicide ideation and hopelessness prior to each therapy session. They may also utilize the Beck Depression Inventory–II (BDI-II; Beck, Steer, & Brown, 1996), which is a 21-item self-report depression instrument. The BDI-II has one specific suicide item (i.e., item 9) that directly assesses for suicidal thoughts. This item, in particular, may be used to monitor changes in suicide ideation throughout the course of treatment. A recent study on the predictive validity of the BDI-II indicated that patients with scores of 2 or above on the

TABLE 7.1. Indicators for Determination of Low and High Suicidal Risk

Indicator	Lower risk	Higher risk
Suicide ideation[a]	SSI item 4 or 5 = 0 or BDI-II Item 9 = 0 or 1	SSI Item 4 or 5 > 0 or BDI-II Item 9 ≥ 2
Depression[a]	BDI-II < 20 (Mild)	BDI-II ≥ 20 (moderate–severe)
Hopelessness[a]	BHS < 9 (Mild)	BHS ≥ 9 (moderate–severe)
Reasons for living	Many	None
Access to lethal methods	None	Immediate
Impulse control	Within normal limits	Poor (e.g., anger outbursts)
Treatment compliance	Within normal limits	Poor (e.g., refuses treatment)
Prior suicide attempts	None	One or more prior attempts
Social support	Perception of available support	Perception of poor support
Alcohol/drug abuse	None	Abuse or dependence
Psychosis or mania	None	Symptoms and/or diagnosis
Recent life stressor(s)	None	Severe recent life stressor(s)

Note. BDI-II, Beck Depression Inventory; BHS, Beck Hopelessness Scale; SSI, Scale for Suicide Ideation.
[a]For further details about these risk factors, refer to Brown, Beck, Steer, and Grisham (2000).

suicide item were 6.9 times more likely to commit suicide than patients who scored below 2 (Brown, Beck, Steer, & Grisham, 2000).

COGNITIVE TREATMENT OF SUICIDE

Theoretical Rationale

Beck's cognitive model of depression and emotional disorders serves as the foundation for the intervention presented in this section (Beck, 1976; Beck, Rush, Shaw, & Emery, 1979). The model posits that activated maladaptive cognitions in the form of automatic thoughts, assumptions, and core beliefs may result in suicide behavior. More specifically, Beck (1996) proposes a theory of "modes," which refers to structural and operational units of personality that consist of a composite of unified and functionally synchronous cognitive, affective, motivational, and behavioral systems. A "suicide mode" can be activated should the patient, for instance, experience loss-related cognitions (e.g., "I have lost all that is important to me"), suicide-related cognitions (e.g., "Life is no longer worth living"), sad or angry affect, passivity in seeking help, and/or increased impulsivity and motivation to plan and subsequently act upon injuring him/herself.

Cognitive Conceptualization of Suicide

In CT, suicide behavior is targeted directly for clinical intervention and is viewed as a maladaptive coping strategy often utilized presumably to solve extreme psychological distress. Suicidal patients are conceptualized as poor problem solvers. The chronic inability to generate or to consider all alternative options, whether available immediately or possibly in the future, is indicative of the serious hopelessness and helplessness experienced by these patients. In particular, patients with a history of prior attempts may require minimal internal or external triggers to reactivate the "suicide mode"; in cases where the mode is highly accessible in memory, automatic behaviors to self-injure may be likely. Subsequently, from the depressed patient's perspective, suicide is seen as the only option, and even as "a rational course of action" (Beck, 1976, p. 123). The desire to die then outweighs the desire to live.

The stepwise approach to CT is, therefore, first to deactivate the suicide mode; second, to modify its structure and content; and third, to construct and practice more adaptive structural modes (Beck, 1996). Patients are helped to challenge their pessimism and high estimations for future negative outcomes, and to transform hopelessness into hopefulness. Patients are taught problem-solving strategies and are assisted in the development and maintenance of healthy coping strategies, so that suicide behavior is no longer the only available option worth considering. In summary, suicide behavior is viewed as a problematic symptom in and of itself that deserves immediate attention, before other therapeutic goals are addressed. Intervention is aimed at utilizing empirically based strategies that minimize the chance of recurrence of suicidal behavior.

We recommend that the cognitive conceptualization of suicide be shared with the patient at the early phase of treatment, preferably during the first therapy session. The clinician explains the specific treatment goals and rationale. The patient is invited to work collaboratively toward increasing his/her desire to live by exploring new coping options. The maladaptive coping behavior of acting out distressing symptoms no longer remains the *only* available option.

Therapeutic Issues in Working with Suicidal Patients

The treatment of suicidal behavior presents many challenges to both the novice and the seasoned clinician. Although standard CT for depression may be applied to this high-risk group, clinicians may utilize a modified, 10-session, empirically based cognitive protocol that is specific to the needs of suicide attempters. The major objective of this intervention is to decrease the recurrence of future suicidal behavior through the use of general CT principles. Additional aims are to reduce psychological risk factors for suicide, such as depression, hopelessness, and suicide ideation. Findings from a recently published controlled clinical trial indicate an overall reduction rate of approximately 50% in subsequent suicide attempts among recent suicide attempters, as well as significant decreases in their levels of depression and hopelessness (Brown et al., 2005).

General Clinical Recommendations

Three clinical issues are reviewed to maximize the effectiveness of the cognitive intervention presented later in this chapter: (1) patient therapy attendance and compliance, (2) a "team" approach to intervention, and (3) attention to sociocultural factors in treatment engagement.

Effective strategies to engage patients in treatment, as well as to increase overall therapy attendance and compliance, need to be implemented. Patient attrition from psychotherapy is a documented problem in suicide attempters (i.e., only 20–40% of patients continue with outpatient treatment following their psychiatric hospitalization; O'Brien, Holton, Hurren, & Watt, 1987).

Therapy compliance can decrease due to factors such as shame about the suicide attempt; stigma and negative, culturally based attitudes about mental health services; poor economic resources; and chronic substance use (Berk, Henriques, Warman, Brown, & Beck, 2004).

When a patient drops out of psychotherapy, especially during the early stages, he or she is not likely to benefit from the delivery of treatment. Because the original reason for referral often has not been addressed, one may even expect that the patient's psychological difficulties, if left untreated, may worsen over time. Therefore, we recommend the implementation of a psychoeducation session before formal onset of CT. During this session, the therapist can directly assess the patient's attitudes and expectations about treatment and readiness for change. The major aims of psychoeducation are threefold: (1) to educate the patient about the nature and rationale for treatment, and his/her role as a participant in CT; (2) to educate the patient about the high attrition rates and the common reasons for treatment failure and/or dropout; and (3) to educate the patient about potential barriers to treatment and to provide the problem-solving skills and resources to address these difficulties.

Management and treatment of suicidal patients require time, effort, careful consideration of complex clinical factors, and decisions about hospitalization and/or breach of patient confidentiality. We advocate a "team" approach to intervention for two reasons: (1) to collaborate with other professionals to maximize quality patient care, and (2) to create a support network for all team members, so that issues such as patient safety, crisis management, and countertransference may be more effectively addressed. Decisions about patient care should be made in collaboration with all other providers (e.g., psychiatrist, substance abuse counselor, social worker) to best serve the needs of the patient.

A final recommendation is for clinicians to pay close attention to factors such as socioeconomic class, religion, culture, and the extent of perceived and actual social support available to the patient. The socially and economically disadvantaged tend to experience long-standing, multiple chronic stressors; consequently, mental health care may be perceived as a low priority. Although the CT protocol presented here is a manualized treatment package, we emphasize the importance of clinician flexibility and consideration of individual factors that may present as treatment obstacles. For instance, following a recent psychoeducation session with a Moslem female suicide attempter with a history of childhood sexual abuse, forced genital mutilation, and subsequent discomfort with male authority figures, a decision was made to assign the case to a female therapist to ensure the patient's early compliance and continuation with treatment. In the case of a patient who could not attend therapy due to transportation difficulties, phone sessions and financial assistance with transportation were considered.

The following clinical practices may increase overall treatment compliance: (1) reminder phone calls, (2) flexible scheduling, (3) willingness to conduct phone sessions, (4) a team approach to tracking the patient and encouraging treatment compliance, and (5) frequent problem-solving sessions to address difficulties in transportation, child care, housing, medication adherence, and follow-up. Although it is understandable that an outpatient therapist may not have the ability to provide all these support services, it is highly recommended that he/she take a more active and directive role in coordinating efforts with an existing case manager or medical provider to increase patient engagement in treatment.

General Cognitive Session Structure

The weekly CT sessions follow a similar structure (for a review of basic CT skills, see J. S. Beck, 1995). The patient is informed about this structure during the psychoeducation meeting held before the commencement of treatment. A typical cognitive session consists of the following weekly components: mood check (including assessment of mood during the past 7 days and completion of the BDI-II and BHS), risk assessment (assessing suicide ideation, intent, and plan[s]), alcohol and substances check (severity, frequency, and duration of usage for each abused substance during the past week), adjunctive treatment and compliance check (type, dosage, and adherence to all medications are noted, in addition to the previous and next medication appointments), agenda setting, bridge from the last session, suicide protocol task (described later in this section), homework review and assignment, and session feedback.

Description of the Cognitive Protocol

The cognitive protocol for treatment of suicidal behavior (Brown, Henriques, Ratto, & Beck, 2002) comprises one 60- to 90-minute psychoeducation session and approximately 10 (45- to 50-minute) weekly psychotherapy sessions. During the psychoeducation session, patients are informed that the offered treatment is short term and time limited. Patients are provided with a copy of *Choosing to Live: How to Defeat Suicide through Cognitive Therapy* (Ellis & Newman, 1996). Treatment is initiated with patient consent and following the psychoeducation session. For patients who have recently experienced a suicide attempt or an interrupted suicide attempt, it is recommended that the first treatment session be scheduled within 72 hours after the attempt or discharge from the hospital.

The cognitive protocol for the treatment of suicide aims to accomplish the following main objectives: (1) decrease patients' severity of depression, hopelessness, and suicide ideation; (2) increase problem-solving and coping skills, especially relative to the problems and stressful life events that preceded and triggered the most recent suicidal behavior; (3) increase patients' gradual establishment and adaptive use of a broad social support network; (4) increase patients' use of and compliance with adjunctive medical, substance abuse, psychiatric, and social interventions; (5) educate patients about the interconnection between feelings, thoughts, and behaviors, so that they fully understand the conceptualization involving the cognitions associated with their suicidal behavior; and (6) prepare patients, family members, and/or friends in implementation of emergency procedures in cases where suicidal behavior may recur.

Treatment is terminated when the patient is able to complete a task of relapse prevention with his or her therapist. In cases where the patient is not ready to complete this exercise successfully, treatment is extended to accommodate the patient. A termination checklist may be used to determine whether a patient is ready to end treatment. For instance, consistently reduced scores on self-report measures such as the BDI-II and the BHS; evidence of improved problem-solving skills; homework compliance; engagement in adjunctive medical, psychiatric, and chemical dependence treatment services; and development of a social support system are all factors that may be considered in assessment of patient readiness for termination.

The remainder of this chapter outlines the stages of CT and its main elements for individuals with suicidal behavior. The intervention is flexible and should not be followed strictly in its sequence of presentation at the expense of therapeutic rapport and clinical judgment. The challenge is for the therapist to develop an *individualized* cognitive conceptualization of the patient for the purposes of treatment planning. An active and directive role is encouraged, with particular attention paid to collaborative work with the patient. We generally conceptualize therapy in three stages: (1) the early phase of treatment (Sessions 1–3) whose aims are to engage the patient, to plan for patient safety, and to develop an initial cognitive conceptualization based on a review of the patient's suicide history or, if applicable, the most recent incident of suicide behavior; (2) the middle phase of treatment (Sessions 4–7) whose aims are to teach various cognitive and behavioral strategies to reconstruct patient's problematic coping style, to build a social support network, and to increase participation in adjunctive medical and psychiatric services; and (3) the final phase of treatment (Sessions 8–10) whose aims are to assess formally the patient's increased cognitive-behavioral skills through a relapse prevention task.

Early Phase of Treatment (Sessions 1–3)

Objective 1: Engaging the Patient in Treatment

Depressed individuals with suicidal behavior may present for treatment due to pressure placed upon them by family members or friends, or they may at times appear apathetic, uninterested, or even hopeless about the therapeutic process. The general clinical recommendations we provided earlier have already emphasized the importance of therapy attendance and compliance, implementing a psychoeducation component, a "team" approach to intervention, and the role of sociocultural factors in treatment engagement. What remains to be discussed is the therapist's mind-set and attitude in working with such a difficult, at-risk patient. The therapist is encouraged to develop a strong early therapeutic alliance with the patient, with the direct aim of transforming hopelessness into hope.

The first step in accomplishing this challenging task is to gain an accurate understanding of the patient's experience, negative thinking, and cognitive distortions. Instead of dismissing the hopelessness felt by the patient and its underlying reasons, one needs to understand how the patient has come to see his/her life situation as utterly hopeless. Once the therapist is able to demonstrate true empathy, the patient may be willing to consider that change is possible. Through cognitive restructuring, a patient can be helped to understand that hopelessness equals inertia and powerlessness, whereas *realistic* hope (i.e., "hoping smart") can result in activity, gained power, and subsequent life change. Hopeless patients commonly demonstrate all-or-none thinking (e.g., "There is absolutely no hope for me"). The therapist's response needs to convey the importance of visualizing a hope continuum for various life domains (e.g., relationship with children, work situation, improved mood).

Objective 2: Generating a Safety Plan

Individuals with suicidal behavior often encounter difficulties in coping effectively with crisis situations and may at such times be prone to experience increased risk for harming themselves. The purpose of safety planning is first to discuss thoroughly the patient's prior experiences, specifically, maladaptive cognitions and behaviors that involve self-injury at times of crises. The second purpose is to provide the patient with an individualized, hierarchically arranged, written list of coping strategies to implement in future distressing circumstances.

The task of generating a safety plan is a collaborative process that is generally completed within the psychoeducation meeting and further solidified during the initial sessions, evaluated for its effectiveness, and further expanded throughout the course of treatment as the patient learns new coping skills. The safety plan (see Figure 7.1) should include the contact information for the therapist; the on-call therapist, if available; a local, 24-hour emergency psychiatric hospital or center; and at least one reliable crisis hotline. Patients are asked to sign the generated safety plan and are provided with additional copies to share with a designated family member and/or friend.

Objective 3: Developing a Cognitive Case Conceptualization for Suicide Behavior

The "cognitive case conceptualization" is an individualized cognitive map of the current automatic thoughts, conditional assumptions, and core beliefs activated before, during, and after suicidal behavior. It is based on collected data about the patient's early childhood experiences, typical activating events, associated automatic thoughts, emotional responses, and subsequent behavior. Figure 7.2 illustrates a completed cognitive case conceptualization diagram for a depressed suicide attempter. We recommend that a cognitive case conceptualization diagram be generated collaboratively with the patient in session. Because the diagram is based on a series of hypotheses, its content should be refined periodically as needed during the course of treatment.

An important clinical task during this early phase of treatment is to provide patients an opportunity to "tell their story" about the most recent suicidal behavior and the specific events leading up to it. This activity is helpful for three reasons: First, this may be the patient's first chance to disclose the details surrounding his/her suicide behavior. By providing the patient with a supportive and nonjudgmental environment, the patient's storytelling can be cathartic. The therapist's ability to communicate empathy and discuss freely or to hear about the details of the suicidal behavior builds a strong alliance with the patient. Second, the patient's suicidal behavior story provides a wealth of information for the purposes of cognitive case conceptualization and treatment planning. For instance, one can collect data about the events surrounding the patient's suicidal behavior and suicide-related beliefs, problem-solving abilities, and implemented compensatory strategies. Third, during the process of generating a cognitive case conceptualization, the patient is educated about the interrelatedness of thoughts, feelings, and behaviors that serves as the foundation for CT. A frequent review of the generated diagram allows the patient to see the patterns of association between specific situational problems and subsequent suicidal behavior. At this point, therapist and the patient can develop a suicide-related problem list, prioritize the problems, and develop a plan for addressing each.

Emergency Numbers

- University of Pennsylvania Hospital—Psychiatry Emergency Evaluation Center (PEEC)
  - 555-555-5555 (24-hour service, 7 days a week)
- National Hopeline Network (24-hour service, 7 days a week)
  - (800) SUICIDE   (800) 784-2433
    Starts with machine saying you're going to be redirected to local call center

Therapist and Case Manager Contact Numbers

Therapist's Name
Address Line 1
Address Line 2
PHONE: (555) 555-5555

Case Manager's Name
Address Line 1
Address Line 2
PHONE: (555) 555-5555

When I notice the following signs:	Having flashbacks, feeling depressed, feeling like I was nothing or nobody—like there is no space here for me in this world, that I would be better off dead . . .
That lead to:	Me staying up all night, obsessing, crying, thinking about hurting myself . . .
I plan to do the following:	1. Get out of the house 2. Go for a walk 3. Call my grandmother 4. Listen to the new country music CD I bought
When others notice the following signs:	I am not talking, I go to my room and I lock the door, I stay in my room for 2 days—not coming out at all, turning my phone off . . .
I would like them to:	Come and talk to me and INSIST to stay until they figure out what is wrong with me. 1. My sister can call and leave a message. 2. My husband can give me a hug.
I am in serious trouble when I or others notice that:	I have psychiatric medications in my possession and I start to count the number of pills I have.
When I am in serious trouble:	I will try to use my safety plan. If this plan does not work, then I will call my therapist (Jane 555-555-5555) or my case manager (Sam 555-555-5555). In case of an emergency, I will call the Psychiatric Emergency Room (555-555-5555) to be evaluated for possible hospitalization. I can also call 911.

Patient Signature: _____   Date: _____

Therapist Signature: _____   Date: _____

FIGURE 7.1. Sample safety plan.

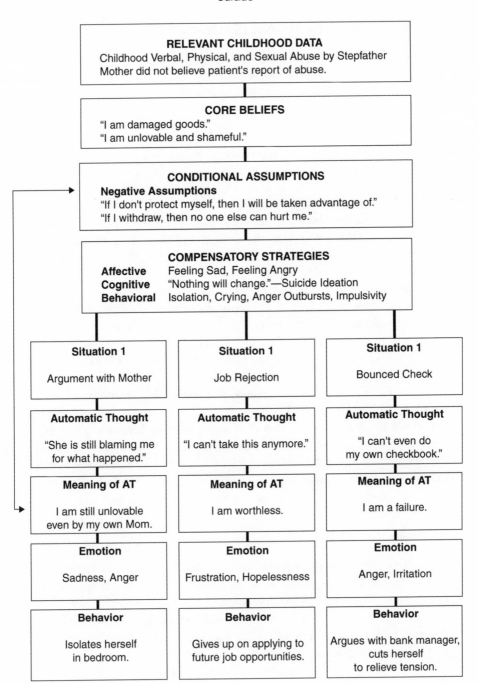

RELEVANT CHILDHOOD DATA
Childhood Verbal, Physical, and Sexual Abuse by Stepfather
Mother did not believe patient's report of abuse.

CORE BELIEFS
"I am damaged goods."
"I am unlovable and shameful."

CONDITIONAL ASSUMPTIONS
Negative Assumptions
"If I don't protect myself, then I will be taken advantage of."
"If I withdraw, then no one else can hurt me."

COMPENSATORY STRATEGIES
Affective   Feeling Sad, Feeling Angry
Cognitive   "Nothing will change."—Suicide Ideation
Behavioral Isolation, Crying, Anger Outbursts, Impulsivity

Situation 1	Situation 1	Situation 1
Argument with Mother	Job Rejection	Bounced Check

Automatic Thought	Automatic Thought	Automatic Thought
"She is still blaming me for what happened."	"I can't take this anymore."	"I can't even do my own checkbook."

Meaning of AT	Meaning of AT	Meaning of AT
I am still unlovable even by my own Mom.	I am worthless.	I am a failure.

Emotion	Emotion	Emotion
Sadness, Anger	Frustration, Hopelessness	Anger, Irritation

Behavior	Behavior	Behavior
Isolates herself in bedroom.	Gives up on applying to future job opportunities.	Argues with bank manager, cuts herself to relieve tension.

FIGURE 7.2. Cognitive Case Conceptualization Diagram.

Middle Phase of Treatment (Sessions 4–7)

The therapeutic work completed during the middle phase of treatment is grounded in the generated cognitive conceptualization. The primary focus is on helping the patient to develop adaptive cognitive and behavioral skills to better manage future suicidal behavior.

Objective 1: Modifying Negative Suicide-Relevant Automatic Thoughts and Core Beliefs

Once the patient's automatic thoughts and core beliefs in relation to his/her suicidal behavior are identified, the therapist first assists the patient in evaluating these cognitions and, second, in modifying them. Patients are initially taught to evaluate their automatic thoughts by gaining an understanding of their most commonly utilized cognitive distortions. A Dysfunctional Thought Record can be used to teach the patient about more effective responses to daily distortions in the form of automatic thoughts. Emphasis is placed on the impact of these cognitive distortions on the accompanying emotional, physiological, and behavioral reactions.

The next step is to educate the patient about his/her core beliefs. What is important for the patient to understand at this stage is that such beliefs are generally rooted in childhood events, not in absolute truth, and can be tested, as well as changed. The therapist hopes that modification of core beliefs results in a lower likelihood of future suicidal behavior. To accomplish this goal, cognitive restructuring techniques such as Socratic questioning, cognitive continuum, historical tests of core beliefs, behavioral experiments, and/or restructuring early memories may be used to help the patient to devise more positive, realistic, and functional core beliefs.

RECOMMENDED ACTIVITY

An activity that helps the patient challenge his/her suicide–activating core beliefs, such as "My life is worthless," or automatic thoughts, such as "I have no reason to live," involves the construction of a hope box. The purpose of the hope box is to help patients directly challenge their maladaptive thoughts by being reminded of previous successes, positive experiences, and current reasons for living, especially at times of extreme distress. The process of constructing the hope box allows patients to work actively on modifying their core beliefs that they are worthless, helpless, and/or unlovable. Patients are encouraged to decorate the hope box with inspiring words and pictures. Items included in the box vary depending on each patient and may consist of pictures of loved ones, a favorite poem, a religious prayer, and/or coping cards. One of our patients, for instance, chose to include a positive work evaluation letter and a picture of herself in her early 20s as a reminder of a very positive and fulfilling time in her life.

Objective 2: Teaching Problem-Solving Skills

Depressed individuals with suicidal behavior usually face daily stressors, in addition to other, more challenging problems. The therapist, during the early stages of treatment, starts to gain an understanding of these problems. The therapist's task at the middle stage is to educate the patient about the direct relation between one's life-problems and perceived inability to solve these problems, and his/her subsequent suicidal behavior. The ultimate goal is to prepare the patient to react differently to future life stressors by learning effective problem-solving strategies. Once this goal is accomplished, the patient no longer relies solely on suicidal behavior as the only preferred means of dealing with problematic situations.

Teaching problem-solving skills comprises the following steps: (1) identifying and listing problems, (2) prioritizing problems, (3) connecting problems in living to suicidality, (4) assessing the functionality and adaptiveness of responses, (5) generating alternatives and plans, (6) weighing pros and cons of proposed solutions, (7) working out discrete tasks to achieve the goal, and (8) reviewing the consequences of the chosen solution(s).

RECOMMENDED ACTIVITY

Therapist and patient collaboratively create a problem list, then rank-order these problems based on their level of impact on the patient's past and/or present suicidal behavior. Once a problem list is generated, each problem is examined. Although the patient is asked to understand that therapy cannot aim to *fix* each problem, he or she learns that various options are available to start a *process* of resolving each problem. The therapist can model, as well as direct the patient to implement, effective problem-solving strategies. For instance, for a patient who is unemployed, one strategy may be to refer him/ her to a community job-counseling program or even to review the patient's résumé in session.

Objective 3: Developing Healthy Behavioral Coping Skills

Individuals with suicidal behavior are likely to have low distress tolerance and poor affective regulation. One goal of therapy is to help these individuals develop healthy coping skills, so that their chances of relying on self-injury and suicidal behavior are minimized. Patients are taught to engage in a variety of activities, such as progressive muscle relaxation, controlled breathing exercises, a regular exercise regimen, and/or distraction in the form of self-soothing strategies, such as taking a bath, imagining a positive scene, or listening to a favorite piece of music.

The development and continual practice of healthy coping strategies are important steps in teaching a patient to "procrastinate" relative to their suicidal impulses, which generally occur in waves. A diagram of a patient's mood and suicidality over time that visually illustrates his/her gradual or sudden increase and subsequent decrease in impulsivity may help the patient understand the one need to "ride out" suicidal urges. Simple coping strategies or delay tactics may include taking a nap, going for a walk, making a phone call, cleaning one's home, or visiting a friend. Another important delay tactic is to remove immediate access to lethal means by safeguarding one's environment. As therapy progresses, the patient can be prepared further to implement long-term coping strategies (e.g., completing college course work to increase job opportunities) in addition to these short-term strategies.

RECOMMENDED ACTIVITY

Coping cards are small, wallet-size cards generated collaboratively in session. They provide the patient an easily accessible way to "jump-start" adaptive thinking during a suicidal crisis. The patient is encouraged to use the coping cards to practice adaptive thinking even when not in crisis. Three types of coping card may be constructed. One way is to place each suicide-relevant automatic thought or core belief on one side of the card and the alternative, more adaptive response on the other. Another way is to write down a list of coping strategies. Still another way is to write a list of instructions to motivate or "activate" the patient toward completing a specific goal.

Objective 4: Increasing Social Support and Compliance with Adjunctive Services

An important goal of therapy is to increase patients' social support networks. A common observed core belief in patients with suicidal behavior is that "no one cares." For patients who already have an existing network of supportive friends, family members, or coworkers, the goal is to increase their perception of social support and to practice communication skills that make future social support likely. Patients may be encouraged, for instance, to share their safety plan with a family member in session or to ask a specific person for assistance with a therapeutic task (e.g., removing lethal means from the premises). For those patients who truly lack an existing social support network, the goal is to establish gradually an adaptive network of accessible social support. Connecting patients to people and resources in the community is a great way to accomplish this task. One patient treated at our program, for instance, currently has developed a relationship with two case managers, several addiction counselors, and two therapists. These newly formed relationships have reinforced the notion that he has a team of professionals "watching out for him."

Another important therapeutic goal is to increase the patient's compliance with adjunctive medical, psychiatric, and chemical dependence treatment services. As mentioned previously, patients with suicidal behavior are likely to experience a host of life problems that are more adequately addressed by a comprehensive range of services. A patient is taught that such services can begin to make a difference only if he/she demonstrates a clear commitment to adhere to treatment recommendations. Of course, this task is not easy, and the therapist's role is to provide encouragement, support, and guidance through this process.

RECOMMENDED ACTIVITY

The patient is helped to generate a comprehensive list of individuals within his/her circle of social support. This list can include members, friends, coworkers, other patients (e.g., Alcoholics Anonymous [AA] or Narcotics Anonymous [NA] sponsor), and/or treatment providers who care. Next, the patient outlines the potential contributions each of these individuals may be asked to make to assist with his/her therapeutic progress. The patient is asked to keep track of positive interactions with each of these individuals and to involve each appropriate person in one aspect of his/her treatment process.

Late Phase of Treatment (Sessions 8–10)

Formal assessment of how well the patient has learned cognitive-behavioral skills is warranted at the final stage of treatment and is accomplished by the patient's completion of a guided imagery exercise, the relapse prevention task (RPT). The purpose of the RPT is twofold. The first aim is to activate images, thoughts, and feelings associated with previous, or the most recent, suicidal behavior in a safe therapeutic environment. The second aim is to evaluate treatment progress by directly assessing the patient's ability to respond adaptively to this activated state. A decision to terminate treatment is appropriate following the successful completion of RPT.

The RPT is completed in five stages. In the first stage, the therapist describes the purpose of this activity and obtains patient feedback and consent to begin the procedure. The patient is informed that because detailed imagery and discussion of previous suicidal behavior may activate strong physiological and emotional responses, full debriefing follows to ensure comfort and safety prior to each session's termination. In the second stage, the patient is asked to imagine the chain of events, thoughts, and feelings leading to his/her most recent suicidal behavior. Basically, the patient is being asked again to share his/her suicide story. The therapist guides the patient through this imagery exercise, scene by scene, using all senses to construct a detailed sequence of events and their meaning to the patient on the specific day of the suicidal behavior. The third stage of the RPT is similar to the second stage. The patient is again taken through the sequence of events leading to the most recent suicidal behavior, but this time he/she is asked to respond actively to maladaptive thoughts and images. The therapist stops the patient as needed and directly questions him/her about alternative ways of thinking, feeling, and behaving. This stage can be repeated if necessary, until the patient is able to demonstrate solid learning of the cognitive-behavioral strategies taught in treatment.

During the fourth stage of RPT, the therapist uses the generated cognitive case conceptualization and overall knowledge about the patient's history and existing situation to create a future scenario that is likely to activate suicidal behavior. The patient is then taken through another imagery exercise, this time, one that involves a future suicidal crisis. The therapist questions the patient about possible coping strategies, provides positive feedback, and proposes additional alternative strategies. The fifth and final stage of RPT involves debriefing the patient. The therapist provides a summary of learned skills in therapy, praises the patient for his/her completion of this final therapeutic task, and assesses his/her overall emotional reaction to this activity. The patient is reminded that mood fluctuations and future setbacks are to be expected. One therapeutic activity may involve the collaborative creation of a coping card that lists a series of strategies for addressing future setbacks instead of automatic reliance on "catastrophic" and "all-or-none" thinking. The patient is given the option of requesting future booster sessions. The necessity and structure of these sessions may be discussed prior to therapy termination.

CASE ILLUSTRATION

Ms. S, a 34-year-old, single African American female with a 10th-grade education, overdosed on her antidepressant medication with a moderate degree of suicide intent and lethality following occupational stressors that led to her job termination. The patient attributed her depressive symptoms to her recurrent poor job evaluations during the past year. In addition, Ms. S had been experiencing significant symptoms of posttraumatic stress disorder (PTSD) due to her history of chronic sexual abuse at the age of 14, and witnessing at the age of 28 the killing of her boyfriend by gang members. Her first and only other reported suicide attempt was at the age of 15, when she confided in her mother about the sexual molestation by the mother's live-in boyfriend. However, her mother reportedly did not believe her daughter's account of the abuse and allowed the perpetrator to remain in the household. The patient had a history of alcohol, marijuana, and cocaine abuse prior to her boyfriend's death 6 years earlier. She has remained clean for the past 5 years. At intake, she presented with severe symptoms of depression and hopelessness (BDI = 41; BHS = 19), and subsequently was diagnosed with MDD, severe, recurrent PTSD, and borderline personality traits.

During the psychoeducation and first therapy session, the patient was informed about the structure and duration of treatment. During the safety planning, Ms. S insisted that she needed help exclusively with her PTSD symptoms; she did not want to talk about her most recent suicide attempt or possible future attempts. The therapist explained the rationale of the current treatment, and provided empathy and direct assistance to Ms. S in obtaining services for all her immediate difficulties, including PTSD symptoms, unemployment, and medication management. The patient was referred to a PTSD treatment program at the University of Pennsylvania, where she was enrolled in a treatment study and received free exposure therapy for her trauma-related symptoms. In addition, Ms. S was assigned a case manager and reconnected with a community psychiatrist she had known previously. Once these arrangements were made, the therapist emphasized the primary goal for Ms. S's treatment at our facility: to decrease the likelihood of future suicidal behavior as a coping response. At this time, Ms. S agreed to share her suicide attempt story with the therapist during an emotionally charged session that was quite distressing for her. Based on the patient's account of internal and external stressors, a cognitive case conceptualization was generated (see Figure 7.2). Three major activating stressors relative to the patient's suicidal behavior were identified: (1) recollection of childhood abuse and activation of core beliefs such as "I am damaged goods"; (2) a conflictual and unsupportive relationship with her mother; and (3) unemployment. At this point, patient and therapist had formed a strong therapeutic alliance, mostly due to the effort put forth by the therapist to help Ms. S with her other problems.

During the middle stages of therapy, the therapist began to teach Ms. S various cognitive-behavioral strategies to increase her overall functioning. Unfortunately, during this time, the patient's cousin committed suicide. Following the suicide, Ms. S refused to attend therapy sessions, ignored all of the therapist's efforts to get in touch with her, and isolated herself in the bedroom at her mother's house. A few weeks later, the patient's mother called our office in a state of crisis and reported that her daughter was experiencing severe symptoms of depression and had expressed a strong desire to kill herself. To maintain patient confidentiality, the therapist asked to speak directly to the patient. Ms. S, crying uncontrollably, reported intense levels of depression and kept asking to be left alone so that she could "end it all." During this crisis call, the patient's brother arrived at the house, and he and the therapist decided that Ms. S should be taken to the emergency department for a psychiatric evaluation. Ms. S was not hospitalized: she later called to thank the therapist for working with her family members to oversee her care on the day of the crisis.

Ms. S returned to therapy shortly after this incident and added her mother and brother to the list of individuals who cared for her safety. She remained compliant with treatment recommendations, learned new skills (e.g., how to communicate better with her mother), and started to look actively for employment. Several therapy sessions were even spent on outlining the steps in the job search process, role-playing job interviews, and problem-solving potential obstacles. The patient's mood dramatically improved as she became more confident with her job search skills; impressively, she began volunteer work at a local church, started to work toward completing her general equivalency degree (GED) requirements, and obtained a part-time paid position. At the time of her therapy termination, Ms. S was still engaged in PTSD treatment. She obtained scores of 0 on both the BDI and the BHS for three consecutive appointments, reported no suicide ideation, and indicated a high commitment to living fully.

REVIEW OF EFFICACY RESEARCH

In a recent study (Brown et al., 2005), adults evaluated at the University of Pennsylvania's Hospital Emergency Department within 48 hours of a suicide attempt were randomized either to receive CT ($N = 60$) or not to receive CT ($N = 60$). Both groups received enhanced usual care that included the assessment and referral services of a study case manager. Follow-up assessments were performed at 1, 3, 6, 12, and 18 months. The primary outcome measure was the incidence of repeat suicide attempts. Secondary outcome measures included suicide ideation, hopelessness, and depression. From baseline to the 18-month assessment, 24.1% of the participants in the CT group, compared to the 41.6% of the participants in the usual care group, made at least one subsequent suicide attempt. Although there were no significant between-group differences on rates of suicide ideation at any assessment point, the severity of depression was significantly lower for the CT group at 6, 12, and 18 months. Significantly reduced levels of hopelessness were observed for the CT group at 6 months. Overall, the results of this randomized clinical trial indicated that a relatively brief cognitive protocol, as presented here, effectively reduced the rate of repeated attempts by 50% in adults who had recently attempted suicide.

Over the years, only a limited number of studies have examined the effectiveness of various psychosocial interventions with suicidal persons. Unfortunately, there is also a paucity of research for specific at-risk populations, such as older adults (Pearson & Brown, 2000) and individuals with substance dependence. Successful interventions with suicide attempters include intensive follow-up treatment or case management (e.g., Van Heeringen et al., 1995), interpersonal psychotherapy (e.g., Guthrie et al., 2001), dialectical behavior therapy (Linehan et al., 2006), and CT (e.g., Brown et al., 2005). Further research that examines the effectiveness of psychosocial interventions for suicide attempters with co-occurring psychiatric and substance use disorders is warranted.

CONCLUSIONS

This chapter has described elements of a cognitive intervention for depressed individuals with suicidal behavior. As indicated earlier, suicide among individuals with depression is a major public health problem. Individuals with MDD are at an increased risk for suicidal behavior, especially during the early years within the course of their illness. Our recommendation is that suicidal behavior itself is indicative of poor problem solving and needs to be targeted directly during treatment. The brief cognitive intervention described here has been examined empirically and found to be effective in preventing future suicidal behavior. Mental health providers who work with depressed individuals who engage in suicidal behavior are encouraged to utilize the information presented here to help patients in the development and maintenance of adaptive coping strategies, so that suicidal behavior is no longer the *only* available option that they consider.

ACKNOWLEDGMENTS

We acknowledge the research assistance of Kathryn Lou, Brian Dearnley, and Daniella Sosdjan. Our thanks to Amy Wenzel for her review of the manuscript. Preparation of this manuscript was supported by grants from the National Institute of Mental Health (Nos. R01 MH067805 and P20 MH072905915) and the Centers for Disease Control and Prevention (No. R49 CCR321714).

REFERENCES

American Psychiatric Association. (2003). *Practice guidelines for the assessment and treatment of patients with suicidal behaviors.* Arlington, VA: Author.

Beck, A. T. (1976). *Cognitive therapy and the emotional disorders.* New York: Meridian.

Beck, A. T. (1996). Beyond belief: A theory of modes, personality, and psychopathology. In M. Salkovskis (Ed.), *Frontiers of cognitive therapy* (pp. 1–25). New York: Guilford Press.

Beck, A. T., Brown, G., Berchick, R. J., Stewart, B. L., & Steer, R. A. (1990). Relationship between hopelessness and ultimate suicide: A replication with psychiatric outpatients. *American Journal of Psychiatry, 147,* 190–195.

Beck, A. T., Brown, G. K., Steer, R. A., Dahlsgaard, K. K., & Grisham, J. R. (1999). Suicide ideation at its worst point: A predictor of eventual suicide in psychiatric outpatients. *Suicide and Life-Threatening Behavior, 29,* 1–9.

Beck, A. T., Kovacs, M., & Weissman, A. (1979). Assessment of suicidal intention: The Scale for Suicide Ideation. *Journal of Consulting and Clinical Psychology, 47,* 343–352.

Beck, A. T., Rush, A. J., Shaw, B. F., & Emery, G. (1979). *Cognitive therapy of depression.* New York: Guilford Press.

Beck, A. T., & Steer, R. A. (1988). *Manual for the Beck Hopelessness Scale.* San Antonio, TX: Psychological Corporation.

Beck, A. T., Steer, R. A., & Brown, G. K. (1996). *Manual for the Beck Depression Inventory* (2nd ed.). San Antonio, TX: Psychological Corporation.

Beck, J. S. (1995). *Cognitive therapy: Basics and beyond.* New York: Guilford Press.

Berk, M. S., Henriques, G. R., Warman, D., Brown, G. K., & Beck, A. T. (2004). A cognitive therapy intervention for suicide attempters: Overview of the treatment and case examples. *Cognitive and Behavioral Practice, 11,* 265–277.

Blair-West, G. W., Cantor, C. H., Mellsop, G. W., & Eyeson-Annan, M. L. (1999). Lifetime suicide risk in major depression: Sex and age determinants. *Journal of Affective Disorders, 55,* 171–178.

Borg, S. E., & Stahl, M. (1982). A prospective study of suicides and controls among psychiatric patients. *Acta Psychiatrica Scandinavica, 65,* 221–232.

Brown, G. K. (2002). *A review of suicide assessment measures for intervention research in adults and older adults.* National Institute of Mental Health, Suicide Research Consortium (*www.nimh.nih.gov/suicideresearch/adultsuicide.pdf*).

Brown, G. K., Beck, A. T., Steer, R. A., & Grisham, J. R. (2000). Risk factors for suicide in psychiatric outpatients: A 20-year prospective study. *Journal of Consulting and Clinical Psychology, 68,* 371–377.

Brown, G. K., Henriques, G. R., Ratto, C., & Beck, A. T. (2002). *Cognitive therapy treatment manual for suicide attempters.* Philadelphia: University of Pennsylvania, unpublished manuscript.

Brown, G. K., Ten Have, T., Henriques, G. R., Xie, S. X., Hollander, J. E., & Beck, A. T. (2005). Cognitive therapy for the prevention of suicide attempts: A randomized controlled trial. *Journal of the American Medical Association, 294,* 563–570.

Cole, T. B., & Glass, R. M. (2005). Mental illness and violent death: Major issues for public health. *Journal of the American Medical Association, 294,* 623–624.

Dahlsgaard, K. K., Beck, A. T., & Brown, G. K. (1998). Inadequate response to therapy as a predictor of suicide. *Suicide and Life-Threatening Behavior, 28,* 197–204.

Ellis, T. E., & Newman, C. F. (1996). *Choosing to live: How to defeat suicide through cognitive therapy.* Oakland, CA: New Harbinger.

Goldstein, R. B., Black, D. W., Nasrallah, A., & Winokur, G. (1991). The prediction of suicide: Sensitivity, specificity, and predictive value of a multivariate model applied to suicide among 1906 patients with affective disorders. *Archives of General Psychiatry, 48,* 418–422.

Guthrie, E., Kapur, N., Mackway-Jones, K., Chew-Graham, C., Moorey, J., Mendel, E., et al. (2001). Randomised controlled trial of brief psychological intervention after deliberate self-poisoning. *British Medical Journal, 323,* 135–138.

Guze, S. B., & Robins, E. (1970). Suicide and primary affective disorders. *British Journal of Psychiatry, 19,* 437–448.

Hoyert, D. L., Kung, H. C., & Smith, B. (2005). Deaths: Preliminary data for 2003. *National Vital Statistics Reports, 53*(15), 1–48.

Inskip, H. M., Harris, E. C., & Barraclough, B. (1998). Lifetime risk of suicide for affective disorder, alcoholism, and schizophrenia. *British Journal of Psychiatry, 172,* 35–37.

Jacobs, D. G. (Ed.). (1999). *The Harvard Medical School guide to suicide assessment and intervention.* San Francisco: Jossey-Bass.

Kessler, R. C., Borges, G., & Walters, E. E. (1999). Prevalence of and risk factors for lifetime suicide attempts in the National Comorbidity Survey. *Archives of General Psychiatry, 56,* 617–626.

Lewis, G., Hawton, K., & Jones, P. (1997). Strategies for preventing suicide. *British Journal of Psychiatry, 171,* 351–354.

Linehan, M. M., Comtois, K. A., Murray, A. M., Brown, M. Z., Gallop, R. J., Heard, H. L., et al. (2006). Two-year randomized controlled trial and follow-up of dia-

lectical behavior therapy vs therapy by experts for suicidal behaviors and borderline personality disorder. *Archives of General Psychiatry, 63,* 757–766.

Malone, K. M., Haas, G. L., Sweeney, J. A., & Mann, J. J. (1995). Major depression
and the risk of attempted suicide. *Journal of Affective Disorders, 34,* 173–185.

Modestin, J., Schwarzenbach, F. A., & Wurmle, O. (1992). Therapy factors in treating
severely ill psychiatric patients. *British Journal of Medical Psychology, 65,* 147–156.

Motto, J., Heilborn, D. C., & Juster, R. P. (1985). Development of a clinical instrument to estimate suicide risk. *American Journal of Psychiatry, 142,* 680–686.

O'Brien, G., Holton, A. R., Hurren, K., & Watt, L. (1987). Deliberate self-harm and
predictors of out-patient attendance. *British Journal of Psychiatry, 150,* 246–247.

Oslin, D. W., Zubritsky, C., Brown, G., Mullahy, M., Puliafico, A., & Ten Have, T.
(2004). Managing suicide risk in late life: Access to firearms as a public health
concern. *American Journal of Geriatric Psychiatry, 12,* 30–36.

Papakostas, G. I., Petersen, T., Pava, J., Masson, E., Worthington, J. J., Alpert, J., et al.
(2003). Hopelessness and suicidal ideation in outpatients with treatment-
resistant depression: Prevalence and impact on treatment outcome. *Journal of
Nervous and Mental Disease, 191,* 444–449.

Pearson, J. L., & Brown, G. K. (2000). Suicide prevention in late life: Directions for
science and practice. *Clinical Psychology Review, 20,* 685–705.

Placidi, G. P. A., Oquendo, M. A., Malone, K. M., Brodsky, B., Ellis, S. P., & Mann, J. J.
(2000). Anxiety in major depression: Relationship to suicide attempts. *American
Journal of Psychiatry, 157,* 1614–1618.

Rudd, M. D., Joiner, T. E., & Rajab, M. H. (2001). *Treating suicidal behavior.* New
York: Guilford Press.

Szanto, K., Reynolds, C. F., Conwell, Y., Begley, A. E., & Houck, P. (1998). High levels of hopelessness persist in geriatric patients with remitted depression and a
history of attempted suicide. *Journal of the American Geriatric Society, 46,* 1401–
1406.

U.S. Public Health Service. (2001). *National strategy for suicide prevention: Goals and
objectives for action.* Rockville, MD: U.S. Department of Health and Human
Services.

Van Heeringen, C., Jannes, S., Buylaert, W., Henderick, H., de Bacquer, D., & Van
Remoortel, J. (1995). The management of non-compliance with referral to
out-patient after-care among attempted suicide patients: A controlled intervention study. *Psychological Medicine, 25,* 963–970.

Vieta, E., Nieto, E., Gasto, C., & Cirera, E. (1992). Serious suicide attempts in affective patients. *Journal of Affective Disorders, 24,* 147–152.

Young, M. A., Fogg, L. F., Scheftner, W., Fawcett, J., Akiskal, H., & Maser, J. (1996).
Stable trait components of hopelessness: Baseline and sensitivity to depression.
Journal of Abnormal Psychology, 105, 155–165.

8

PANIC DISORDER
AND SOCIAL PHOBIA

Michael W. Otto
Mark B. Powers
Georgia Stathopoulou
Stefan G. Hofmann

Social phobia

Given the chronic avoidance, social isolation, role impairment, and disrupted quality of life associated with the anxiety disorders (e.g., Rubin et al., 2000; Schneier, Johnson, Hornig, Liebowitz, & Weissman, 1992), it is not surprising that anxiety comorbidity exacts a toll on the treatment of major depression. For example, a prospective study of 85 primary care patients showed that anxiety predicts persistence of depression 1 year later (Gaynes et al., 1999), with an 82% rate of depression at 1-year follow-up in the comorbid group compared to 57% in the noncomorbid group. Moreover, although at baseline the two groups did not differ in the severity of depressive symptoms, by 3-month follow-up the comorbid group exhibited greater depressive severity, indicated by an average 54.9 annual disability days over the follow-up period compared with an average of 19.8 days for the noncomorbid group (see also Fava et al., 2004; Frank et al., 2000). These results extend to psychosocial treatment. For example, Brown, Schulberg, Madonia,

Shear, and Houck (1996) found that although patients with a history of anxiety disorders made significant gains in psychotherapy, they were less likely to complete the treatment study and showed less improvement overall than patients with major depression only.

The negative effects of anxiety comorbidity appear to extend to bipolar disorder as well. In a large, prospective study, Otto and associates (2006) found that anxiety comorbidity predicted a worse course of bipolar disorder, with fewer days of relative euthymia over a year of study, poorer quality of life and role functioning, greater risk of relapse for those patients starting the study period in relative euthymia, and a slower rate of recovery for patients already depressed. Greater anxiety comorbidity (two or more disorders) predicted an intensification of these negative outcomes, and among individual anxiety disorders, social phobia and posttraumatic stress disorder had prominent influences. These findings and data from other studies indicated a worse course, poorer response to treatment, greater role dysfunction, greater substance use disorder comorbidity, and greater suicidality for patients with bipolar disorder with comorbid anxiety and panic spectrum disorders (McElroy et al., 2001; Simon et al., 2004).

Our purpose in this chapter is to provide a broader account of the rates and nature of the co-occurrence between anxiety disorders and major depression. In particular, we examine the influence of anxiety comorbidity on the nature and outcome of depression, with a focus on panic disorder and social phobia. Given this information, we then discuss treatment considerations that evolve from the partial guidance offered by the empirical literature. Although anxiety comorbidity is high in bipolar disorder, linked to a poorer course, and targeted in cognitive-behavioral therapy (CBT) protocols for bipolar disorder (Henin, Otto, & Reilly-Harrington, 2001), currently there is an absence of published treatment outcome studies of anxiety comorbidity in these samples. Accordingly, our chapter focuses only on treatment issues concerning the co-occurrence of anxiety and unipolar depression.

COMORBIDITY OF DEPRESSION AND ANXIETY

The National Comorbidity Survey (NCS) showed dramatically higher rates of panic disorder in individuals with a history of depression (Kessler et al., 1998). Chronologically, primary depression predicted the first onset of subsequent panic attacks but not of panic disorder. Chronologically, primary panic attacks, with or without panic disorder, predicted a first onset of subsequent major depression. Data from the NCS also indicate increased clinical severity when depression and panic disorder co-occur. Comorbid depression and panic disorder was associated with greater symptom severity, persistence, role impairment, suicidality, and help seeking (Roy-Byrne et al., 2000). Findings did not differ according to which disorder was chronologically primary.

There is also strong evidence for a high co-occurrence of major depression and social phobia (Magee et al., 1996; Rush et al., 2005), with even greater rates of depression among individuals with more social fears and among individuals seeking treatment (Kessler, Stang, Wittchen, Stein, & Walters, 1999). For example, in a sample of 449 outpatients with a lifetime diagnosis of social phobia, Brown and colleagues (2001) found a 60% rate of lifetime major depression and a 20% rate of lifetime dysthymia. The onset of social phobia typically occurs prior to the onset of depression (e.g., Brown et al., 2001; van Ameringen, Mancini, Styan, & Donison, 1991), and evidence suggests that social phobia increases the risk of subsequent depression (e.g., Stein et al., 2001).

Shared Psychopathology

According to Clark and Watson's (1991) tripartite theory, high negative affect is a common factor shared by both anxiety and depression, whereas low positive affect and high autonomic arousal are uniquely characteristic of depression and anxiety, respectively. Research testing the validity of the tripartite model in outpatients with anxiety and mood disorders has found that social phobia and depression are both distinguished by high negative affect and low positive affect, and that neither is characterized uniquely by physiological hyperarousal (Brown, Chorpita, & Barlow, 1998). Furthermore, psychopathology research indicates that social phobia and depressive disorders are characterized by some of the same exaggerated beliefs about the costs of negative social performance. For example, Wilson and Rapee (2005) found that individuals with social phobia tend to believe that social errors result in negative evaluations from others, and that the negative evaluations both reflect negative personal characteristics and herald long-term negative consequences. Moreover, depression is associated with an intensification of many of these beliefs. These findings are consistent with earlier reports of an intensification of core fears of negative evaluation in individuals with comorbid social phobia and major depression (Ball, Otto, Pollack, Uccello, & Rosenbaum, 1995).

Given the overlap in latent higher-order trait dimensions between social phobia and depression, as well as the ubiquity of negative self-related cognitions in both disorders, the unitary view of anxiety and depression might predict that CBT would target shared elements of affective and cognitive distress in anxiety and depression, leading to reciprocal and simultaneous changes in both. However, the results by Moscovitch, Hofmann, Suvak, and In-Albon (2005) suggest that in patients with social phobia, the treatment response to CBT is characterized by early, specific improvements in social phobia symptoms, which in turn leads to improvements in symptoms of depression. Therefore, although depression and social anxiety show considerable overlap in their psychopathology, the mechanisms of treatment change for the two syndromes appears to be separate, and CBT for social anxiety only indirectly targets depressive symptoms. Similar findings suggest that depression enhances core fears associated with panic disorder—fears of the somatic sensations of anxiety. Specifically, Otto, Pollack, Fava, Uccello, and Rosenbaum (1995) reported that depression was linked to moderate elevations on the anxiety sensitivity index, and that these scores dropped significantly with treatment of the depression. In addition, depression appears to sap coping resources, so that depressed patients are less able to buffer stress and engage adaptive problem-solving skills; many of these difficulties resolve with treatment of the depression (Otto et al., 1997). Finally, depression can be expected to sap energy and motivation while providing the neurovegative symptoms and dysfunctional attitudes that define depressive states.

Together, studies of depression and depression comorbidity relative to core fears associated with social phobia and panic disorder suggest that depression may well enhance these fears in a state-dependent fashion, while also decreasing coping skills and problem solving. One implication of these findings is that individuals with comorbid depression and anxiety disorders may present with greater phobic severity. Indeed, depression comorbidity with anxiety disorders is associated with increased symptom severity and disability (e.g., Fava et al., 2004; Katzelnick et al., 2001; Schneier et al., 1992). Furthermore, an association between panic disorder and suicide appears to be linked exclusively with the effects of comorbidity, including depression comorbidity, instead of being a direct risk associated with panic disorder itself (Vickers & McNally, 2004).

ASSESSMENT OF SOCIAL PHOBIA AND PANIC DISORDER IN DEPRESSION

Social anxiety and social phobia can be assessed with behavioral observation methods (see for a review, Glass & Arnkoff, 1989); interview rating scales, such as the Liebowitz Social Anxiety Scale (LSAS) and the Brief Social Phobia Scale (BSPS; Davidson et al., 1991; Liebowitz, 1987); and many self-report measures of social anxiety and avoidance, including the Fear of Negative Evaluation scale (FNE; Watson & Friend, 1969) and the Social Avoidance and Distress Scale (SADS) by Watson and Friend (1969), the Social Phobia Scale (SPS) and the Social Interaction Anxiety Scale (SIAS) by Mattick and Clarke (1998), and the Social Phobia and Anxiety Inventory (SPAI) for adults (Turner, Beidel, Dancu, & Stanley, 1989) and children (Beidel, Turner, & Morris, 1995) (for a more comprehensive review, see Hofmann & Barlow, 2002). For panic disorder, core fears associated with the disorder can be assessed with the Anxiety Sensitivity Index (ASI; Reiss, Peterson, Gursky, & McNally, 1986). A popular clinician-rated instrument that nicely captures the range of distress and disability associated with panic disorder—anticipatory anxiety, panic frequency, panic severity, fear of symptoms, avoidance behaviors—is the Panic Disorder Severity Scale (PDSS; Shear et al., 1997).

COMMONALITIES IN THE TREATMENT OF MOOD AND ANXIETY DISORDERS

In treating comorbid conditions, clinicians need to consider the degree to which strategies used in one problem area may be utilized in the treatment of other areas of distress. This approach not only holds the potential for more efficient treatment but also may be useful for honing a patient's own skills in applying principles of treatment to new problem areas—skills that are important for relapse prevention efforts.

Cognitive interventions are, of course, ubiquitous in empirically supported treatments for mood and anxiety disorders. In both anxiety and mood disorders, cognitive interventions include, for example, informational interventions, Socratic questioning, self-monitoring, and behavioral experiments (J. S. Beck, 1995). In general, for the anxiety disorders, these strategies often target the overestimations of the probability or degree of catastrophe of feared outcomes (cf. Barlow & Craske, 2000; Hope, Heimberg, Juster, & Turk, 2000). Moreover, in our experience, the content of cognitions encountered in depression is similar to that encountered in social phobia. In both disorders, restructuring efforts are likely to target beliefs about personal inadequacy and unlovability, perhaps related to self-imposed perfectionistic standards. Hence, because of this shared content of dysfunctional thoughts, cognitive interventions for one disorder may easily be extended to the other.

Compared to comorbid social phobia, cognitive interventions for panic disorder, although using the same strategies, are likely to involve cognitive content that is more distinct from depression. In panic disorder, core dysfunctional cognitions focus on catastrophic misinterpretations of the meaning and consequences of anxiety symptoms ("Am I having a heart attack?"; "What if I lose control?"; "I am going to be humiliated"; for recent study, see Raffa, White, & Barlow, 2004). Nonetheless, the negative and self-punitive cognitions that follow the avoidance of desired activities ("I can't believe I didn't go; I am such a loser"; "I just can't do things that others do") appear to be more similar to the cognitive content frequently encountered in depression (e.g., Beck, Rush, Shaw, & Emery, 1987).

In the treatment of comorbid conditions, clinicians can teach patients the method, style, and results of cognitive restructuring, then apply it to the symptom domains identified as most important for a coherent ordering of treatment, while keeping in mind the complications brought by the comorbid condition. For example, Otto and Gould (1996) have suggested that if panic disorder is selected as a primary focus of treatment, three areas for cognitive restructuring are important in addressing the impact of depression on this treatment. First, as we discuss further below, depression is likely to enhance fears of anxiety sensations and negative evaluations of others (Otto et al., 1995; Wilson & Rapee, 2005). Accordingly, during presentation of the model of the disorder, we believe the mood-state-dependent aspects of anxiogenic thoughts should be emphasized. Patients need to be informed of the degree to which negative thoughts "feel truer" when affect is strong; that is, worries about negative outcomes in the future *feel* as if they will come true, concerns about negative evaluations from others *feel* more like they are happening, and worries about health or the meaning of symptoms *feel* more dire when depression is present. Patients need to be made aware of this phenomenon and to be vigilant, as part of cognitive restructuring efforts, to challenging these thoughts when mood is low.

Second, patients should be prepared for their tendency to evaluate progress negatively (e.g., "This isn't working; I am not like other patients that can get better; I am failing"), and to practice recognizing and confronting these cognitions *before* they encounter them during exposure assignments. In particular, we believe it is important for therapists to troubleshoot homework assignments and, when depression is present, to review explicitly common negative reactions to progress that may occur during the week between sessions. The aim is to help patients identify these cognitions (e.g., "My therapist told me I might be thinking that") as a way to nullify the emotional impact of these thoughts and to occasion cognitive restructuring efforts.

Third, due to motivational issues, patients may require additional attention to homework adherence, including perhaps clearer and more objective self-monitoring of progress and cognitive restructuring interventions focused on motivation for homework completion. This involves more troubleshooting relative to homework assignments when they are made, as well as stronger efforts to acknowledge progress when it occurs. Again, we recommend that therapists rehearse common negative motivational responses when assigning homework (e.g., "Given that your mood is low, what are you going to think when you do your exposure practices this week?") and rehearse alternative responses (e.g., "When you are at home, feeling like exposure practice is pointless, what do you think might help you?"). For patients with strong impairments in motivation, we make all assignments especially stepwise (with multiple small steps geared toward success) and attend to ways we can chain together behaviors to place patients in the right context for an exposure (e.g., the first step is to get patients out of the house and active, so that exposure assignments seem relevant). This process is aided by the natural synergy between emphasis on stepwise exposure to feared situations and events in the anxiety disorders and its counterpart in behavioral activation treatments for depression.

Behavioral activation approaches to depression emphasize the role of depression-related inactivity and withdrawal as maladaptive coping strategies that isolate individuals from opportunities for positive affect and propagate depression (for review, see Hopko, Lejuez, Ruggiero, & Eifert, 2003). Accordingly, treatment emphasizes step-by-step reemergence into meaningful work, social, and leisure activities. A focus on the return to meaningful activities is synergistic with the goals of exposure interventions, although when applied to the treatment of anxiety disorders, greater emphasis is devoted to teaching strategies to manage anxious apprehension and to accept the anxious affect likely to be evoked as part of exposure (see Otto, Powers, & Fischman, 2005). The potential confluence of goals for behavioral activation interventions is nicely illustrated in a case example by Hopko, Lejuez, and Hopko (2004), who applied behavioral activation interventions in a 10-session, stepwise exposure format to patients with both depression and panic disorder.

When a therapist arranges treatment to focus first on depression, we encourage attention to three sources of negative affect that are likely to be driven by a comorbid anxiety disorder. First, fears of anxiety sensations or avoided situations (social or agoraphobic) make participation in a wide variety of activities especially difficult (with frequent distress and/or avoidance). Second, self-perceived failures in these situations/activities (at times defined simply by the reoccurrence of anxiety and avoidance) may intensify negative self-evaluations and depressed affect, and compromise the positive affect that would otherwise be generated by these activities. Third, cognitive responses to social and role failures due to anxiety and avoidance may intensify patients core beliefs that they are flawed or incompetent. Accordingly, activity assignments for depression may require careful troubleshooting to assess the degree to which anxiety and avoidance will be elicited, and adoption of a stepwise exposure approach, with anxiety-specific cognitive preparation (e.g., Barlow & Craske, 2000; Hope et al., 2000; Otto, Jones, Craske, & Barlow, 1996) to address these issues proactively. The degree to which anxiety and panic responses are directly punishing to patients and retard their efforts to return to enjoyable activities (i.e., the anxiety makes potentially enjoyable events feel like failure experiences) may be one reason why anxiety disorders appear strongly to reduce the efficacy of treatments for major depression (see below).

The degree to which emotional acceptance is promoted by CBT is an additional common factor that deserves attention in the treatment of comorbid conditions. For example, study of the relapse prevention effects of cognitive therapy for depression suggests that the degree to which these techniques enhance metacognitive awareness (a cognitive set in which negative thoughts and emotions are viewed as passing mental events rather than characteristics of the self; e.g., "I am my affect") is linked to a reduced risk of relapse (Teasdale et al., 2002). Likewise, at their core, exposure-based treatments for anxiety disorders, and panic disorder in particular, provide training to reduce fears of anxiety sensations and to respond adaptively despite the presence of these sensations (Otto et al., 2005). Patients in exposure-based treatments learn to respond differently to anxiety sensations; specifically, to learn to do nothing special to manage the sensations (stopping all the effort to avoid, protect against, or otherwise stop emotional sensations, and instead learning to become more comfortable with this affect). In panic disorder in particular, when patients learn to react differently to anxiety sensations, the regular evocation of panic attacks ceases. Indeed, this sort of promotion of emotional acceptance/tolerance may be a general factor in treatment that helps patients break the link between negative affect and dysfunctional responses to that affect (e.g., avoidance in anxiety disorders, and inactivity in depression) that propagates disorders (Barlow, Allen, & Choate, 2005). As discussed by Barlow et al., therapeutic packages that emphasize the replacement of the action tendencies driven by negative affect with actions consistent with alternative emotions have shown efficacy for a variety of disorders, including depression, anxiety disorders, and borderline personality disorder. This conceptualization is also consistent with "acceptance" models of change that emphasize adaptive pursuit of goals regardless of the presence of aversive thoughts or emotions (see Hayes, Strosahl, & Wilson, 1999). Accordingly, in the treatment of comorbid conditions, clinicians may want to underscore this ability. Working to extend this communality across the affective patterns under treatment (extending emotional acceptance skills that patients learn from exposure also to responses to the negative affect of depression) may prove useful for efficient treatment of comorbid conditions and/or provide broader skills for relapse prevention.

At a clinical level, it accordingly seems important for cognitive therapists to help patients at a level beyond detection and correction of specific cognitive errors: helping them to develop a more general capacity to take their thoughts less seriously, while working to become more comfortable with their experience of affect in the context of working to meet personal goals (e.g., completing events that provide a sense of both mastery and pleasure in relation to depression, or meeting goals in social situations rather than being vigilant to symptoms or fears about evaluations from others).

Ordering Treatment

In addition to maximizing the common application of component interventions that are useful in both anxiety and depressive disorders, the therapist must decide how to order their treatment. Should the anxiety disorder or the depression be targeted first? Compared to the anxiety literature, the depression literature does not provide much empirical guidance other than to document a poorer outcome for pharmacological and cognitive-behavioral treatment when comorbid anxiety is present (e.g., Brown et al., 1996; Gaynes et al., 1999). In contrast, a growing body of research suggests that CBT for anxiety disorders is fairly resilient with respect to the effects of depression. These data, presented in some detail below, have been influential at the clinical level to motivate us frequently to target anxiety disorders rather than depression as the first phase of treatment. Accordingly, we provide in these sections more details on issues of attending to comorbid depression rather than the reverse when treating anxiety disorders. However, we realize that such general guidance is challenging given the complexity of individual cases; hence, we also offer the following considerations on the ordering of treatment (see Table 8.1).

First, because research indicates that a match between the patient's expectations and treatment methods is important for treatment adherence (Eisenthal, Emery, Lazare, & Udin, 1979; Grilo, Money, Barlow, Goddard, Gorman, et al., 1998; Schulberg et al., 1996), treatment selection should be informed by both the patient's primary areas of distress and his/her beliefs about what is needed in therapy. These considerations on the patient's side should be complemented on the therapist's side by a functional analysis of the controlling relations between the anxiety and depression. Does the situa-

TABLE 8.1. Considerations in the Ordering of Treatment Interventions

Considerations	Comments
Ensure that treatment offers a match with patient expectations.	In addition to eliciting the patient's sense of which symptom clusters are the primary source of distress and disability, devote effort to helping the patient see controlling relations between the symptoms.
Ensure that the ordering of treatment makes sense relative to a functional analysis of the links between the patient's anxiety, depression, and avoidance.	Patient expectations need to be balanced against the therapist's analysis of how one set of symptoms may limit progress on other sets of symptoms.
Beware of overattending to in-session distress relative to maintaining a step-by-step focus on core maladaptive patterns.	Ensure that progress from the last session is consistently reviewed, and that any new distress is integrated within the general model of change to help the therapy stay on track.
Attend to early gains as a strategy to promote motivation for treatment.	At every stage of treatment, help the patient see the links between his/her efforts in and out of therapy, and changes in symptoms and disability.

tional distress and avoidance from the anxiety disorder limit the affective benefit that a patient may derive from a more primary focus on depressed mood? Are the anxiety, avoidance, and dysfunction from the anxiety disorder used as evidence for core beliefs underlying depression? Alternatively, is the depressed mood strong enough to compromise the patient's motivation or willingness to complete exposure exercises, or his/her ability to judge or utilize the success of these exercises?

In completing this functional analysis, we caution therapists against overattention to insession, weekly depressive distress to the exclusion of out-of-session dysfunctional patterns. Depressive symptoms, particularly in-session sadness and tearfulness, are often more salient to clinicians than the anxiety and avoidance symptoms that tend to occur outside rather than inside the clinician's office. Indeed, treatment of the anxiety disorder in patients with comorbid depression requires that the clinician focus on what is most *useful* to the patient over the interval between sessions instead on what is most obviously *comforting* within the session. This difficult process requires the clinician to judge what is in the patient's best interest—whether to focus on the affective distress of the moment or on a broader agenda that may offer earlier relief from punishing anxiety that may be fueling affective distress more broadly. Certainly the clinician is aided in this process by the collaborative relationship with the patient, balancing the patient's own sense of which disorder deserves primary attention and the clinician's perspective on which affective patterns appear to be most central to maintenance of the disorders.

As a final point on the ordering of interventions, we also encourage therapists to provide patients with early evidence that treatment *can* lead to beneficial change; that is, the most central problem does not always need to be the first treatment target. Research suggests that early gains in treatment can boost motivation and therapeutic alliance (see Tang & DeRubeis, 1999). Accordingly, we encourage therapists to focus attention on the interventions that might offer the earliest, noticeable benefit to the patient, using initial treatment gains as (1) a way to boost the patient's momentum in therapy, and (2) establish efficacy with a therapeutic strategy that can be applied to other problem areas.

Nonetheless, the outcome literature suggests that treatment of comorbid conditions may need a longer course of treatment, and we encourage clinicians to be resilient in pursuing full remission of mood and anxiety disorders. Treatment of comorbid anxiety and depression may require more sessions of treatment, because (1) some patients may require additional treatment to reach remission given their greater illness severity; (2) the comorbid condition may not resolve, and may require additional treatment once the other disorder has been treated; or (3) the selected treatment may fail outright. Residual symptoms tend to be predictors of relapse; hence, additional treatment targeting full remission offers not only the short-term benefits of better quality of life but also a better long-term outcome.

CASE ILLUSTRATION

J. L., a 32-year-old, single, African American woman employed as a temporary office assistant, sought help for extreme anxiety in a variety of social situations. When describing her difficulties, J. L. reported that she had had "problems with people" ever since she was teased and taunted in junior high school. She reported that she had had few friends and felt continuously uneasy, alone, and terrified in school. In addition, she feared parties; public speaking; participating in meetings and classes; speaking with unfamiliar people and authority figures; being assertive; maintaining a conversation; entering public places, such as restaurants, coffee shops, and stores; and dating. She reported that she never had a serious romantic relationship. J. L. stated that she feared all of these situations because she was worried that people were evaluating her negatively. She noted, "I just have a huge fear of people. I always think that I will not be liked." She further stated, "Initiating anything with people is difficult. I get immediately nervous." J. L. reported that her fear in social situations had resulted in a pattern of avoidance that had significantly interfered with her life. When describing the level of interference her social discomfort has caused, J. L. said: "I feel that I have missed my whole life. I just want to be able to communicate with others." J. L. revealed that she wished she could feel more relaxed in these situations and not be concerned about whether others were evaluating her.

In addition, J. L. reported long-standing difficulties with depressed mood. More often than not, she felt down and had difficulty engaging in activities. Along with her depressed mood, she reported that she had sleeping problems, low self-esteem, poor concentration, and a sense of hopelessness about the future. J. L.'s symptoms had been present since she was approximately 15 years old. Her depression appeared to have been a direct consequence of her social anxiety.

Her ultimate referral to CST was preceded by an acute worsening of both her social concern and her depression. J. L. had returned to school, taking evening classes. With her return to a classroom setting, her memories of her early teasing were enlivened, and she reported fearful ruminations on a daily basis. J. L. described being so nervous that she walked a greater distance to her class so that she could avoid crowds of people, including unexpectedly coming upon her classmates out of class. Her distress about her social concerns reached a peak around a class presentation where a mock interview had to be completed in front of the class. During her part of the interview, she felt her anxiety reach panic proportions, and she was sure that the whole class was riveted to her halting speech and trembling hands. After the class was over, she heard a student comment that the interview went poorly. She described this incident as the last straw. She drove home choking back tears and resolving that she would not be humiliated again. She described her thoughts as racing as she vowed not to go back to school or allow such feelings of humiliation to be elicited again. On the way home, she stopped at a drugstore and bought over-the-counter sleeping pills. Once home she searched the medicine cabinet for any pills she could take, and came away with a bottle of ibuprofen. She took handfuls of both the ibuprofen and the sleeping pills, thinking all the time of the need to escape from school, from humiliation, from her life. She covered herself with a blanket, began feeling sleepy, and waited to die. At this time her roommate came home from work, discovered her in this state, and called for an ambulance. With brief inpatient treatment, her acute suicidal intent resolved. Her chronic depressed mood—meeting criteria for major depression—her fears of humiliation, and her ongoing social anxiety disorder did not resolve. She was subsequently referred to outpatient treatment.

At the time of the interview, J. L. endorsed symptoms of depression and passive suicidal ideation. She stated that although she often "wishes for relief" from her current state of social anxiety, she did not feel that she was a danger to herself at the present time. On the basis of the information obtained during the diagnostic interview, a principal diagnosis of social phobia (generalized subtype) with avoidant personality disorder was assigned. In addition, she received the diagnoses of major depressive disorder, recurrent, moderate.

As a result of her suicide attempt at age 19, J. L. was hospitalized. She subsequently received individual psychotherapy and psychiatric treatment for a period of 5 years following this incident. At the time of the assessment, J. L. was taking Dexedrine, 5 mg/day; Klonopin, 1 mg/day; and Wellbutrin, 200 mg/day.

Shortly after this assessment, J. L. was invited to participate in a free treatment trial at an anxiety specialty clinic. As part of this study, she received 12 weekly sessions of CBT in a group format. J. L. responded very positively to the intervention. Her level of social anxiety, as measured with the Difference score of the SPAI, dropped from 158.2 to 133.6 at posttreatment (15.6% reduction from pretest), and further decreased to 110.4 6 months after the end of treatment (32.1% reduction from pretest). Although the treatment did not address specifically her symptoms of depression, her Beck Depression Inventory (BDI) score dropped from 26 before treatment to 9 at the end of treatment, which is a 65.4% reduction from the level at pretest (no information on her BDI score was available for the 6-month follow-up assessment).

REVIEW OF EFFICACY RESEARCH

There are a number of reasons to expect poorer outcomes among patients with depression and comorbid anxiety disorders. Indeed, investigators have suggested that comorbid depression may reduce patient motivation to conduct self-directed exposures (Marks, 1987), may affect habituation patterns (Abramowitz, Franklin, Street, Kozak, & Foa, 2000; Abramowitz & Foa, 2000; Foa, 1979; Mills & Salkovskis, 1988), and may lead patients to minimize new (safety) learning from exposure interventions (Telch, 1988). Fortunately, there is some evidence that anxiety treatment effects may be more robust than expected. Indeed, early indications that severe depression may interfere with within- or between-session extinction in the treatment of obsessive–compulsive disorder (Foa, 1979) have not been particularly evident in later studies. As Abramowitz et al. (2000) and Abramowitz and Foa

(2000) noted, depressed patients with obsessive–compulsive disorder achieve treatment gains in exposure-based CBT, albeit at a lower magnitude than less depressed patients. Studies of the efficacy of CBT for other anxiety disorders provide an expanded account of the resilience of treatment when depression comorbidity is confronted.

Treatment of Panic Disorder in Individuals with Depression

In a review of CBT for panic disorder, Mennin and Heimberg (2000) described the minimal impact of comorbid mood disorders, particularly at follow-up assessments. Dimensional studies of depressive symptoms at baseline do not reliably predict outcome of CBT treatment of panic disorder (Basoglu et al., 1994; Black, Wesner, Gabel, Bowers, & Monahan, 1994; Jansson, Öst, & Jerremalm, 1987). Likewise, categorical analysis of the presence or absence of comorbid major depression suggested similar efficacy of CBT treatment of panic disorder (Brown, Antony, & Barlow, 1995; Laberge, Gauthier, Cote, Plamondon, & Cormier, 1993; McLean, Woody, Taylor, & Koch, 1998). For example, McLean et al. compared 37 patients with comorbid panic disorder and major depression to 53 patients with panic disorder only. All patients received 10 sessions of CBT for panic disorder; comorbid depression had no effect on treatment outcome for panic disorder.

Treatment outcome studies also indicate that depression symptoms often improve with panic treatment (e.g., Clark et al., 1994; Öst, Thulin, & Ramnerö, 2004; Tsao, Mystkowski, Zucker, & Craske, 2002). For example, Tsao and associates investigated the effects of CBT for panic disorder on comorbid conditions, including depression. They found that comorbid diagnoses in general declined from 60.8% at pretreatment to 37.3% at posttreatment. They also found that a comorbid diagnosis of clinical depression (major depression and dysthymia) declined from 18% pretreatment to 6% posttreatment. This study demonstrated that not only did a comorbid diagnosis of depression not interfere with panic treatment, but also that CBT treatment for panic significantly reduced clinical depression. However, cautionary evidence is provided by Maddock and Blacker (1991). Although they found that secondary depression (depression emerging after the onset of panic disorder) did not predict negative treatment outcome, primary depression was linked to poorer outcome. Depression chronicity tends to be a reliable predictor of poorer outcome in studies of depression treatment (e.g., Keller et al., 1992); hence, this effect may have less to do with the order of onset of the disorders, and more with the relatively early onset and duration of the depression.

Nonresponse of depression in panic treatment also has been studied. Woody, McLean, Taylor, and Koch (1999) compared 49 outpatients with major depression and no panic disorder to 37 outpatients who had received CBT for panic disorder without resolution of their depression. All patients received 10 sessions of CBT for depression; results indicated that both groups improved equally on depression outcome measures, with no significant effect for previous panic disorder comorbidity. Accordingly, if depression does not improve during panic treatment, there are indications that subsequent CBT targeting depression leads to anticipated levels of improvement.

In summary, current research on panic disorder indicates that brief programs of CBT targeting panic disorder lead to strong treatment effects regardless of the presence of depression. In some cases, comorbid depression does improve with the treatment of the panic disorder, but if this is not the case, initial study indicates that subsequent CBT targeting the depression can help to resolve it. Similar encouraging evidence is also available for the CBT of social phobia.

Treatment of Social Phobia in Individuals with Depression

Despite the high frequency and clinical severity of the co-occurrence of social phobia and major depression, many studies have excluded depression in clinical trials. For example, a meta-analysis of 30 cognitive and/or behavioral treatments of social phobia, published from 1996 to 2002, found that only 11 studies included patients with social phobia and comorbid depression (Lincoln & Rief, 2004). In this meta-analysis, the impact of comorbid depression could be examined only by comparing studies that did or did not exclude comorbid depression. The results indicated that inclusion of at least some patients with comorbid depression appeared to make little difference in the overall study findings, with near identical estimates of mean pre- to posttreatment effect sizes for studies that did ($d = 0.91$) or did not ($d = 0.92$) exclude patients with depression.

Clinical trials examining the impact of comorbid depression on the treatment of social phobia have produced equivocal results. Van Velzen, Emmelkamp, and Scholing (1997) found that comorbid anxiety or depression did not affect treatment outcome of exposure treatment for social phobia. Their comprised sample 18 patients with social phobia, with either comorbid anxiety or depression, compared to 43 individuals without these comorbidities. Likewise, Turner, Beidel, Wolff, Spaulding, and Jacob (1996) found no differences in treatment outcomes for social phobia treatment among 13 patients with social phobia with Axis I comorbidity (dysthymia, generalized anxiety disorder, or simple phobia) and 8 patients without comorbidity. These promising results, based on small studies that did not differentiate between anxiety and mood comorbidity, received additional support from a larger scale (N = 141) study by Erwin, Heimberg, Juster, and Mindlin (2002). The authors compared the response to 12 sessions of cognitive-behavioral group therapy (CBGT) in three groups of patients with social phobia: those with a primary diagnosis of social phobia and no comorbid diagnoses, those with a primary diagnosis of social phobia and an additional anxiety disorder diagnosis, and those with a primary diagnosis of social phobia and an additional mood disorder diagnosis. Their findings showed that patients with social phobia and comorbid mood disorders, but not comorbid anxiety disorders, were more severely impaired than patients with no comorbid diagnosis, both before and after CBGT. However, the rate of improvement in therapy was the same in both groups.

In contrast to these studies, the negative impact of depression on social phobia treatment outcome was shown in studies by Chambless, Tran, and Glass (1997) and Scholing and Emmelkamp (1999). Chambless et al. (1997) examined the prognostic value of pretreatment depression, as well as personality disorder traits, patients' expectations of treatment, clinician-rated breadth and severity of impairment, and frequency of negative thoughts for CBGT of 62 outpatients with social phobia. The findings indicated that pretreatment depression was the most consistent predictor of poorer treatment outcome for measures of anxious apprehension and anxiety. Scholing and Emmelkamp (1999), in a partial replication of the Chambless et al. (1997) study, examined the role of pretreatment depression, personality disorder traits, clinician-rated severity of impairment, and frequency of negative self-statements during social interactions among 50 patients with generalized social phobia and 26 patients with somatic fears in social situations. In agreement with Chambless et al., they found a significant correlation between pretreatment depression and residual gain scores (r = .20, p < .05). At an 18-month follow-up assessment, however, depression had no significant predictive value for treatment outcome.

An additional perspective on the influence of comorbidity on social phobia treatment is provided by studies offering more detailed analyses of changes in symptoms across treatment. For example, Persons, Roberts, and Zalecki (2003) examined session-by-session symptom changes in anxiety and depression among 58 outpatients who received individual CBT for a variety of anxiety and mood disorders, although not specifically for social phobia. The authors showed that self-reported symptoms of anxiety and depression were highly predictive of one another and correlated more strongly when measured in the same session than when measured at different session-by-session time points. Based on these findings, the authors argued that anxiety and depression change together during the course of CBT, and that these nosologically distinct diagnoses may actually represent variants of a unitary, underlying disorder.

Preliminary evidence against this hypothesis comes from a more recent study that also investigated the interactive process of changes in social anxiety and depression during treatment (Moscovitch et al., 2005). This study examined the effects of CBT for social phobia on changes in depression. The authors gathered weekly measures of anxiety and depression in 66 adult outpatients with social phobia who participated in CBGT. Multilevel mediation analyses revealed that improvements in social anxiety mediated 91% of the improvements in depression over time. Conversely, decreases in depression only accounted for 6% of the decreases in social anxiety over time. Moreover, changes in social anxiety fully mediated changes in depression during the course of treatment. These findings suggest that in patients with social phobia, secondary symptoms of depression are ameliorated via effective CBT that targets primary symptoms of social anxiety. In other words, in patients with social phobia, secondary symptoms of depression are ameliorated via effective CBT that targets primary symptoms of social anxiety. It is possible that social anxiety blocks the path to positive reinforcement of attachment relationships (Eng, Heimberg, Hart, Schneier, & Liebowitz, 2001) and reducing social anxiety may lead to improvements in depression through the mechanism of increased positive reinforcement in interpersonal domains. Therefore, depending on the level of depressive symptoms, it might not be necessary to target depression initially or simultaneously when treating social phobia. Instead, we recommend that clinicians first target the principal social phobia diagnosis of individuals with mild to moderate depression, then reassess the depression status after a successful social phobia treatment.

In summary, studies suggest that outpatients with social phobia and comorbid depression are likely to present with more severe symptoms at pretreatment and to retain some of this severity at posttreatment, but in general they are likely to improve at the same rate as their nondepressed counterparts. Also, response to treatment of social phobia may well drive improvement in comorbid depression. Accordingly, these data provide clinicians with some confidence that for patients with comorbid social phobia and depression, brief CBT targeting social phobia has a good chance of success despite the presence of depression.

CONCLUSIONS

As clinicians well know, psychiatric comorbidity tends to be the rule rather than the exception for patients presenting for clinical treatment. For anxiety patients with comorbid depression, the clinical trial literature provides encouraging evidence for the degree to which anxiety treatments may be resilient to the influence of depression comorbidity. In comparison, available evidence for the resilience of depression treatment to the effects of anxiety comorbidity is less encouraging, although both areas of inquiry are clearly in need of further controlled study. In this chapter, we have discussed principles that may aid the selection of the appropriate initial targets and strategies for treatment in individuals with co-occurring anxiety and depression. As always, in this enterprise, the clinician and patient are aided by a careful and collaborative functional analysis of the controlling links between negative affective, avoidant, and other maladaptive patterns that can maintain disorders.

REFERENCES

Abramowitz, J. S., & Foa, E. B. (2000). Does comorbid major depressive disorder influence outcome of exposure and response prevention for OCD? *Behavior Therapy, 31*, 795–800.

Abramowitz, J. S., Franklin, M. E., Street, G. P., Kozak, M. J., & Foa, E. B. (2000). Effects of comorbid depression on response to treatment for obsessive–compulsive disorder. *Behavior Therapy, 31,* 517–528.

Ball, S. G., Otto, M. W., Pollack, M. H., Uccello, R., & Rosenbaum, J. F. (1995). Differentiating social phobia and panic disorder: A test of core beliefs. *Cognitive Research and Therapy, 19*, 473–482.

Barlow, D. A., Allen, L. B., & Choate, M. L. (2005). Toward a unified treatment for emotional disorders. *Behavior Therapy, 35*, 205–230.

Barlow, D. H., & Craske, M. G. (2000). *Mastery of your anxiety and panic (MAP-3): Therapist guide for anxiety, panic, and agoraphobia* (3rd ed.). Oxford, UK: Oxford University Press.

Basoglu, M., Marks, I. M., Swinson, R. P., Noshirvani, H., O'Sullivan, G., & Kuch, K. (1994). Pre-treatment predictors of treatment outcome in panic disorder and agoraphobia treated with alprazolam and exposure. *Journal of Affective Disorders, 30,* 123–132.

Beck, A. T., Rush, A. J., Shaw, B. F., & Emery, G. (1987). *Cognitive therapy of depression.* New York: Guilford Press.

Beck, J. S. (1995). *Cognitive therapy: Basics and beyond.* New York: Guilford Press.

Beidel, D. C., Turner, S. M., & Morris, T. L. (1995). A new inventory to assess childhood social anxiety and phobia: The Social Phobia and Anxiety Inventory for Children. *Psychological Assessment, 7,* 73–79.

Black, D. W., Wesner, R. B., Gabel, J., Bowers, W., & Monahan, P. (1994). Predictors of short-term treatment response in 66 patients with panic disorder. *Journal of Affective Disorders, 30,* 233–241.

Brown, C., Schulberg, H. C., Madonia, M. J., Shear, M. K., & Houck, P. R. (1996). Treatment outcomes for primary care patients with major depression and lifetime anxiety disorders. *American Journal of Psychiatry, 153,* 1293–1300.

Brown, T. A., Antony, M. M., & Barlow, D. H. (1995). Diagnostic comorbidity in panic disorder: Effect on treatment outcome and course of comorbid diagnoses following treatment. *Journal of Consulting and Clinical Psychology, 63,* 408–418.

Brown, T. A., Campbell, L. A., Lehman, C. I., Grisham, J. R., & Mancill, R. B. (2001). Structural relationships among dimensions of the DSM-IV anxiety and mood disorders and dimensions of negative affect, positive affect, and autonomic arousal. *Journal of Abnormal Psychology, 110,* 585–599.

Brown, T. A., Chorpita, B. F., & Barlow, D. H. (1998). Structural relationships among dimensions of the DSM-IV anxiety and mood disorders and dimensions of negative affect, positive affect, and autonomic arousal. *Journal of Abnormal Psychology, 107,* 179–192.

Chambless, D. L., Tran, G. Q., & Glass, C. R. (1997). Predictors of response to cognitive-behavioural group therapy for social phobia. *Journal of Anxiety Disorders, 11,* 221–240.

Clark, D. M., Salkovskis, P. M., Hackmann, A., Middleton, J., Pavlos, A., & Gelder, M. (1994). A comparison of cognitive therapy, applied relaxation, and imipramine in the treatment of panic disorder. *British Journal of Psychiatry, 164,* 759–769.

Clark, L. A., & Watson, D. (1991). Tripartite model of anxiety and depression: Psychometric evidence and taxonomic implications. *Journal of Abnormal Psychology, 100,* 316–336.

Davidson, J. R. T., Potts, N. L. S., Richichi, E. A., Ford, S. M., Krishnan, R. R., Smith, R., et al. (1991). The Brief Social Phobia Scale. *Journal of Clinical Psychiatry, 52,* 48–51.

Eisenthal, S., Emery, R., Lazare, A., & Udin, H. (1979). "Adherence" and the negotiated approach to patienthood. *Archives of General Psychiatry, 36,* 393–398.

Eng, W., Heimberg, R. G., Hart, T. A., Schneier, F. R., & Liebowitz, M. R. (2001). Attachment in individuals with social anxiety disorder: The relationship among adult attachment styles, social anxiety, and depression. *Emotion, 1,* 365–380.

Erwin, B. A., Heimberg, R. G., Juster, H., & Mindlin, M. (2002). Comorbid anxiety and mood disorders among persons with social anxiety disorder. *Behaviour Research and Therapy, 40,* 19–35.

Fava, M., Alpert, J. E., Carmin, C. N., Wisniewski, S. R., Trivedi, M. H., Biggs, M. M., et al. (2004). Clinical correlates and symptom patterns of anxious depression among patients with major depressive disorder in STAR*D. *Psychological Medicine, 34,* 1299–1308.

Foa, E. (1979). Failure in treating obsessive–compulsives. *Behaviour Research and Therapy, 17,* 169–176.

Frank, E., Cyranowski, J. M., Rucci, P., Shear, M. K., Fagiolini, A., Thase, M. E., et al. (2002). Clinical significance of lifetime panic spectrum symptoms in the treatment of patients with bipolar I disorder. *Archives of General Psychiatry, 59,* 905–911.

Frank, E., Shear, M. K., Rucci, P., Cyranowski, J. M., Endicott, J., Fagiolini, A., et al. (2000). Influence of panic–agoraphobic spectrum symptoms on treatment response in patients with recurrent major depression. *American Journal of Psychiatry, 157,* 1101–1107.

Gaynes, B. N., Magruder, K. M., Burns, B. J., Wagner, H. R., Yarnall, K. S., & Broadhead, W. E. (1999). Does a coexisting anxiety disorder predict persistence of depressive illness in primary care patients with major depression? *General Hospital Psychiatry, 21*(3), 158–167.

Glass, C. R., & Arnkoff, D. B. (1989). Behavioral assessment of social anxiety and social phobia. *Clinical Psychology Review, 9,* 75–90.

Grilo, C. M., Money, R., Barlow, D. H., Goddard, A. W., Gorman, J. M., et al. (1998). Pretreatment patient factors predicting attrition from a multicenter randomized controlled treatment study for panic disorder. *Comprehensive Psychiatry, 39,* 323–332.

Hayes, S. C., Strosahl, K. D., & Wilson, K. G. (1999). *Acceptance and commitment therapy.* New York: Guilford Press.

Henin, A., Otto, M. W., & Reilly-Harrington, N. A. (2001). Introducing flexibility in manualized treatment: Application of recommended strategies to the cognitive-behavioral treatment of bipolar disorder. *Cognitive and Behavioral Practice, 8,* 317–328.

Hofmann, S. G., & Barlow, D. H. (2002). Social phobia (social anxiety disorder). In D. H. Barlow (Ed.), *Anxiety and its disorders: Second edition: The nature and treatment of anxiety and panic* (pp. 454–476). New York: Guilford Press.

Hope, D. A., Heimberg, R. G., Juster, H. A., & Turk, C. L. (2000). *Managing social anxiety: A cognitive-behavioral therapy approach.* Oxford, UK: Oxford University Press.

Hopko, D. R., Lejuez, C. W., & Hopko, S. D. (2004). Behavioral activation as an intervention for co-existent depressive and anxiety symptoms. *Clinical Case Studies, 3,* 37–48.

Hopko, D. R., Lejuez, C. W., Ruggiero, K. J., & Eifert, G. H. (2003). Contemporary behavioral activation treatments for depression: Procedures, principles, and progress. *Clinical Psychology Review, 23,* 699–717.

Jansson, L., Öst, L.-G., & Jerremalm, A. (1987). Prognostic factors in the behavioral treatment of agoraphobia. *Behavioral Psychotherapy, 15,* 31–44.

Katzelnick, D. J., Kobak, K. A., DeLeire, T., Henk, H. J., Greist, J. H., Davidson, J. R., et al. (2001). Impact of generalized social anxiety disorder in managed care. *American Journal of Psychiatry, 158,* 1999–2007.

Keller, M. B., Lavori, P. W., Mueller, T. I., Endicott, J., Coryell, W., Hirschfeld, R. M., et al. (1992). Time to recovery, chronicity, and levels of psychopathology in major depression: A 5-year prospective follow-up of 431 subjects. *Archives of General Psychiatry, 49,* 809–816.

Kessler, R. C., Stang, P., Wittchen, H. U., Stein, M., & Walters, E. E. (1999). Lifetime comorbidities between social phobia and mood disorders in the U.S. National Comorbidity Survey. *Psychological Medicine, 29,* 555–567.

Kessler, R. C., Stang, P. E., Wittchen, H. U., Ustun, T. B., Roy-Burne, P. P., & Walters, E. E. (1998). Lifetime panic–depression comorbidity in the National Comorbidity Survey. *Archives of General Psychiatry, 55,* 801–808.

Laberge, B., Gauthier, J. G., Cote, G., Plamondon, J., & Cormier, H. J. (1993). Cognitive-behavioral therapy of panic disorder with secondary major depression: A preliminary investigation. *Journal of Consulting and Clinical Psychology, 61,* 1028–1037.

Liebowitz, M. R. (1987). Social phobia. *Modern Problems in Pharmacopsychiatry, 22,* 141–173.

Lincoln, T. M., & Rief, W. (2004). How much do sample characteristics affect the effect size?: An investigation of studies testing the treatment effects for social phobia. *Journal of Anxiety Disorders, 18*(4), 515–529.

Maddock, R. J., & Blacker, K. H. (1991). Response to treatment in panic disorder with associated depression. *Psychopathology, 24,* 1–6.

Magee, W. J., Eaton, W. W., Wittchen, H. U., McGonagle, K. A., & Kessler, R. C. (1996). Agoraphobia, simple phobia, and social phobia in the National Comorbidity Survey. *Archives of General Psychiatry, 53,* 159–168.

Marks, I. M. (1987). *Fears, phobias, and rituals.* New York: Oxford University Press.

Mattick, R. P., & Clarke, J. C. (1998). Development and validation of measures of social phobia scrutiny fear and social interaction anxiety. *Behaviour Research and Therapy, 36,* 455–470.

McElroy, S. L., Altshuler, L. L., Suppes, T., Keck, P. E., Jr., Frye, M. A., Denicoff, K. D., et al. (2001). Axis I psychiatric comorbidity and its relationship to historical illness variables in 288 patients with bipolar disorder. *American Journal of Psychiatry, 158,* 420–426.

McLean, P. D., Woody, S., Taylor, S., & Koch, W. J. (1998). Comorbid panic disorder and major depression: Implications for cognitive-behavioral therapy. *Journal of Consulting and Clinical Psychology, 66,* 240–247.

Mennin, D. S., & Heimberg, R. G. (2000). The impact of comorbid mood and personality disorders in the cognitive-behavioral treatment of panic disorder. *Clinical Psychology Review, 20,* 339–357.

Mills, I., & Salkovskis, P. (1988). Mood and habituation to phobic stimuli. *Behaviour Research and Therapy, 26,* 435–439.

Moscovitch, D. A., Hofmann, S. G., Suvak, M., & In-Albon, T. (2005). Mediation of changes in anxiety and depression during treatment for social phobia. *Journal of Consulting and Clinical Psychology, 75*, 945–952.

Öst, L.-G., Thulin, U., & Ramnerö, J. (2004). Cognitive behavior therapy vs exposure in vivo in the treatment of panic disorder with agoraphobia. *Behaviour Research and Therapy, 42*, 1105–1127.

Otto, M. W., Fava, M., Penava, S. A., Bless, E., Muller, R. T., & Rosenbaum, J. F. (1997). Life event and cognitive predictors of perceived stress before and after treatment for major depression. *Cognitive Therapy and Research, 21*, 409–420.

Otto, M. W., & Gould, R. A. (1996). Maximizing treatment–outcome for panic disorder: Cognitive-behavioral strategies. In M. H. Pollack, M. W. Otto, & J. F. Rosenbaum (Eds.), *Challenges in clinical practice: Pharmacologic and psychosocial strategies* (pp. 113–140). New York: Guilford Press.

Otto, M. W., Jones, J. C., Craske, M. G., & Barlow, D. H. (1996). *Stopping anxiety medication: Panic control therapy for benzodiazepine discontinuation (therapist guide).* Oxford, UK: Oxford University Press.

Otto, M. W., Pollack, M. H., Fava, M., Uccello, R., & Rosenbaum, J. F. (1995). Elevated Anxiety Sensitivity Index scores in patients with major depression: Correlates and changes with antidepressant treatment. *Journal of Anxiety Disorders, 9*, 117–123.

Otto, M. W., Powers, M. B., & Fischman, D. (2005). Emotional exposure in the treatment of substance use disorders: Conceptual model, evidence, and future directions. *Clinical Psychology Review, 25*, 824–839.

Otto, M. W., Simon, N. S., Wisniewski, S. R., Miklowitz, D. J., Kogan, J. N., Reilly-Harrington, N. A., et al. (2006). Prospective 12–month course of bipolar disorder in outpatients with and without comorbid anxiety disorders. *British Journal of Psychiatry, 189*, 20–25.

Persons, J. B., Roberts, N. A., & Zalecki, C. A. (2003). Anxiety and depression change together during treatment. *Behavior Therapy, 34*, 149–163.

Raffa, S. D., White, K. S., & Barlow, D. H. (2004). Feared consequences of panic attacks in panic disorder: A qualitative and quantitative analysis. *Cognitive and Behavioral Therapy, 33*, 199–207.

Reiss, S., Peterson, R. A., Gursky, D. M., & McNally, R. J. (1986). Anxiety sensitivity, anxiety frequency and the prediction of fearfulness. *Behaviour Research and Therapy, 24*, 1–8.

Roy-Byrne, P. P., Stang, P., Wittchen, H. U., Ustun, B., Walters, E. E., & Kessler, R. C. (2000). Lifetime panic–depression comorbidity in the National Comorbidity Survey: Association with symptoms, impairment, course and help-seeking. *British Journal of Psychiatry, 176*, 229–235.

Rubin, H. C., Rapaport, M. H., Levine, B., Gladsjo, J. K., Rabin, A., Auerbach, M., et al. (2000). Quality of well being in panic disorder: The assessment of psychiatric and general disability. *Journal of Affective Disorders, 57*, 217–221.

Rush, J. A., Zimmerman, M., Wisniewski, S. R., Fava, M., Hollon, S. D., Warden, D., et al. (2005). Comorbid psychiatric disorders in depressed outpatients: Demographic and clinical features. *Journal of Affective Disorders, 87*, 43–55.

Schneier, F. R., Johnson, J., Hornig, C. D., Liebowitz, M. R., & Weissman, M. M. (1992). Social phobia: Comorbidity and morbidity in an epidemiologic sample. *Archives of General Psychiatry, 49,* 282–288.

Scholing, A., & Emmelkamp, P. M. G. (1999). Prediction of treatment outcome in social phobia: A cross-validation. *Behaviour Research and Therapy, 37,* 659–670.

Schulberg, H. C., Block, M. R., Madonia, M. J., Scott, C. P., Rodriguez, E., Imber, S. D., et al. (1996). Treating major depression in primary care practice: Eight-month clinical outcomes. *Archives of General Psychiatry, 53,* 913–919.

Shear, M. K., Brown, T. A., Barlow, D. H., Money, R., Sholomskas, D. E., Woods, S. W., et al. (1997). Multicenter collaborative Panic Disorder Severity Scale. *American Journal of Psychiatry, 154,* 1571–1575.

Simon, N. S., Otto, M. W., Wisniewski, S. R., Fossey, M., Sagdayu, K., Frank, E., et al. (2004). Anxiety disorder comorbidity in bipolar disorder: Data from the first 500 STEP-BD participants. *American Journal of Psychiatry, 161,* 2222–2229.

Stein, M. B., Fuetsch, M., Müller, N., Höfler, M., Lieb, R., & Wittchen, H.-U. (2001). Social anxiety disorder and the risk of depression: A prospective community study of adolescents and young adults. *Archives of General Psychiatry, 58,* 251–256.

Tang, T. Z., & DeRubeis, R. J. (1999). Sudden gains and critical sessions in the cognitive-behavioral therapy for depression. *Journal of Consulting and Clinical Psychology, 67,* 894–904.

Teasdale, J. D., Moore, R. G., Hayhurst, H., Pope, M., Williams, S., & Segal, Z. V. (2002). Metacognitive awareness and prevention of relapse in depression: Empirical evidence. *Journal of Consulting and Clinical Psychology, 70,* 275–287.

Telch, M. J. (1988). Combined pharmacological and psychological treatments for panic sufferers. In S. Rachman & J. D. Maser (Eds.), *Panic: Psychological perspectives* (pp. 167–187). Hillsdale, NJ: Erlbaum.

Tsao, J. C. I., Mystkowski, J. L., Zucker, B. G., & Craske, M. G. (2002). Effects of cognitive-behavioral therapy for panic disorder on comorbid conditions: Replication and extension. *Behavior Therapy, 33,* 493–509.

Turner, S. M., Beidel, D. C., Dancu, C. V., & Stanley, M. A. (1989). An empirically derived inventory to measure social fears and anxiety: The Social Phobia and Anxiety Inventory. *Psychological Assessment, 1,* 35–40.

Turner, S. M., Beidel, D. C., Wolff, P. L., Spaulding, S., & Jacob, R. G. (1996). Clinical features affecting treatment outcome in social phobia. *Behaviour Research and Therapy, 34,* 795–804.

Van Ameringen, M., Mancini, C., Styan, G., & Donison, D. (1991). Relationship of social phobia with other psychiatric illness. *Journal of Affective Disorders, 21,* 93–99.

Van Velzen, C. J., Emmelkamp, P. M., & Scholing, A. (1997). The impact of personality disorders on behavioral treatment outcome for social phobia. *Behaviour Research and Therapy, 35,* 889–900.

Vickers, K., & McNally, R. J. (2004) Panic disorder and sucide attempt in the National Comorbidity Survey. *Journal of Abnormal Psychology, 113,* 582–591.

Watson, D., & Friend, R. (1969). Measurement of social–evaluative anxiety. *Journal of Consulting and Clinical Psychology, 33,* 448–457.

Wilson, J. K., & Rapee, R. M. (2005). The interpretation of negative social events in social phobia with versus without comorbid mood disorder. *Journal of Anxiety Disorders, 19,* 245–274.

Woody, S., McLean, P. D., Taylor, S., & Koch, W. (1999). Treatment of major depression in the context of panic disorder. *Journal of Affective Disorders, 53,* 163–174.

9

GENERALIZED ANXIETY DISORDER, OBSESSIVE–COMPULSIVE DISORDER, AND POSTTRAUMATIC STRESS DISORDER

Alisa R. Singer
Keith S. Dobson
David J. A. Dozois

Generalized anxiety disorder (GAD), obsessive–compulsive disorder (OCD), and posttraumatic stress disorder (PTSD) are challenging to treat, especially when these disorders are comorbid with depression. Consequently, clinicians must be familiar with a number of issues specific to each disorder and their comorbid condition, including epidemiological considerations, assessment strategies, case conceptualization, and intervention techniques. In this chapter, we present the challenges of treating patients with these complex conditions and highlight strategies for overcoming barriers. A case example illustrates the various points made throughout this chapter.

COMORBIDITY AMONG DEPRESSION, GAD, OCD, AND PTSD

Clinical and Epidemiological Studies

Epidemiological and clinical studies support a strong association between depression and GAD, OCD, and PTSD. The National Comorbidity Survey (NCS) demonstrated that 58% of primarily depressed patients also experienced an anxiety disorder, estimating the rate of comorbidity between depression and GAD to be 17.2% (Kessler et al., 1996). The NCS found that of those individuals with a primary diagnosis of current GAD, 39% had current major depression and 22% had current dysthymia (Judd et al., 1998). Studies also suggest comorbidity rates of 21–54% between depression and OCD (Abramowitz, 2004). Epidemiological and clinical studies also indicate that up to 56% of individuals have concurrent PTSD and depression, and that as many as 95% of individuals with PTSD have a lifetime history of major depression (Bleich, Koslowsky, Dolev, & Lerer, 1997).

In clinical studies, an association between depression and anxiety is also supported. Brown and Barlow (1992), for example, found that 55% of patients with an anxiety or mood disorder met the diagnostic criteria for an additional concurrent anxiety or depressive disorder. The rate was even higher when lifetime diagnoses were examined. Major depressive disorder (MDD), dysthymia, PTSD, and GAD were the most highly comorbid disorders.

Research suggests that an anxiety disorder is more likely to precede a mood disorder than the reverse (Mineka, Watson, & Clarke, 1998). The risk of MDD within a given year increases significantly during the year after first onset of an anxiety disorder, with an odds ratio (OR) of 62.0 for GAD (Kessler et al., 1996). Similarly, In the case of PTSD, studies suggest that in the majority of cases depression is secondary to the PTSD (Shalev et al., 1998). Retrospective data from the NCS, for example, suggest that 78.4% of individuals with comorbid depression and PTSD experienced clinically significant depression after the onset of the PTSD (Kessler, Sonnega, Bromet, Hughes, & Nelson, 1995). However, a 1-year prospective study showed that depression and PTSD can also occur simultaneously upon exposure to trauma (Shalev et al., 1998). Comorbid depression was present in 44.5% of patients with PTSD at 1 month, and 43.2% of patients at 4 months following the traumatic event.

Comorbidity is also associated with greater severity of symptomatology and functional impairment (Brown, Schulberg, Madonia, Shear, & Houck, 1996). Patients with depression and anxiety, for instance, frequently respond less well to treatment (Nutt, 2000) and accrue more demands on the health care system than do individuals with either disorder alone (Tylee, 2000). Compared to patients with depression alone, individuals with anxious depression also tend to have more severe symptoms and pose a greater risk for suicide (Stein, 2001). Shalev et al. (1998) also found that, relative to individuals with PTSD, those with comorbid depression had more severe symptomatology and lower levels of functioning.

Diagnostic Features

Diagnostically, GAD, PTSD, and OCD share a number of common features with depression. Repetitive, negative thinking is common to both depression and GAD. The repetitive thinking in GAD is in the form of worry, the content of which typically regards possible negative outcomes for future events (Dozois, Dobson, & Westra, 2004). In depression, the repetitive thinking is in the form of "rumination" which has been defined as behaviors and thoughts that focus the individual's attention on his/her depressive symptoms, and the implications and consequences of these symptoms (Nolen-Hoeksema, 1991). Individuals tend to negatively appraise themselves, their feelings, behaviors, situations, life stresses, and ability to cope. Depression and OCD also share the common feature of negative repetitive thinking. However, the main distinction is that the obsessions are "ego-dystonic" in OCD, which means that the thoughts are mood-incongruent and cause the individual distress, whereas the negative thinking is generally mood-congruent in depression. PTSD and MDD also have a common feature, in that exposure to a traumatic event or significant stressor is associated with the onset of both disorders (Shalev et al., 1998). The central feature of PTSD is that the symptomatology develops following an acute, extreme traumatic event. Similarly, in depression, negative life events have been implicated in the onset of depressive episodes; however, the accumulative effect of several negative life events or of chronic stress has also been associated with depression onset (Rowa, Beiling, & Segal, 2005).

One important issue concerns whether comorbidity among depressive and anxiety disorders should be diagnosed as distinct entities or as a mixed anxiety–depressive disorder (Zinbarg & Barlow, 1991). At present, there is a paucity of research to support mixed anxiety–depression as a distinct diagnostic category that would better account for the symptom picture, although it currently exists in the section on criteria sets and axes for further study in the text revision of the fourth edition of the *Diagnostic and Statistical Manual of Mental Disorders* (DSM-IV-TR; American Psychiatric Association, 2000). In addition, there is literature to suggest that the anxiety and mood disorders share common features, as well as features that are unique from one another (cf. Brown, Chorpita, & Barlow, 1998; Dozois et al., 2004). Specific diagnostic issues are beyond the scope of this chapter, but we note that diagnostic overlap continues to be debated. However, for treatment, there are a number of advantages for conceptualizing these disorders as separate entities. A DSM-IV diagnosis can not only aid in the communication with other professionals but also assist in the identification of the appropriate scientific base regarding the disorder and its treatment options.

The Effect of Comorbidity on the Process and Outcome of Cognitive Therapy

Most of the literature regarding cognitive therapy (CT) of GAD, OCD, and PTSD describes treatments in which the disorders are considered in isolation. Most well-controlled, randomized clinical trials have focused on "pure" cases of anxiety or depression and have shown promising outcomes in the treatment of these conditions (Chambless & Ollendick, 2001). Yet the samples utilized in the empirically supported treatment literature include few (if any) participants who have comorbid depression and anxiety (e.g., Ladouceur et al., 2000).

Few researchers have examined the impact of coexisting anxiety disorders on CT for depression, and studies that do exist have yielded conflicting results (Rowa et al., 2005). Some studies have investigated the general role of comorbid anxiety disorders in treatment outcome in depression. In a study of a manualized group therapy, in comparison to patients without comorbid disorders, depressed individuals with comorbid anxiety presented with more severe depression at pretest and continued to exhibit residual symptoms at posttest, suggesting that comorbidity contributed to poorer therapeutic effectiveness (Gelhart & King, 2001).

In a study of an individualized case formulation approach to CT, Persons, Roberts, and Zalecki (2003) investigated whether both anxiety and depressive symptoms would improve over the course of treatment. Both anxious and depressive symptoms improved by at least 50% or more in 31.6% of patients. However, less optimistic results were that 35.1% of patients showed improvement on only one set of symptoms, and 33.3% of patients showed no improvement on either anxiety or depression.

There is some preliminary research on the impact of depression in the treatment of specific anxiety disorders. In one study, patients with OCD, who were initially in the severe range of depression, showed significantly lower rates of improvement with standard treatment for OCD (exposure and response prevention), than did individuals with no, mild, or moderate depression (Abramowitz, Franklin, Street, Kozak, & Foa, 2000). Other studies indicate that nontargeted depressive symptoms improve as a result of treatment aimed at GAD and PTSD. Meta-analytic data indicate that depressive symptoms also improve with CT aimed at treating GAD (cf. Chambless & Gillis, 1993). In addition, depressive symptoms appear to improve following CT for PTSD (Ehlers, Clark, Hackmann, McManus, & Fennell, 2005).

Given that comorbid depression and anxiety is associated with increased symptom severity and functional impairment, treatment of the comorbid patient is especially challenging. As such, we contend that the strategy for CT of comorbid conditions should involve a comprehensive and idiographic approach to assessment, followed by a case conceptualization that is tailored to the individual patient.

ASSESSMENT OF COMORBIDITY OF GAD, OCD, AND PTSD

Due to the high rate of current co-occurrence between depression and anxiety, it is *always* important for the clinician to inquire about anxiety disorders when interviewing patients who present for treatment of depression. However, the need to inquire is accentuated when "soft signs" are present. For example, a patient with a history of abuse would prompt a clinician to inquire about PTSD. A history of unreasonable fears, such as those related to contamination, would indicate the need to screen for OCD. A patient who repeatedly discusses worries regarding the future may prompt the clinician to inquire about GAD.

Due to time pressures of managed care, an assessment of comorbidity that includes both diagnostic precision and the information needed to develop a treatment plan likely requires more than one or two assessment sessions. It is important first to establish that the individual meets, for example, the DSM-IV diagnostic criteria (American Psychiatric Association, 2000). The incorporation of a structured diagnostic interview, such as the Structured Clinical Interview for DSM-IV Axis I disorders (SCID; First, Gibbon, Spitzer, & Williams, 1996) or the Anxiety Disorders Interview Schedule for DSM-IV (ADIS-IV; Di Nardo, Brown, & Barlow, 1994), can assist in a thorough assessment and is generally more reliable than a clinical interview in diagnosing comorbidity (Zimmerman & Mattia, 1999). One possible reason for the poor comorbidity detection rate in unstructured interviews is that clinicians often focus on the chief complaint and neglect to broaden the assessment to include other areas of functioning.

The temporal relationship between the depression and the comorbid anxiety disorder ought to be assessed to establish primary and secondary diagnoses. A longitudinal history is critical in understanding the development of the comorbid conditions and assists in developing a case formulation. It is important to assess the age of onset for each condition and the context in which each set of symptoms developed. In addition, it is important to inquire about early childhood experiences and traumas, as well as relationship and work/school history. This information helps the clinician understand factors that may have fostered the belief system that underlies the patient's psychological vulnerability, and leads to the development of a CT treatment plan.

The clinician should also gather a thorough list of the patient's reported anxiety and depressive symptoms. From this list, the clinician can inquire about how the anxiety and depressive symptoms relate to each other, which aids in understanding the patient's situation, to guide choices for the selection of psychotherapy and medication if needed (Belzer & Schneier, 2004). It has been recommended that clinicians inquire about the relationship between the symptoms (Belzer & Schneier, 2004). Did one set of symptoms clearly emerge, or was onset of both conditions simultaneous? For example, one patient reported that his OCD contamination fears emerged first, then the depression followed as a result of the impairments caused by the OCD. Do symptoms wax and wane concurrently? Individuals with comorbid depression and PTSD may report that as the severity of intrusive thoughts increases, they notice that their mood lowers and they begin to feel more hopeless about their future. Does one symptom seem to lead to the other or does each seem to exist on its own? What role do stressors play in the fluctuation or recurrence of each set of symptoms over time? For example, an individual with comorbid GAD and depression may report a tendency to ruminate about past mistakes but when engaged in a future-oriented task, worry about potential negative outcomes and his/her ability to cope. In addition, we recommend that clinicians assess for maladaptive coping strategies, including the abuse of substances.

The clinician can enhance rapport with the patient while also gathering information that assists in the formulation and treatment plan by inquiring about the patient's own perception of the etiological relationship between his/her anxiety and depression (Belzer & Schneier, 2004). Such information can assist clinician and patient in establishing which disorder is the most distressing and ought to be the focus, at least initially, of treatment.

In addition to interview methods, numerous self-report measures are available for assessing general psychopathology and specifically GAD, OCD, and PTSD. The findings from self-report can be integrated with the results from a structured or clinical interview, as well as with other depression-related self-report inventories. There are two major advantages to incorporating quantitative measures of the severity of symptoms. First, pretreatment measures of the severity of symptoms can be used to gauge which disorder is more severe and ought to be the initial focus of treatment. Even though one disorder may be temporally primary, a secondary disorder that is of greater severity and more distressing needs to be managed before treating the primary condition. Alternatively, the clinician may choose to target the less severe problem that may lead to the quickest success, thus increasing patient motivation for addressing more severe difficulties later. Another advantage is that self-report inventories can be administered repeatedly over the course of therapy to track changes in both conditions and to monitor treatment progress. A detailed list of the available inventories is beyond the scope of the chapter (see Antony & Barlow, 2002; Nezu, Ronan, Meadows, & McClure, 2000).

To aid in treatment planning, it may also be necessary to gather information regarding the cognitive and behavioral features of the disorders. Campbell and Brown (2002) suggest that individuals with GAD may engage in habitual "worry behaviors," such as making extensive and detailed lists, seeking reassurance from loved ones to ascertain their safety, and forgetting to do important tasks. These behaviors may relieve the anxiety in the short term by creating a greater sense of control over feared outcomes, but they serve to maintain the anxious belief that something terrible will happen. Such behaviors prevent the patient from learning that these fears are unfounded. Also, avoidance can increase depression because of a reduction in reinforcement secondary to the avoidance (e.g., an individual who avoids activities that involve other people fails to receive positive reinforcement from others, which leads to the emergence of depression). Thus, it is important to ask patients about the behaviors that they do to reduce their anxiety. Individuals with GAD also tend to have time-management and problem-solving deficits that result from, as well as exacerbate, their worry and tension. They may worry so much about a problem that they fail to engage in the tasks needed to fulfill other obligations. The clinician may need to ask whether worry ever interferes with the ability to complete tasks. To inquire about problem-solving deficits, the clinician can ask whether worrying leads to effective solutions to problems, or whether the patient has other ways of solving problems when they arise. "Meta-worry" (Wells & Carter, 1999) is a cognitive process that involves appraisals of the functions and consequences of worry. An individual with GAD may hold positive and negative beliefs about worrying. Understanding the beliefs that an individual holds about worry is important for treatment planning. For example, it would be difficult to attempt to reduce worry if a patients holds illogical positive beliefs about the benefits of worrying.

For OCD, it may be necessary to collect detailed information regarding the specific cues that cause the patient's distress, patterns of avoidance, rituals, and feared consequences (Foa & Franklin, 2001). Information is also needed regarding the environmental cues (e.g., bathroom floors, toilets, going to bed) and the internal threat cues (e.g., images, impulses, or abstract thoughts) that trigger compulsions. In addition, it is important to gather details pertaining to the feared consequence(s). For example, a patient may perform washing rituals due to a fear that someone else will become ill. It is also important to investigate the strength of the individual's belief in the obsessions and compulsions, and the degree to which he/she recognizes that these thoughts and behavior are irrational. It is also essential to assess the degree to which a patient feels responsible for his/her thoughts (Salkovskis, 1985). Finally, the clinician ought to gather information regarding the patient's patterns of avoidance, both subtle and obvious.

PTSD has a number of features that warrant assessment consideration. Avoidance, shame, and embarrassment are common features in PTSD, and many patients are reluctant to discuss the details of the trauma they endured. Thus, it is important that the clinician be especially mindful of the potential to "retraumatize" during a detailed assessment of the patient's experience (Litz, Miller, Ruef, & McTeague, 2002). It is especially recommended that clinicians create an interpersonal context of safety and trust during the assessment of PTSD. Therapists should pay attention to emotional reactions during the discussion of trauma and gather only the information that is needed to establish a diagnosis. Because incompletion of treatment is common (Ehlers et al., 2005), building trust and rapport with patients with PTSD increases the likelihood that they will return to treatment.

Because of the complexity of comorbidity, self-monitoring homework may be especially useful in the assessment and treatment planning stages. At the end of the initial assessment session, the clinician can assign homework in which the patient is asked to rate depression and anxiety levels three times per day. The patient's situational details, and any feelings and thoughts that occur, can also be monitored at each recording. By reviewing the patterns of recordings, the clinician can determine the relative severity of each condition, and this information can assist him/her in both understanding the nature of the comorbidity and determining how best to treat it. In addition, the relationship between symptoms can be investigated in a detailed manner, leading to a better understanding of the situation for both the patient and therapist.

CASE CONCEPTUALIZATION OF COMORBIDITY OF GAD, OCD, AND PTSD

The case conceptualization of comorbidity is crucial in treatment. The approach described in this section is adapted from Persons and Davidson (2001). The case formulation needs to be modified to account for comorbidity between depression and GAD, OCD, or PTSD.

For the patient with comorbidity, the problem list likely includes difficulties related to both depression and the anxiety disorder. Some of these problems may result from the depression, the anxiety, or both disorders. The patient's mood, cognitive, behavioral, situational, and interpersonal difficulties need to be described in concrete terms. For GAD, OCD, and PTSD, avoidance may be a particularly prominent problem. Patients with GAD may use worry as a way to avoid more salient emotional topics (Borkovec, 1994), whereas patients with OCD may avoid stimuli that trigger their obsessions and compulsions, and patients with PTSD may avoid situations that trigger their intrusive thoughts related to the traumatic event. Unique problems for patients with GAD might include uncontrollable worry, muscle tension, interpersonal problems as a result of reassurance-seeking behavior, time-management problems or poor problem-solving skills.

In the case of comorbidity, a working hypothesis needs to adapt cognitive theory to describe the relationship between problems on the patient's individual problem list. A working hypothesis based on a cognitive theory describes the relationship between the precipitants and the schemas (core beliefs about self, world, and others) and processes that, when activated, led to the disorders. The working hypothesis statement is an attempt to understand how the comorbid conditions developed and relate to one another, and it is continually refined and reformulated throughout treatment as additional information is gathered.

The case formulation also includes a postulation of how early childhood–adulthood experiences may have contributed to a psychological vulnerability that, when activated by life stressors, led to the emergence of each condition. Early experiences of uncontrollability may represent the psychological vulnerability for anxiety disorders, particularly for GAD (Barlow, 1991). Borkovec (1994) has suggested that childhood histories of psychosocial trauma (e.g., death of a parent, physical/sexual abuse) and insecure attachment to primary caregivers may be childhood origins that lead to the development of a psychological vulnerability for GAD. For PTSD, prior negative experiences and traumas may exert influence and give additional negative meaning to the traumatic event (Ehlers & Clark, 2000). Clinicians should consider life experiences when developing a working hypothesis about a case of comorbidity.

Barlow (1991) suggested that the onset of depression in the context of a primary anxiety disorder is dependent on the extent of one's psychological vulnerability, the severity of the current stressor, and the coping mechanisms available. Comorbidity arises when psychological vulnerability is high, the current stressor is of greater severity, and there are few coping mechanisms. It has been postulated that "pure" anxiety is the result of perceptions of uncertainty and helplessness, whereas comorbid anxiety and depression arise when helplessness is prolonged and the individual eventually gives up, loses hope, and becomes depressed (Mineka & Nugent, 1995). To illustrate this concept, Barlow (1991, p. 14) suggested that, in the face of life stress, the anxious individual thinks, "That terrible event is not my fault but it may happen again, and I may not be able to cope with it but I've got to give it a try," whereas the anxious–depressed individual might think, "That terrible event may happen again and I won't be able to cope with it, and it's probably my fault anyway so there's really nothing I can do."

The case conceptualization should also include core beliefs that are hypothesized to lead to the manifestation of the disorders. It has been theorized that pathological worry in GAD is associated with perceptions that the world is a threatening place, and that one will not be able to cope with or control future negative events (Brown, O'Leary, & Barlow, 2001). A number of obsessive–compulsive beliefs have also been identified; in particular, individuals with OCD tend to have an inflated sense of responsibility for their intrusive thoughts (Salkovskis, 1985). In addition, beliefs about the over-importance of thoughts, such as the belief that thoughts are morally equivalent to actions, otherwise known as thought–action fusion, may be present (Rachman, 1993). Metacognitive beliefs (i.e., beliefs about the importance of controlling one's thoughts) have also been proposed to be a core dysfunction in OCD (Clark & Purdon, 1993). Beliefs in relation to perfectionism and excessive concern over mistakes have also been implicated in OCD (Frost & Steketee, 1997). Ehlers and Clark (2000) proposed that individuals with PTSD hold dysfunctional external beliefs ("The world is a dangerous place") and internal beliefs (the view that one's capability, acceptability, or survivability has been threatened).

In addition to specific cognitive content, most anxiety disorders also involve a process of attentional bias, which is thought to maintain the disorder (Clark, 1999); thus, this may also need to be considered in the development of a case formulation of comorbidity. "Low tolerance of uncertainty," defined as the way in which an individual perceives and responds to information in uncertain or ambiguous situations, is also a central feature in GAD (Dugas, Gagnon, Ladouceur, & Freeston, 1998) and is thought to exacerbate the "what if . . . ?" thought processes that arise in GAD. Individuals with OCD tend to conclude that situations are dangerous based on the absence of evidence for safety, but fail to conclude from information about the absence of danger that a situation is safe. Rituals are performed in attempt to reduce the likelihood of harm but never provide evidence of safety, and therefore, need to be repeated (Foa & Franklin, 2001). In addition, patients with PTSD may overgeneralize from the original event, consequently, perceiving a range of normal events as more dangerous than they really are (Ehlers & Clark, 2000).

It is especially helpful to explain in a manner that the patient understands that the two conditions exist and how they may have developed. The case conceptualization should be discussed in a collaborative way to foster trust and rapport, by eliciting feedback from the patient regarding his/her own perceptions of the problems. From the problem list generated by the clinician and patient, goals for treatment and a treatment plan can be derived.

TREATMENT OF DEPRESSION COMORBID WITH GAD, OCD, AND PTSD

In the treatment of comorbidity, the clinician has to choose whether to treat the disorders simultaneously or sequentially. Few guidelines exist for the treatment of comorbidity between depression and GAD, OCD, and PTSD, although it has been suggested that depression should be treated prior to treatment of OCD (Abramowitz, 2004). In addition, results from treatment outcome research suggest that if the primary anxiety disorder is treated, depressive symptoms do improve (i.e., Ehlers et al., 2005).

Irrespective of whether the disorders are treated simultaneously or sequentially, it is important to monitor both conditions consistently throughout treatment to gauge the progress of therapy and to reconsider the plan if treatment progress is not optimal. We recommend that whether to treat the disorders concurrently or sequentially be decided on a case-by-case basis, based on the case formulation. For example, if the assessment suggests that the anxiety disorder is primary and of greater severity than the depression, then incorporating CT protocols developed for the treatment of GAD (i.e., Brown et al., 2001), OCD (i.e., Salkovskis, 1999), or PTSD (i.e., Ehlers & Clark, 2000) is warranted.

Modifying Standard CT for Depression and Comorbid GAD, OCD, and PTSD

If the clinician determines that the depression should be treated first, we recommend that he/she administer standard CT for depression, while remaining cognizant of the potential effects that the comorbid anxiety disorder may have on treatment. If the comorbid condition negatively impacts treatment progress, then the interventions may need to be modified.

To treat comorbid depression, it is recommended that behavioral activation be emphasized, with the goals of decreasing depressed mood and increasing hopefulness and motivation for therapy. It is important that the clinician first provide a conceptualization of the link between behavior and feelings, emphasizing the role of avoidance in maintaining depressed mood. Techniques such as goal setting and scheduling of pleasurable and mastery activity can facilitate self-activation. In the first phase of treatment, patients are asked to monitor their daily activities and mood, to increase their awareness of the connection between behaviors and feelings. Next, patients are asked to select and to schedule alternative behaviors, which can include pleasurable activities (e.g., taking a bath, engaging in hobbies) and mastery activities (e.g., washing dishes, paying bills). Patients are then encouraged to try the new behaviors and to observe the effect on their mood. In recent years, a treatment for depression that emphasizes primarily behavioral activation (with less emphasis on cognitive restructuring) has been developed and refined (Martell, Addis, & Jacobson, 2001). A self-help workbook is also available for the general public (Addis & Martell, 2004). Once the depression has decreased, and if patient and therapist mutually agree, the therapy can then shift to treatment of the anxiety disorder.

When conducting standard CT for depression, the therapist can anticipate that an individual with comorbid GAD might be prone to overestimate the likelihood of a negative outcome in an impending behavioral experiment designed to treat depression. The therapist should pay attention to "what if . . . ?" thinking when discussing behavioral experiments with a patient with GAD. It is important to use Socratic questioning to explore the patient's catastrophic beliefs about the anticipated outcome of a behavioral experiment and to challenge the patient's estimate of the likelihood that a negative outcome will occur. It is also important to generate possible coping strategies and solutions in the event that a negative outcome occurs. It may also be helpful to ask the patient to make predictions and to monitor the outcome of a behavioral experiment to determine whether his/her negative predictions do indeed come true.

In the case of PTSD, clinicians may need to slow the pace of therapy, because patients may be at risk of dissociation when discussing traumatic events. It will likely be difficult to use cognitive restructuring techniques designed to challenge the content of cognitions (e.g., "What is the evidence for [a negative event?]?"), because these patients' histories include exposure to a traumatic event; thus, they may have real-life evidence to support their cognitive distortions (e.g., a rape victim may believe that "all men are dangerous"). When engaging in cognitive restructuring, it is important for the clinician not only to acknowledge the evidence from a traumatic event but also to assist the patient in acknowledging evidence that does not support the cognitive distortions (e.g., "It is true that I am the survivor of rape, but there are men in this world who are not dangerous"). Furthermore, it may be more helpful to engage in interventions designed to modify the process of thinking, for example, by exploring the advantages and disadvantages of holding onto a particular thought and gently guiding the patient toward more helpful way of thinking.

When treating depression in patients who also have comorbid obsessions, it is also recommended that clinicians use cognitive interventions designed to alter cognitive processes rather than challenge the content of patients' thinking. Patients with obsessions, in particular, need psychoeducation regarding the lack of dangerousness associated with obsessions, because their catastrophic interpretations of the obsessional thoughts or images lead to increased anxiety and distress. Metacognitive beliefs (i.e., beliefs about the importance of controlling one's thoughts) have also been proposed to be a core dysfunction in OCD (Clark & Purdon, 1993). In addition, deficits in metacognitive processing, or thinking about thinking, have been implicated in both depression and GAD; thus, interventions designed to increase metacognitive awareness and control may effectively treat both the anxiety and the depression. For example, monitoring of automatic thoughts and identifying common themes can be helpful in increasing awareness of thought processes. In addition, helping patients to generate a list of metacognitive statements (e.g., "Thoughts are just thoughts and I do not have to pay attention to them") may also aid in reducing distress associated with worry, obsessions, and depressive thinking.

In the next section, we discuss specific interventions to treat the anxiety disorder that may be needed as adjuncts to standard CT for depression.

Education

Psychoeducation regarding the nature of anxiety, including the physiological, behavioral and cognitive aspects (Brown et al., 2001), is likely to be beneficial. Patients may express that they are aware that they have disorders in addition to depression, but they lack knowledge regarding the disorders. Thus, it is recommended that clinicians name the conditions and present a model that describes how the disorders are related. Furthermore, it is important to provide psychoeducation for the treatment rationale.

Behavioral Interventions

To address behavioral avoidance, the addition of exposure interventions may be especially helpful. For example, in the case of PTSD, patients have difficulty retrieving a complete memory of the trauma, although they involuntarily experience recurrent thoughts and images of the event in a very vivid and emotional way. PTSD is believed to arise because of the poor elaboration and incorporation of the memory of the trauma into autobiographical memory, leading to poor voluntary recall and cueing of intrusions by stimuli that may be temporarily associated with the trauma: thus, one target of PTSD treatment is the patient's systematic exposure to the memory of the event through recall with a therapist (Ehlers & Clark, 2000). *In vivo* exposure is also used to target avoidance of the current life triggers of PTSD symptoms (Ehlers & Clark, 2000) and to obtain data to disconfirm the misappraisals.

CT for OCD, called exposure and response prevention, includes prolonged exposure to obsessional cues, coupled with procedures to prevent rituals (Foa & Franklin, 2001). Repeated prolonged exposure to the feared thoughts and situations is believed to provide information that disconfirms the mistaken associations and promotes habituation. Exposure is conducted gradually as the patient tackles situations that are increasingly more distressing. The efficacy of exposure plus response prevention has been demonstrated in numerous treatment outcome studies (for a review, see Chambless & Ollendick, 2001).

An intervention also used for GAD, known as worry exposure, involves identifying two or three spheres of worry that are ordered hierarchically. Patients are then instructed to hold the catastrophic images in their minds for 20–30 minutes, then to generate as many alternative outcomes as they can to the worst possible outcome (Brown et al., 2001).

Avoidance can also take the form of safety behaviors that prevent or minimize the feared catastrophe (Clark, 1999). For example, a car accident survivor, extremely vigilant for possible dangerous situations, might drive slowly or avoid crowded streets (Ehlers & Clark, 2000). An individual with GAD may seek reassurance from loved ones regarding their safety. Therapy can also target safety behaviors by teaching the patient to enter the feared situation, while purposefully not using the safety behaviors. To target arousal and physiological symptoms, relaxation training and breathing retraining might also be incorporated.

Cognitive Interventions

Cognitive restructuring can be used to modify dysfunctional cognitions relevant to the anxiety disorder (e.g., faulty appraisals of threat from intrusive thoughts), as well as those relevant to depression (e.g., "I can't ever be happy again"). Thus, patients learn to use the same skills to reduce both their depressive and anxious thinking (Abramowitz, 2004). Individuals with anxiety problems often overestimate the probability and severity of various threats (risks), and underestimate their ability to cope with them (resources) (Beck & Emery, 1985). Thus, the goal of cognitive restructuring is to help patients to develop healthier and more evidence-based thoughts—to help them to adjust the imbalance between perceived risk and resource (Beck & Emery, 1985).

Specific cognitive distortions may need to be identified and challenged through cognitive restructuring. For example, common distortions in GAD include "probability overestimation" and "catastrophic thinking." To counter catastrophic thoughts, patients are asked to imagine the worst possible feared outcome actually happening, then to evaluate critically the severity of the impact of the event. Cognitive restructuring in the treatment of comorbid depression and PTSD may need to target the negative appraisals of the traumatic event and its sequelae, which lead to a sense of recurrent threat.

Cognitive interventions can also be applied to the core beliefs that underlie depression, anxiety disorders, or both. For example, standard cognitive restructuring interventions can be applied to test the validity of (and modify) beliefs about one's inflated responsibility for intrusive thoughts, thought–action fusion, perfectionism, and excessive concern over mistakes that may be present in patients with OCD. Cognitive restructuring may be needed to address dysfunctional beliefs in patients with PTSD regarding the dangerousness of the world and their capability, acceptability, or survivability. Finally, cognitive restructuring may also need to address the positive or negative beliefs about worry that are present in patients with GAD, as well as the core beliefs that they have little or no control over perceived threats.

Finally, individuals with comorbid disorders may present with a number of problems related to interpersonal or occupational functioning. Therapy may need to include problem-solving interventions designed to identify a problem, generate a list of potential solutions, choose from the list of alternatives, and implement the solution to the problem (D'Zurilla & Nezu, 2001).

Adjunct Therapies

Treatment with psychotropic medication may also be needed in conjunction with CBT for patients with comorbid depression and anxiety disorders (Belzer & Schneier, 2004). The medication classes of selective serotonin reuptake inhibitors (SSRIs) or selective norepinephrine reuptake inhibitors (SNRIs) may have potential efficacy with both depressive and anxious symptoms; thus, monotherapy is recommended (Belzer & Schneier, 2004). In particular, medication is recommended for treating comorbid OCD and depression, and it is also important that the depressive symptoms be addressed sufficiently prior to commencing exposure and response prevention (Abramowitz, 2004). Patients may need to be encouraged to stay on a medication, even if they fail to see improvement in their anxiety symptoms. For example, OCD has been shown to have a delayed response to psychotropic medication, and there is some evidence of the need for higher SSRI doses for superior efficacy with OCD (Belzer & Schneier, 2004).

CASE ILLUSTRATION

Referral Route and Presenting Problems

Mary, a 45-year-old, unemployed European American woman, was referred to an outpatient service by her psychiatrist for CT for depression. At the time of the initial assessment, Mary tended to make vague statements that lacked emotional details, although she appeared visibly upset and tearful. She reported feeling depressed and hopeless for the last 3 years. She requested therapy for her depression. Based on the results from a SCID-I interview, Mary met MDD criteria (depressed mood, lack of motivation, appetite disturbance, difficulty concentrating, and feelings of worthlessness). She denied having suicidal ideation. She also met the criteria for PTSD (e.g., recurrent thoughts, avoidance of thoughts and people, diminished range of affect, irritability, and sleep disturbance) in response to a hostage taking that had taken place 3 years earlier. Her score on the PTSD Checklist (PCL; Weathers, Litz, Huska, & Keane, 1991) indicated that she met the criteria for PTSD. A score of 33 on the Beck Depression Inventory–II (BDI-II; Beck, Steer, & Brown, 1996) suggested that she was experiencing severe depressive symptoms. Mary was taking Effexor at the time of the initial interview.

Current Situation

Mary lived with her common-law partner of 4 years. Her partner was employed as a store manager. Mary has sporadic contact with her 25-year-old son from her first marriage. Other than seeing her immediate family, Mary reports significant social isolation. She reports that "everything" is a stress, due to her tendency to avoid problems and encounters with other people. She also indicates that she is under significant financial stress, and that her partner recently declared bankruptcy. Mary also avoids conversations with other people due to potential interpersonal conflict. Throughout her day, thoughts of the robbery enter her mind, but she tries to suppress them through distraction methods, such as listening to the radio. She tends to ruminate about the effect that the robbery has had on her life and often feels hopeless about the future.

Relevant History

Mary was held up at gunpoint 3 years earlier, while working as a bank teller. During the event, she responded with intense fear and helplessness, because she felt physically threatened. The robbery was interrupted by police, who later determined that the weapon was in fact a toy gun. In the months following the incident, Mary described symptoms of reexperiencing the event, avoidance, and arousal that continued to worsen. One year later, she went to the emergency department complaining of an exacerbation of depression precipitated by the criminal proceedings against the assailant. Mary was discharged with unremitted depressive and posttraumatic stress symptoms that have persisted for the past 3 years.

Distal History

Mary, born and raised in England, was the third of five children. Her father worked as a store manager, and her mother was a homemaker. She described a happy childhood, and that she got along well with her parents and siblings. In her elementary years, Mary described a period of poor academic performance. However, in later years, her grades improved significantly and she eventually graduated from a 2-year college program in retail. Mary worked in several management positions until the age of 41, when she was let go from her company due to downsizing. Unable to obtain employment in retail, Mary began working at a bank. At the time of the robbery, she was under considerable financial strain due to her child care responsibilities. Mary was married for 4 years to her first husband, but the marriage ended due to his infidelity. She met her current common-law partner at the age of 37. She described their relationship as mistrustful, due to an affair that he had had 4 years earlier and he had agreed to end.

Formulation/Working Hypothesis

Mary's relationship history, including a failed marriage, may have fostered her beliefs regarding mistrust of others and her vulnerability to harm. Furthermore, at the time of the robbery, she was under financial strain, which may have further threatened Mary's view of herself and led her to question her own competence. This conflict between her expectation and life circumstances may have led to a heightened general arousal even prior to the robbery. The belief that others are mistrustful and that she was vulnerable to harm, along with the concomitant anxiety, likely predisposed Mary to react in intense fear to the perceived threat during the hostage incident. The hostage taking likely reinforced her beliefs about mistrusting others; thus, posttraumatic stress symptoms emerged, including recurrent thoughts of the incident. To cope with her symptoms, Mary generally has avoided other people and situations where conflict with others might occur, which has resulted in significant isolation. Since the trauma, Mary has also experienced a number of negative life events, including bankruptcy and a decline in her relationship with her children. These failures may have led her to doubt her abilities. To the extent that the core belief that she is a failure exists, it may predispose Mary to depressed mood and feelings of worthlessness and hopelessness. Her pattern of behavioral avoidance has likely led to an unremitting course of depressive and posttraumatic symptoms.

Treatment Plan

It was decided that individual CT interventions would address Mary's depressive symptoms, avoidance behaviors, as well as her sense of mistrust of others and vulnerability to harm. Initially, treatment was intended to focus on Mary's depression, which she reported as her primary concern. The clinician would initially address her depressive symptoms with behavioral activation interventions to increase Mary's social involvements and pleasurable activities. At the beginning of treatment, the clinician decided that, should posttraumatic stress symptoms arise as Mary became more behaviorally active, therapy would also focus on imaginal exposure to the traumatic event, as well as *in vivo* exposure to her daily triggers. Cognitive interventions would also be employed to treat the PTSD by helping Mary to challenge her negative perceptions of her own behavior during the event, its sequelae, and any self-blame or shame that might exist. The clinician anticipated that Mary's avoidance of emotionally salient material would be a possible road block to treatment; thus, the pace of therapy would be adjusted to increase rapport and trust. Because Mary's current life circumstances (financial and family problems) also had the potential to become issues in therapy, the clinician would employ problem-solving interventions if needed.

Treatment Interventions and Outcome

Mary completed 14 cognitive-behavioral therapy sessions. In the first treatment session, the clinician provided feedback in a collaborative manner regarding the assessment and diagnostic findings. Mary agreed with the conceptualization, and she and her clinician discussed her goals for therapy. Mary reported that her main objective was to be less depressed. The clinician suggested that therapy begin with an increase in Mary's social involvements and pleasurable activities. A schedule of pleasurable activities was generated, which included walking her dog, going to the store, and making phone calls to friends. Mary was reluctant, because socialization triggered PTSD symptoms, but she was hopeful about the potential benefits. Her homework was to keep a daily record of her activities and to monitor her mood and anxiety three times per day.

By the third session, it became clear that the treatment of Mary's depression was affected by her PTSD symptoms. She had attempted to go to public places, which led to initial feelings of being overwhelmed and subsequent feelings of despair. Mary also expressed her concerns about the helpfulness of therapy. The therapist made the decision that behavioral activation interventions were negatively impacted by intrusive thoughts and avoidance related to PTSD; thus, treatment needed to shift to PTSD.

The subsequent sessions of Mary's treatment involved a protocol of PTSD treatment, adapted from Ehlers and Clark (2000). Initial sessions included psychoeducation regarding the nature of PTSD and its treatment. A strong rationale was provided for the treatment of PTSD and the key element of thinking about the trauma more and discussing it in detail. In addition, thoughts of the trauma were triggered by current events, because the details of the event have become associated in Mary's mind with terror. Thus, neutral stimuli, such as public places, banks, and other people, triggered her anxiety. An important component of treatment included exposure to both the memory of events and current triggers.

Some sessions were devoted to relaxation and breathing exercises to reduce her state of arousal, and she reported benefits. Two sessions focused on reliving the experience of the traumatic event by recalling the details of it. Mary was reluctant to recall the details of the robbery; however, the solid rationale for treatment increased her willingness. As recommended by Ehlers and Clark (2000), she was instructed to recall the event in her mind's eye, making the image as realistic as possible, and included her thoughts and feelings about what was happening. She was asked to recall the event in the present tense. The therapist asked probing questions to help Mary stay with the memory. Cognitive restructuring was used to identify and discuss problematic thoughts and beliefs regarding the trauma.

The remaining sessions focused on *in vivo* exposure to the real-life triggers of Mary's anxiety. A hierarchical list of triggers was generated in session that included loud voices, customer service lines, and interpersonal situations in which tension may occur. Each week Mary chose an exposure situation of moderate difficulty to try on her own. Instructions were provided about the length of time she should spend in the situation, as well as coping strategies (e.g., breathing exercises, positive coping statements) for dealing with her anxiety. A record form was developed to assist Mary with this task. For example, Mary's first exercise was to return an item she had purchased from a store. Because she tended to avoid listening to strangers out of fear they would say something harmful to her, Mary was instructed to pay attention to the voices she heard while standing in line. Each week exposure was reviewed and any troubleshooting addressed. Mary began entering situations that she had previously avoided, including volunteering at a market, which resulted in a significant improvement in her depression.

The next stage of therapy was intended to address Mary's dysfunctional core beliefs, but treatment was terminated prematurely, because the robber's prison sentence ended and he was released. Mary and her common-law partner moved to another city due to her fear of encountering the perpetrator. At discharge, Mary's anxiety and depressive symptoms had improved with the treatment focused on her PTSD. At discharge, her BDI-II score was 23, suggesting that Mary was experiencing moderate depression. Her score on the PCL was 45, suggesting that she continued to experience some symptoms of PTSD but she did meet the criteria for the disorder.

CONCLUSIONS

In this chapter, we have reviewed the treatment of comorbid depression and GAD, PTSD, and OCD. Epidemiological and clinical studies support a strong association between these conditions, yet there is generally a paucity of research regarding the treatment of these disorders when they co-occur. It is recommended that clinicians use a comprehensive and idiographic approach to assessment, followed by a case conceptualization tailored to the individual patient. Our case example illustrates how comorbidity can significantly impact treatment and the need for the clinician to be flexible and willing to modify interventions when the outcome is not optimal. Our review also suggests the need for further scientific study in the role of comorbid anxiety and depression in psychological assessment and treatment.

REFERENCES

Abramowitz, J. S. (2004). Treatment of obsessive–compulsive disorder in patients who have comorbid major depression. *Journal of Clinical Psychology, 60,* 1133–1141.

Abramowitz, J. S., Franklin, M. E., Street, G., Kozak, M., & Foa, E. B. (2000). Effects of comorbid depression on response to treatment for obsessive compulsive disorder. *Behavior Therapy, 31,* 517–528.

Addis, M. E., & Martell, C. E. (2004). *Overcoming depression one step at a time: The new behavioral activation approach for getting your life back.* Oakland, CA: New Harbinger.

American Psychiatric Association. (2000). *Diagnostic and statistical manual* (4th ed., text rev.). Washington, DC: Author.

Antony, M. M., & Barlow, D. H. (Eds.). (2002). *Handbook of assessment and treatment planning for psychological disorders.* New York: Guilford Press.

Barlow, D. H. (1991). The nature of anxiety: Anxiety, depression, and emotional disorders. In R. M. Rapee & D. H. Barlow (Eds.), *Chronic anxiety, generalized anxiety disorder, and mixed anxiety–depression* (pp. 1–28). New York: Guilford Press.

Beck, A. T., & Emery, G. (1985). *Anxiety disorders and phobias: A cognitive perspective.* New York: Basic Books.

Beck, A. T., Steer, R. A., & Brown, G. K. (1996). *Beck Depression Inventory* (2nd ed.). San Antonio, CA: Psychological Corporation.

Belzer, K., & Schneier, F. R. (2004). Comorbidity of anxiety and depressive disorders: Issues in conceptualization, assessment, and treatment. *Journal of Psychiatric Practice, 10,* 296–306.

Bleich, A., Koslowsky, M., Dolv, A., & Lerer, B. (1997). Post-traumatic stress disorder and depression. *British Journal of Psychiatry, 170,* 479–482.

Borkovec, T. D. (1994). The nature, functions, and origins of worry. In G. Davey & F. Tallis (Eds.), *Worrying: Perspectives on theory assessment, and treatment* (pp. 5–33). New York: Wiley.

Brown, C., Schulberg, H. C., Madonia, M. J., Shear, M. K., & Houck, P. R. (1996). Treatment outcomes for primary care patients with major depression and lifetime anxiety disorders. *American Journal of Psychiatry, 153,* 1293–1300.

Brown, T. A., & Barlow, D. H. (1992). Comorbidity among anxiety disorders: Implications for treatment and DSM-IV. *Journal of Consulting and Clinical Psychology, 60,* 835–844.

Brown, T. A., Chorpita, B. F., & Barlow, D. H. (1998). Structural relationships among dimensions of the DSM-IV anxiety and mood disorders and dimensions of negative affect, positive affect, and autonomic arousal. *Journal of Abnormal Psychology, 107,* 179–192.

Brown, T. A., O'Leary, T. A., & Barlow, D. H. (2001). Generalized anxiety disorder. In D. H. Barlow (Ed.), *Clinical handbook of psychological disorders* (pp. 154–208). New York: Guilford Press.

Campbell, L. A., & Brown, T. A. (2002). Generalized anxiety disorder. In M. M. Antony & D. H. Barlow (Eds.), *Handbook of assessment and treatment planning for psychological disorders* (pp. 147–182). New York: Guilford Press.

Chambless, D. L., & Gillis, M. M. (1993). Cognitive therapy of anxiety disorders. *Journal of Consulting and Clinical Psychology, 61,* 248–260.

Chambless, D. L., & Ollendick, T. H. (2001). Empirically supported psychological interventions: Controversies and evidence. *Annual Review of Psychology, 5,* 685–716.

Clark, D. A., & Purdon, C. (1993). New perspectives for a cognitive theory of obsessions. *Australian Psychologist, 28,* 161–167.

Clark, D. M. (1999). Anxiety disorders: Why they persist and how to treat them. *Behaviour Research and Therapy, 37,* S5–S27.

Di Nardo, P. A., Brown, T. A., & Barlow, D. H. (1994). *Anxiety Disorders Interview Schedule for DSM-IV: Lifetime Version.* San Antonio, TX: Psychological Corporation.

Dozois, D. J. A., Dobson, K. S., & Westra, H. A. (2004). The comorbidity of anxiety and depression, and the implications of comorbidity for prevention. In D. J. A. Dozois & K. S. Dobson (Eds.), *The prevention of anxiety and depression: Theory, research, and practice* (pp. 261–280). Washington, DC: American Psychological Association.

Dugas, M. J., Gagnon, F., Ladouceur, R., & Freeston, M. H. (1998). Generalized anxiety disorder: A preliminary test of a conceptual model. *Behaviour Research and Therapy, 36,* 215–226.

D'Zurilla, T. J., & Nezu, A. M. (2001). Problem-solving therapies. In K. S. Dobson (Ed.), *Handbook of cognitive behavioral therapies* (pp. 211–245). New York: Guilford Press.

Ehlers, A., & Clark, D. M. (2000). A cognitive model of posttraumatic stress disorder. *Behaviour Research and Therapy, 38,* 319–345.

Ehlers, A., Clark, D. M., Hackmann, A., McManus, F., & Fennell, M. (2005). Cognitive therapy for post-traumatic stress disorder: Development and evaluation. *Behaviour Research and Therapy, 43,* 413–431.

First, M. B., Spitzer, R. L., Gibbon, M., & Williams, J. B. W. (1996). *Structured Clinical Interview for DSM-IV Axis I Disorders.* New York: Biometrics Research Department.

Foa, E. B., & Franklin, M. E. (2001). Obsessive–compulsive disorder. In D. H. Barlow (Ed.), *Clinical handbook of psychological disorders* (pp. 209–263). New York: Guilford Press.

Forbes, D., Creamer, M., & Biddle, D. (2001). The validity of the PTSD Checklist as a measure of symptomatic change in combat related PTSD. *Behaviour Research and Therapy, 39,* 977–986.

Frost, R. O., & Steketee, G. (1997). Perfectionism in obsessive compulsive disorder patients. *Behaviour Research and Therapy, 35,* 291–296.

Gelhart, R. P., & King, H. L. (2001). The influence of comorbid risk factors on the effectiveness of cognitive-behavioral treatment of depression. *Cognitive and Behavioral Practice, 8,* 18–28.

Judd, L. L., Kessler, R. C., Paulus, M. P., Zeller, P. V., Wittchen, H. U., & Kunovac, J. L. (1998). Comorbidity as a fundamental feature of generalized anxiety disorders: Results from the National Comorbidity Study (NCS). *Acta Psychiatrica Scandinavica Supplementum, 393,* 6–11.

Kessler, R. C., Nelson, C. B., McGonagle, K. A., Liu, J., Swartz, M., & Blazer, D. G. (1996). Comorbidity of DSM-III-R major depressive disorder in the general population: Results from the US National Comorbidity Survey. *British Journal of Psychiatry, 168*(Suppl. 30), 17–30.

Kessler, R. C., Sonnega, A., Bromet, E., Hughes, M., & Nelson, C. B. (1995). Posttraumatic stress disorder in the National Comorbidity Study. *Archives of General Psychiatry, 52,* 1048–1060.

Ladouceur, R., Dugas, M. J., Freeston, M. H., Leger, E., Gagnon, F., & Thibodeau, N. (2000). Efficacy of cognitive behavioral treatment for generalized anxiety disorder: Evaluation in a controlled clinical trial. *Journal of Consulting and Clinical Psychology, 68,* 957–964.

Litz, B. T., Miller, M. W., Ruef, A. M., & McTeague, L. M. (2002). Exposure to trauma in adults. In M. M. Antony & D. H. Barlow (Eds.), *Handbook of assessment and treatment planning for psychological disorders* (pp. 215–258). New York: Guilford Press.

Martell, C. R., Addis, M. E., & Jacobson, N. S. (2001). *Depression in context: Strategies for guided action.* New York: Norton.

Mineka, S., & Nugent, K. (1995). Mood-congruent memory biases in anxiety and depression. In D. Schacter (Ed.), *Memory distortion: How minds, brains and societies reconstruct the past* (pp. 173–193). Cambridge, MA: Harvard University Press.

Mineka, S., Watson, D., & Clark, L. A. (1998). Comorbidity of anxiety and unipolar mood disorders. *Annual Review of Psychology, 49,* 377–412.

Nezu, A. M., Ronan, G. F., Meadows, E. A., & McClure, K. S. (2000). *Practitioner's guide to empirically-based measures of depression* (Clinical assessment series, Vol. 1). New York: Kluwer Academic/Plenum Press.

Nolen-Hoeksema, S. (1991). Responses to depression and their effects on the duration of depressive episodes. *Journal of Abnormal Psychology, 100,* 569–582.

Nutt, D. (2000). Treatment of depression and concomitant anxiety. *European Neuropsychopharmacology, 10*(Suppl. 14), S433–S437.

Persons, J. B., & Davidson, J. (2001). Cognitive behavioral case formulation. In K. S. Dobson (Ed.), *Handbook of cognitive-behavioral therapies* (pp. 86–110). New York: Guilford Press.

Persons, J. B., Roberts, N. A., & Zalecki, C. A. (2003). Anxiety and depression change together during treatment. *Behavior Therapy, 34,* 149–163.

Rachman, S. (1993). Obsessions, responsibility and guilt. *Behaviour Research and Therapy, 31,* 149–154.

Rowa, K., Bieling, P., & Segal, Z. (2005). Depression. In M. A. Antony, D. R. Ledley, & R. G. Heinberg (Eds.), *Improving outcomes and preventing relapse: Practical strategies for overcoming challenges in CBT* (pp. 204–245). New York: Guilford Press.

Salkovskis, P. M. (1985). Obsessional–compulsive problems: A cognitive-behavioral analysis. *Behaviour Research and Therapy, 23,* 571–583.

Salkovskis, P. M. (1999). Understanding and treating obsessive–compulsive disorder. *Behaviour Research and Therapy, 37,* S29–S52.

Shalev, A. Y., Freedman, S., Peri, T., Brandes, D., Sahar, T., Orr, S. P., et al. (1998). Prospective study of posttraumatic stress disorder and depression following trauma. *American Journal of Psychiatry, 155,* 630–637.

Stein, D. J. (2001). Comorbidity in generalized anxiety disorder: Impact and implications. *Journal of Clinical Psychiatry, 62*(Suppl. 11), 29–34.

Tylee, A. (2000). Depression in Europe: Experience from the DEPRES II survey. *European Neuropsychopharmacology, 10*(Suppl. 4), S445–S448.

Weathers, F. W., Litz, B. T., Huska, J. A., & Keane, T. M. (1991). *The PTSD Checklist (PCL).* Boston: National Center for PTSD/Boston VA Medical Center.

Wells, A., & Carter, K. (1999). Preliminary tests of a cognitive model of generalized anxiety disorder. *Behaviour Research and Therapy, 37,* 585–594.

Zimmerman, M., & Mattia, J. I. (1999). Psychiatric diagnosis in clinical practice: Is comorbidity being missed? *Comprehensive Psychiatry, 40,* 182–191.

Zinbarg, R. E., & Barlow, D. H. (1991). Mixed anxiety–depression: A new diagnostic category? In R. M. Rapee & D. H. Barlow (Eds.), *Chronic anxiety, generalized anxiety disorder, and mixed anxiety–depression* (pp. 136–152). New York: Guilford Press.

10

SUBSTANCE USE DISORDERS

Cory F. Newman

Depressed individuals who also have problems with alcohol and other drugs face an uphill climb in getting and adhering to the treatment they need to manage and overcome this formidable combination of clinical issues. From a treatment systems standpoint, there has been a historical division between mental health and substance abuse treatment services (Evans & Sullivan, 2001; Mueser, Noordsby, Drake, & Fox, 2003). Until recently, it was fairly common for patients with this comorbidity (often known as "dual diagnosis") to be denied an integrative treatment (Carroll, 2004). Instead, patients were instructed to receive treatment for either the mood disorder or the substance-related problem as a prerequisite to receiving care for the other. Anecdotally, patients have lamented that they tried to seek help, only to be told that their alcohol and drug use precluded them from involvement in the "depression program," or that their depression needed to be "resolved" before they could gain admission into the "drug and alcohol group." The result was that these patients too often fell through the cracks in the mental health care system, feeling shut out from treatment.

Additionally, patients themselves often posed challenges to their own prospects for remission and recovery from either the mood or the substance problems. For example, depressed patients who abused alcohol and other drugs were more apt to find that their trials on antidepressant medications

(ADMs) were unsatisfactory, inasmuch as their recreational and/or addictive use of substances interacted unfavorably with their prescription medications, hindered their cognizance of following directions for proper dosing and scheduling, and may have damaged the liver's ability to metabolize the ADM properly, to name but a few of the difficulties. Similarly, patients may have reasoned to themselves that they "needed" to continue drinking or engaging in related drug abuse to "cope" with their feelings of loneliness, ennui, and/or despair. This sort of maladaptive belief about the role of alcohol and illicit drugs in their lives interfered with these patients' ability to benefit from talk therapy for depression, in that they were poor attenders, were often neglectful in doing therapy homework, and contributed to the decline of the quality of their lives regardless of the quality of their therapy. The patients' faulty beliefs about their "relationship" with alcohol and illicit substances are extremely important targets for intervention in cognitive therapy (CT; Beck, Wright, Newman, & Liese, 1993).

EPIDEMIOLOGY

To date, the largest study of the prevalence and co-occurrence of alcohol, drug, mood, and anxiety disorders is the National Epidemiologic Survey on Alcohol and Related Conditions (NESARC; Grant et al., 2004). The NESARC included 43,000 adult, noninstitutionalized, civilian citizens of the United States, utilizing the fourth edition of the *Diagnostic and Statistical Manual of the Mental Disorders* (DSM-IV: American Psychiatric Association, 1994) definitions of the aforementioned disorders. Findings of the NESARC are striking and informative, showing that 9.4% of the population (or approximately 19.4 million persons) met clinical criteria for either an alcohol or drug use disorder, or both, and that 9.2% of this same sample (or about 19.2 million adult Americans) met diagnostic criteria for independent mood disorders (including major depression, dysthymia, and bipolar spectrum disorders) not accounted for by intoxication or withdrawal from alcohol or other drugs. Furthermore, associations between most substance use disorders and independent mood disorders were positive and highly significant. About 20% of participants with at least one current (i.e., within the past year) independent mood disorder had a comorbid substance use disorder. Likewise, approximately 20% of the general population with a current substance use disorder had at least one independent mood disorder. Although the NESARC study does not resolve questions about causal mechanisms that may underlie relationships between DSM-IV substance use and mood disorders (Grant et al., 2004), it highlights the importance of

assessing and treating these two major problems areas simultaneously in clinical practice.

CONCEPTUALIZATION AND ASSESSMENT

The "Primary versus Secondary Disorder" Problem

When a clinician uses the Structured Clinical Interview for DSM-IV (e.g., SCID-IV: First, Spitzer, Gibbon, & Williams, 1995) to interview a patient, the interviewer is encouraged to indicate the *primary, secondary,* and *tertiary* disorders, as well as their temporal primacy (chronological appearance) in the patient's life. Accordingly, it seems fitting and proper to try to ascertain the following: Which came first (and which is more clinically relevant), the alcohol and/or substance problem, or the depression? However, in the case of mutually interacting disorders such as depression and alcohol and other drug abuse or dependence, attempts to disentangle the causes and effects without a longitudinal assessment are often difficult (e.g., Ramsey, Kahler, Read, Stuart, & Brown, 2004) and may erroneously minimize the clinical significance of the disorder deemed to be secondary. For example, even when there is clear evidence that the depressive disorder predated the sub-stance use problem, and the substance use problem is not officially diagnosed as being severe, some research has suggested that this "secondary" substance use problem is still a top clinical priority. Relatively lesser amounts of alcohol and other drugs can have particularly deleterious effects on individuals who are clinically depressed (e.g., Mueser, Drake, & Wallach, 1998), includ-ing an increase in the risk of suicide (e.g., Cornelius et al., 1995). Therefore, one school of thought (from a treatment standpoint) is to consider *both disor-ders to be primary* (Mueser et al., 2003). Thus, therapists can tell these patients that the goal of therapy entails "dual recovery" (Evans & Sullivan, 2001), in which both the mood disorder and the substance use disorder are of central importance.

Functional Assessment and Functional Analysis

Assessment is a longitudinal process. New data that come to light as patients go through therapy have implications for adjusting and updating the specific diagnoses, and for solidifying or revising the treatment plan. Early assessment often involves open-ended questioning about the patient's functioning in everyday life, specially noting areas of impairment. A comprehensive intake ideally involves the administration of the SCID (e.g., First et al., 1995), dur-ing which the patient's mood disorder and substance abuse or dependence may be identified. In addition to ascertaining the patient's formal diagnoses, the clinician also does a functional assessment and analysis of the role of alcohol and other drugs in the patient's life. The functional *assessment* examines the patient's adjustment across a number of important life domains, including schooling and/or employment, health and safety, interpersonal relationships, legal involvement, and further areas of psychiatric symptomatology. The functional *analysis* examines the factors pertinent to the development and maintenance of the patient's use of alcohol and other drugs. These factors include high-risk situations (e.g., feeling lonely, getting paid, going to a bar), faulty beliefs (e.g., "I *only* drink beer, so there's no way that I can have an alcohol problem"), and reinforcement contingencies (e.g., a patient feels less anxious in social situations when he/she drinks, but then experiences negative consequences when he/she arrives late and hung over at work). Treatment planning develops as an outgrowth of these and other data (Newman, 2004).

The "Soft Signs" of Alcohol and Other Drug Involvement

Patients with comorbid depression and substance abuse are generally more likely to complain about their depression than to express concern about their use of alcohol and other drugs (see Evans & Sullivan, 2001). Some of the "soft signs" of comorbid substance abuse in a patient who otherwise does not volunteer much information about this problem are as follows (the patient may exhibit several of these signs):

1. The patient's attendance is poor. He/she fails to show up for sessions, has flimsy excuses for postponing appointments, and cannot provide convincing answers as to why it took so long to return the therapist's phone calls.
2. After many sessions, the therapist still does not have a clear picture of how the patient occupies his/her time on a daily basis. Upon further questioning, the patient remains vague.
3. A patient who is on prescribed medications for depression complains that the medication is "not working," and that he/she wishes to be off it. The patient summarily blames symptoms such as hypersomnia and general feelings of malaise on the pharmacotherapy.
4. The patient demonstrates odd changes in vocal quality and/or verbal content on the phone, either in live conversation or on voice mail.

5. The patient is surprisingly reluctant to invite a family member to a therapy session, even when the therapist provides a strong rationale to explain the potential utility of eliciting the family members' observations about the patient.

6. The patient seems impaired in the sessions themselves. He/she may be drowsy, slur words, and demonstrate inappropriate, shifting, and/or incongruous affect.

These are the sorts of problems to which therapists can allude when they make their gambit to communicate that the patient's depression may actually be complicated by a substance abuse issue. The astute clinician is ever-mindful of drawing data-based conclusions; therefore, endeavors to obtain corroborating evidence before assuming that the apparent signs of substance abuse indeed reflect a verifiable problem with alcohol and other drugs.

Specific Assessment Measures

Perhaps the most practical means by which the typical outpatient therapist can assess for the depressed patient's use of, abuse of, or dependence on alcohol and other drugs is to use a self-report screening instrument. Mueser at al. (2003) note that many such extant measures developed for the general population often lack strong predictive utility for identifying substance use disorders in clinical populations. A notable exception is the Alcohol Use Disorder Identification Test (AUDIT; Saunders, Aasland, Babor, De La Fuente, & Grant, 1993), "which has shown good sensitivity and specificity in detecting alcohol use disorders in persons with severe mental illness" (Mueser et al., 2003, p. 56). Another useful measure, the Dartmouth Assessment of Lifestyle Instrument (DALI; Rosenberg et al., 1998), is a brief, convenient screening device that can be used as a self-report questionnaire on paper or on computer, and may also be used in clinical-based interview form. The DALI has been found to have high specificity and sensitivity for the detection of alcohol, cannabis, cocaine, and other substance use disorders in clinical populations. Mueser et al. (2003) provide a copy of the DALI, along with scoring instructions, and note that a "positive score on the DALI indicates a high probability (80–90%) that the patient meets DSM criteria for a recent substance use disorder" (p. 56).

Once a depressed patient has been assessed to have a problem with alcohol or other drugs (regardless of whether he/she meets full criteria either for abuse or dependence), additional measures may be used to investigate related variables pertinent to the patient's functioning. One such measure is the Addiction Severity Index (ASI: McLellan et al., 1992), a structured interview that assesses the levels of functioning and impairment across numerous life domains in patients who experience problems with alcohol and other drugs. These domains include medical status, extent of alcohol and other drug use, employment, family and social relationships, legal involvement, and psychological status (including formal psychiatric diagnoses; e.g., depression). As is the case for most standardized instruments, the ASI is best administered periodically to measure the patient's progress over the course of treatment.

TREATMENT ISSUES

The more complicated the clinical picture, the more important the therapeutic relationship and a well-formulated case conceptualization in maximizing the utility of the structure and techniques that comprise CT. This point is quite salient with depressed patients who also have problems with alcohol and other drugs, many of whom may be put off by the therapist's focusing on their drinking and/or drugging, thinking it is accusatory, irrelevant, stigmatizing, and a sign that the therapist "doesn't understand." The therapist often has to engage in a delicate balancing act, on the one hand being tactful, caring, and cautious in bringing up "hot topics" such as chemical dependence, and on the other hand being flexible enough to respect the patient's alternative agenda to preserve the ongoing working relationship. Because premature dropping out of treatment is a significant problem in a substance-abusing population (Siqueland et al., 2002), the therapist has to develop a repertoire of assessment questions and interventions that are empathic, clear, and collaborative, and that give the message that the patient's problems are understood well, without personal judgment.

The specific techniques of CT for depression (e.g., Moore & Garland, 2003) and for substance-related disorders (Beck et al., 1993), are well-articulated in a comprehensive fashion elsewhere and are beyond the scope of this chapter. However, it is important to note some of the particular adaptations to CT for depression that clinicians must consider to deal effectively with dually diagnosed individuals, as summarized below.

Adapting Standard CT for Depression

As one would expect, the application of CT for depression with comorbid substance abuse/dependence entails certain considerations that go beyond the treatment methods for depression alone. Some of these considerations have to do with a patient's (1) aversion to admitting, discussing, or otherwise ameliorating the substance abuse problem; (2) markedly reduced ability to utilize the psychological skills learned in session when he/she is chemically impaired outside of the session; (3) maladaptive belief that alcohol and other drugs are effective and necessary palliatives for his/her depression; and (4) misuse of 12-step principles to counteract some of the tenets of CT. These four considerations, which do not represent an exhaustive list, are expounded upon below.

Patient Aversion to Discussing the Substance Abuse Problem

Many patients who are willing to discuss their clinical depression openly with their therapists are far less eager to address their use of alcohol and other substances. For example, I once treated a patient who proclaimed vehemently that she would leave therapy if I "got on a high horse" and brought up her use of alcohol. Rather than insist on talking about her alcohol abuse on the spot, or (conversely) capitulate to a countertherapeutic demand to remain indefinitely silent about an important clinical issue, I tried to find an entry point into a productive therapeutic dialogue. Thus, I commented on the patient's *assumption* that I would "get on a high horse," noting how acting in such a manner would be at odds with the collaborative spirit of CT to which I was committed, and explaining that I was prepared to discuss all the patient's agenda items respectfully, with the intent of improving her overall functioning and quality of life.

Some patients are unmoved by such comments, and may in fact abandon therapy rather than face an issue they would prefer to avoid. This puts the therapist in a bind, because it is not a good idea to collude with a potentially dangerously incomplete therapeutic agenda, nor is it favorable to lose the chance to establish a productive working relationship with the patient, and have him/her leave therapy and receive no treatment whatsoever. At such times, it is useful to refer to the "stages of change" model in the field of addictions treatment (Prochaska, DiClemente, & Norcross, 1992), which spells out the methods of working with patients in a "precontemplative" stage (before patients even consider changing their behavior) or a "contemplative" stage (when patients start to think about changing but are not yet taking active steps). The goal involves "meeting the patients where they are," such that a therapeutic relationship can be established and strengthened. In doing so, therapists increase the likelihood that the work of CT will move toward successively later stages of change (e.g., preparation, action, maintenance), enabling both parties to deal actively with the problems related to patients' chemical dependence.

This is an imperfect solution, because there is no guarantee that patients will advance in their level of readiness to discuss their substance abuse, and the damage caused by their addiction may be worsening in the meantime. Nevertheless, for patients who are steadfast in their wish to talk only about their depression, and not about alcohol and other drug use, the stages of change approach may offer the best hope of breaking through, so that all topics may eventually be put on the table. In the early stages, the therapist can tread lightly, while recommending that the patient keep a log of his/her drinking or use of other drugs, "just to take some data," with no explicit demand for reductions. The automatic thoughts elicited by this self-monitoring exercise (or by its being assigned) can further serve as useful points of intervention, even if the overtly stated goal does not specifically target changing the patient's addictive behaviors.

Patient Impairment Interferes with Utilization of CT

As psychoactive chemicals alter executive cognitive functioning, patient's ability to use the psychological skills they learned in CT is likely hindered when they are actively drinking and using. For example, the patient who is able to complete a Dysfunctional Thought Record (DTR; see J. S. Beck, 1995) in session may be helpless to generate alternative responses to depressogenic thoughts while sitting at home in an inebriated state. Similarly, the patient who is able to use problem-solving skills in session to weigh the pros and cons of an important decision may impulsively act unwisely when high on drugs during the weekend. Most dangerously, the suicidal patient who—while sober in session—agrees to a set of therapeutic strategies to keep him/her safe may be rendered incapable of staying with this critical program when drunk, or when coming down off a cocaine or amphetamine high. As one therapist told his patient, "I trust your sober mind, but if you're drinking or drugging, I have much less confidence in your brain functioning, and in your ability to stick to our agreements for safety."

One of the ways to increase the likelihood that a chemically impaired patient will be able to use his or her CT skills in the midst of a depressive crisis is to prepare self-help materials in advance of such a situation. For example, patients can make audiotapes in which they give themselves well-reasoned instructions on what to think about to resist doing any number of tempting but harmful things. This tape can also include words of encouragement to stay the course of treatment, even under adverse circumstances and when experiencing cognitive impairment and emotional dyscontrol while under the influence. This method is based on the principle that passive recognition of the proper course of action requires less concentration and focus than the free recall of such complex information. Patients should have their audiotapes, written reminders, important phone numbers (for emergency contacts), and other such therapeutic "props" out in the open, so that they are easily spotted. Adding to the self-help materials on a regular basis makes them an ever-expanding "rainy day journal."

Patients' Use of Substances to Self-Medicate Their Depression

Some patients express the belief that alcohol and other drugs are "the only things that work to help me cope with my depression." They resist the idea that the substances are part of the problem, and defend their need to drink and use to "take the edge off" their sadness and forget about their problems, even if just for a little while. Therapists can empathize with patients' desire to use whatever palliative they can find to alleviate their emotional suffering, but they also offer psychoeducation about the vicious cycle of mood disorders and chemical dependence. A patient might argue that if the therapist's point of view about chemical substances has merit, then ADM should also be seen as problematic in dealing with depression. The therapist can quickly point out that ADM does not impair the patient's judgment and behaviors, but does improve the patient's mood in a steady, gradual, nonaddictive way, and is designed to improve the patient's health, satisfaction, and ability to interact effectively with family and society at large.

Of course, therapists cannot simply suggest that patients give up their preferred method of coping without working with them toward new, healthier means of dealing with the depression. Therapists can acknowledge that the noticeable effects of these new methods may not be as immediate as (for example) taking a shot of whiskey, but that they are more enduring, less problematic, and more able to engender an increase in self-efficacy, which has been found to be associated with positive outcome in treatment (Ramsey, Brown, Stuart, Burgess, & Miller, 2002).

Patients' Misuse of 12-Step Principles to Counter the Spirit of CT

Patients with comorbid depression and chemical dependence sometimes attend a 12-step facilitation group (12SF) in conjunction with their CT. By and large, this can be a very positive thing, because 12SF (e.g., Alcoholics Anonymous [AA], 1976) offers valuable social support to people who often feel alone or believe they have burned their bridges with others. Unfortunately, there are times when patients engage in all-or-none thinking about the tenets of AA and similar groups, to the detriment of their participation in CT.

For example, Step 1 involves admitting powerlessness in the face of the addiction. The purpose of this step is to break through denial and to humble oneself in the presence of a problem whose scope must be acknowledged in order to be overcome. Unfortunately, some people take this "powerlessness" concept to its extreme, to the point of dismissing the idea of learning coping skills and building self-efficacy as a sort of self-delusion that is at odds with an honest admission of having an addiction. Cognitive therapists help their patients to think more creatively and flexibly about how the concepts of "powerlessness" and "self-efficacy" actually can be *complementary*. The powerlessness has to do with the old methods of supposed coping that have failed again and again, such that the objective evidence cries out for broad, sweeping change. The self-efficacy skills are about having the courage to change, and to learn new ways of coping. There is nothing inherently contradictory about respecting the overwhelming power of an addiction, while also striving to grow, to learn, and to gain well-founded confidence in living effectively.

Another way that patients spuriously pit 12SF against CT is by implicitly rejecting the importance and relevance of concepts such as "harm reduction" (Marlatt, 1998) and "the abstinence violation effect" (Marlatt & Gordon, 1985). Such patients fear that their cognitive therapists are missing the point when they try to help them decatastrophize their lapses into substance use. These patients believe that any slip into drinking and drugging is in fact a straight path to catastrophe, and these patients bristle at the notion that they can learn from the slip, contain the scope of the lapse, and stay committed to abstinence as the ultimate goal. In such cases, the cognitive therapist can confirm that they too believe that abstinence is the preferred outcome of treatment. However, there is little evidence that engaging in catastrophic, all-or-none thinking is beneficial to treatment of clinical depression, and to one's sense of hope in continuing to "fight the good fight" toward sobriety. In fact, some patients who adhere to the all-or-none model actually *pervert* the spirit of the 12 Steps by *giving themselves permission* to go on a binge or a bender in response to a minor slip, reasoning maladaptively that they have blown their sobriety, period, and that degree is immaterial. Thus, we have a self-fulfilling prophecy of "one drink equals a drunk."

By contrast, the cognitive model posits that patients who experience a slip do not have to fall prey to the abstinence violation effect (Marlatt & Gordon, 1985), in which their distress over breaking their abstinence leads to further self-medication, thus worsening the slip and leading to a downward spiral. Instead, patients can view each incremental use of the drink or other drug *as a new decision*, which may at any time be "no more using" (Beck et al., 1993). Thus, the vicious cycle of using, hopelessness, self-reproach, self-medication, and further hopelessness can be broken before too much damage is done. When this occurs, the similarity and congruity between 12SF and CT in response to a lapse are readily apparent: Both models now view the patient as being in a "high-risk situation," in which a renewed commitment to getting help for the addiction is the highest priority.

Supplementation of Standard CT for Depression

Additional intervention modalities (beyond CT) for the depressed patient with a substance use disorder include pharmacotherapy, detoxification (either outpatient or inpatient), family interventions, and group therapy, including 12SF. All of these modalities are compatible with outpatient CT, provided that the various clinicians involved do not denigrate each other's treatment approach to the patients, even subtly.

Pharmacotherapy for Depression

Some patients who are in CT for their depression are concurrently on ADM. Patients receiving psychopharmacotherapy are typically told that it is best that they not consume alcohol (or, at the very least, that they restrict their drinking to a minimum) while taking ADM. Unfortunately, patients with depression comorbid with alcohol and other substance abuse are prone to disregard such medical advice. The likely result is that the medication(s) will be rendered less effective, and/or that there will be potentially harmful pharmacological interactions (Evans & Sullivan, 2001). Either way, patients may grow disenchanted with their ADM and assume that it is not working, or that it is causing even more physiological distress.

All too commonly, therapists are taken by surprise upon learning that a patient has discontinued his/her ADM, often well after the fact. To safeguard against this, a therapist can routinely inquire about the patient's use of the ADM and ask sympathetically about any difficulties, while also assessing whether the patient is actually adhering to the prescribed regimen.

Some patients harbor maladaptive beliefs about their ADM. Thus, cognitive therapists should inquire about patients' views about their pharmacotherapy, and highlight any problematic assumptions patients may be making that may interfere with treatment. For example, when "Len" flatly stated that his ADM was "useless," his therapist noted that it would be possible to give the ADM a fair assessment only after Len discontinued use of all other psychoactive chemicals (in his case, alcohol and marijuana), then observe his response to the ADM over a period of weeks and months. Len did not immediately get the point—that what he viewed as *recreational substances* were actually central nervous system depressants, and that he was not giving his ADM a fair chance to play a positive, therapeutic role. Len's therapist said, "I am deeply concerned that you are willing to give up taking the chemicals that are potentially therapeutic, while you are determined to continue taking the chemicals that are worsening your psychological and physiological condition."

Although a review of the specific psychotropic medications that are appropriate for depressed patients with substance use disorders is beyond the scope of this chapter, a few general comments are pertinent. For example, Evans and Sullivan (2001) emphasize that these patients are not good candidates for sedating medications, whether they be benzodiazepines or ADMs with soporific qualities. Among the medications that do not pose the risk of abuse, SSRIs are often a popular choice, because they are very safe in case of overdose and are easy to use. Presenting an alternative view, Rounsaville (2004) reviewed the extant randomized controlled trials on ADM for comorbid depression and cocaine use, and found more favorable results for medications such as desipramine and bupropion than for SSRIs.

Pharmacotherapy for the Substance Use Problem Per Se

For alcohol use disorders, disulfiram (Antabuse) can be an important part of the treatment regimen (Carroll, Nich, Ball, McCance, & Rounsaville, 1998). Disulfiram treatment generally requires direct supervision by either a clinician or a close family member of the patient. In the early years of disulfiram use some fatalities occurred, such as when a patient would engage in binge drinking while taking high doses of the medication. Today, the standard doses have been lowered considerably, thus reducing the risk to negligible levels. When the treatment is working properly, the patient is deterred from drinking alcohol because of the expected, noxious physiological effects produced by its interaction with disulfiram.

Opiate antagonists, such as naltrexone, can also be helpful adjuncts for the dually diagnosed, depressed individual who is seriously committed to sobriety and wishes to reduce the cravings (for alcohol, opiates, and other drugs) that produce high risk for relapse (Anton et al., 1999; Petrakis et al., 2005). As with disulfiram, naltrexone has the best chance of success if its use is supervised. A further pharmacological option for the patient who is dependent on opiates is methadone maintenance therapy. Although data are lacking as to the efficacy of this treatment with dually diagnosed patients, there are no well-established contraindications (Mueser et al., 2003).

Pharmacological detoxification is an additional option for those patients who seem unlikely to stop their use of alcohol and other drugs, even when motivated to change and given adequate social support. This can be performed on an outpatient basis or, alternatively, in an inpatient setting, especially when detoxification entails medical risks. When benzodiazepines are used, doses need to be kept moderate.

Support Groups, 12SF, and Family Interventions

People with substance abuse or dependence often find that there is subtle (and not-so-subtle) social pressure to continue drinking and drugging. Even when persons who use alcohol and other drugs receive disapproval at home, they often find acceptance in a peer group that collectively "gives permission" for such behavior (Alverson, Alverson, & Drake, 2001). Patients sometimes complain that if they relinquish their substance use, then they will no longer have friends (Beck et al., 1993). Thus, it can be very useful for patients to take part in support groups (e.g., 12SF; National Alliance for the Mentally Ill; Rational Recovery, Trimpey, 1996) or more formal therapy groups designed to provide social support and psychological tools for achieving and maintaining sobriety (see Mueser et al., 2003). Groups that are not developed in an inpatient setting often have flexible schedules, so that people can attend sessions even if they work full time, and provide a rational answer to those patients who state that they "don't have time" to ·take part.

Although the 12SF has not been subject to empirical evaluation for the depressive aspect of the dual diagnosis, there has been some support for its effectiveness in reducing the addictive behaviors, thus making it a viable supplemental treatment to CT (Morgenstern, Labouvie, McCrady, Kahler, & Frey, 1997; Ouimette, Finney, & Moos, 1997).

Families play an important role in the lives of persons with dual disorders, for better or worse. For example, the family can serve as vital sources of support for a patient who is feeling ashamed and hopeless. There is ample evidence that the adverse effects of family stress and conflict (centering on a person's mental illness and/or chemical dependence) are bidirectional, with both the patient and the family exhibiting deterioration in functioning and quality of life (e.g., Dixon, McNary, & Lehman, 1995; Fichter, Glynn, Weyer, Liberman, & Frick, 1997). Thus, there is much at stake in trying to help coordinate care between patients and their families in an optimal way.

Descriptions of family-based treatment approaches along with supporting empirical evidence, can be found in Mueser and Glynn (1999).

CASE ILLUSTRATION

Although a brief case summary cannot capture the complexities, the ebb and flow, and the important session-by-session details of an actual course of treatment, the following vignette provides a sample of how a cognitive therapist might initiate a discussion about an alcohol problem with a reluctant, depressed patient.

Drake, a 38-year-old married man working as an insurance agent, sought CT for his chronic depression and intermittent suicidality. At the initial diagnostic interview, Drake was very open about his emotional misery, but he was tight-lipped about alcohol and other substance use, often answering assessment questions with the pat answer, "No more than most people." The therapist decided not to press Drake for further details at that time, because he noticed that Drake was becoming visibly perturbed, and might decide not to follow through with therapy. Instead, the therapist silently decided that he would "flag" the issue of chemical dependence in his notes and come back to it at a more favorable moment.

In the first therapy session, Drake's score on the Beck Depression Inventory (BDI; Beck, Steer, & Garbin, 1988) was 40, indicating a severe level of depression. He endorsed marked sleep disturbance, self-reproach, and suicidal ideation, among other symptoms. The first part of the session focused on Drake's thoughts about suicide. When the therapist was satisfied that the patient did not pose an imminent threat to himself or others, he asked about Drake's use of alcohol and other substances. The following is a condensed facsimile of the dialogue that ensued:

THERAPIST: I remember something you said last week about your drinking alcohol "no more than most people," but I'm wondering whether your alcohol use may be interfering with your sleep. Can we talk about this?

DRAKE: It's a nonissue. (*Long pause, but does not continue.*)

THERAPIST: Meaning?

DRAKE: I can't sleep because I can't shut off my thoughts about how much I hate my life, not because I choose to relax with a few beers when I get home from work, like anybody else.

THERAPIST: Well, one thing we definitely want to talk about is those thoughts that keep you up at night, and how you can manage them more favorably rather than letting them plague you. But I think we should cover all our bases, because your depression is severe, and we don't want to miss any factors that could be inadvertently making your depression worse, such as a few beers after work every day.

DRAKE: Hey, I'm not paying you to imitate my wife. I can hear all this at home for no charge. (*Laughs loudly and nervously, then retreats into a long, awkward silence.*)

THERAPIST: I hit a nerve, didn't I? Sorry about that. I didn't know that your wife was concerned about your alcohol consumption.

DRAKE: Doc, you're getting the wrong idea. Here's the deal. My wife doesn't like the fact that I tune her out when I get home, and she blames the beer for that. She's not worried about me being some kind of alcoholic or something. She just wants me to have stupid conversations with her about stuff I'm in no mood to hear.

THERAPIST: It sounds like you've got some resentment toward your wife, and I certainly don't want you to resent therapy as well. (*Waits for Drake to respond, but Drake just looks away and remains silent.*) I gather that drinking beer has been a means of escape for you—a way to drown out the stresses and strains of your everyday life. What I worry about is the inadvertent *depressive* effect of your drinking beer every day. I am concerned about how drinking could disturb your sleeping too, which you noted was a big concern of yours.

DRAKE: Tell you what. If it will make you happy, I'll give up the beer. I'll switch to wine and Jack Daniels. (*Lets out a hearty laugh, but his face is turning red.*)

THERAPIST: (*Recognizing that Drake is angry, he just looks at Drake sympathetically for a while, and then weighs his words very carefully.*) I know I'm not winning any popularity points with you right now, Drake. I'm trying to offer you my best professional judgment. I think I owe that to you. What are your thoughts right now?

DRAKE: This isn't going to work.

THERAPIST: You mean *therapy* isn't going to work?

DRAKE: Therapy, the medication, the whole nine yards. And you're trying to get me to stop doing the one thing that helps me.

THERAPIST: You mean the drinking?

DRAKE: (*Shoots back a look that seems to say "What else?"*)

THERAPIST: I'm starting to "get it," Drake. You're deeply depressed, you're resentful about your home life and your job, you're trying to cope the best that you can, you're willing to try pharmacotherapy and cognitive therapy, but you're not very hopeful about the results, and the idea that you should give up drinking seems to miss the mark and really ticks you off. How close am I to being on target?

The therapist recognized that Drake was ambivalent about staying in treatment, and that if he insisted that the patient stop drinking, he might drop out of therapy altogether. At the same time, he realized that it would be potentially hazardous to ignore Drake's use of alcohol, and would send the wrong message about how therapy should proceed. Thus, the therapist opted to engage Drake in the collection of data, as the following dialogue illustrates.

THERAPIST: I'm interested in what you said about the alcohol being "the only thing" that makes your mood less depressed. I wonder if we can make a more objective study of this hypothesis. (*Looks at Drake to gauge his body language before taking the risk of proceeding further.*) If you're willing to be a social scientist, with yourself as the subject, I think we can take a closer look at this phenomenon.

DRAKE: What, that beer is my best medicine?

THERAPIST: Exactly.

DRAKE: So what am I supposed to do?

THERAPIST: You collect data on yourself, every day.

DRAKE: How?

THERAPIST: There are a few ways, but here's one idea, for starters. First, you'll have to keep a logbook of your moods, your alcohol intake, and your associated thoughts. (*Explains the nuts and bolts of how this would look in practice.*) I would suggest that you use a scale of 0 to 100 to chart your mood when you get home from work, then after you've had your final beer or any other alcoholic beverage for the evening.

DRAKE: Assuming I'm still conscious. (*Laughs out loud.*)

THERAPIST: (*Thinks that Drake is giving away more hints that his alcohol use is in fact excessive, and that it is important to make the reduction of alcohol consumption a high-priority goal for therapy.*) Well, I guess we'll find out, won't we? But that's not all. I wonder if you can log your mood rating the next morning, right before you leave for work. That will give you three mood ratings per 24 hours—one before you drink, another after you drink, and the final rating the morning after. Oh, and one more thing—could you jot down how many drinks you have each day, just so we can see how this goes together with your mood ratings?

DRAKE: Didn't you say something about writing down my thoughts too?

THERAPIST: That's pretty ambitious for now, but if you want to start doing that, I'm all for it. (*Goes on to explain the concept of self-monitoring one's automatic thoughts.*)

The upshot of this dialogue is that the issue of alcohol was now firmly placed on the therapeutic agenda and would be brought up routinely each session. Drake was willing to come back for further sessions, and he and the therapist began to develop rapport.

As one might predict, Drake had difficulty completing the assignments on a regular basis, but the data he managed to collect were sufficient to advance the cause of understanding the relationship between his moods, his alcohol intake, his thought patterns, and how he felt "the morning after." This set the stage for further interventions, such as experimenting with "an evening of sobriety," so that Drake could collect data on his moods, his thoughts, his quality of sleep, and his feelings the next morning on those days he chose not to drink when he arrived home from work. Such an assignment was a "win–win" proposition. If Drake succeeded in not drinking, the therapist lauded it as a triumph. Furthermore, he took the opportunity to focus Drake's attention on the positive effects of sobriety, such as more pleasant interactions with his wife, a lesser caloric intake (Drake had stated that he wanted to lose 10–20 pounds), saving money, and the chance to focus on productive activities he had abandoned. If, on the other hand, Drake had difficulty in enacting the sobriety experiment, the therapist would note how this was evidence that the drinking had become "habit-forming," thus warranting more attention in treatment. Either way, something productive would come out of the assignment.

Drake's course of therapy was typified by discrete "bunches" of sessions separated by absences of various lengths, some planned and others based on Drake's avoidance of treatment. The patient's condition was at its best when both his drinking and his depressive symptoms decreased significantly, at which time Drake usually wanted to terminate therapy. The therapist often agreed with this plan, provided that Drake continue to take his ADM and to meet as scheduled with his psychiatrist. Almost without exception, Drake's worst times were typified by the following scenario—he would call the therapist "out of the blue," after an unscheduled absence from CT, asking to be seen again following a significant recurrence of binge drinking and related dysphoria.

Drake reluctantly acknowledged that he tended to blame his depressive relapse on his ADM "no longer working" rather than to examine his increase in alcohol use. Drake would then seek CT to improve his mood, but was more ambivalent about addressing the alcohol issue. By the time Drake had reentered CT for the third time following a relapse, the therapist advised Drake also to attend AA as a way to address his alcohol use continuously, irrespective of his current and future involvement in CT. Thus, AA became the "bridge" between Drake's successive trials of CT.

REVIEW OF EFFICACY RESEARCH

Despite the paucity of efficacy research on cognitive-behavioral treatments for dually diagnosed depression and substance use problems (see O'Brien et al., 2004; Rounsaville, 2004), at least two rigorous studies suggest that CT demonstrates superior efficacy in treating substance abuse and dependence compared to alternative treatment approaches, *specifically when the patients are also clinically depressed* (Carroll et al., 1994; Maude-Griffin et al., 1998). Another study compared a cognitive-behavioral intervention and relaxation training for alcoholics with depressive symptoms (who were simultaneously receiving "standard alcohol treatment"). The cognitive-behavioral treatment had superior results on multiple measures of decreased alcohol consumption at follow-up, suggesting better staying power than relaxation training (Brown, Evans, Miller, Burgess, & Mueller, 1997). In a similarly designed study, alcohol-dependent individuals with elevated depressive symptoms who received cognitive-behavioral therapy had better outcomes on alcohol use when they experienced an increased sense of self-efficacy in coping with negative mood states (Ramsey et al., 2002), the likes of which have been known to trigger substance use episodes (Brown et al., 1998).

In an uncontrolled study of parolees receiving mandated treatment for substance abuse relapse prevention, the patient population was divided (post hoc) into those who showed low distress versus high distress on measures of depression and anxiety at intake (Nishith, Mueser, Srsic, & Beck, 1997). The authors report that patients in the high-distress group showed significant decreases in substance use, whereas those in the low-distress group did not. Nishith and her colleagues conclude that these data support the hypothesis that CT may be a more potent intervention for substance-abusing patients whose depression is prominent.

On a broader scale, Mueser et al. (2003) summarized a number of studies that seem to suggest an integrative treatment package for patients with dual disorders requires a long-term program with extended follow-up, which, the authors argue, is superior to a short-term intensive approach to care. Mueser and his colleagues went on to state that much more research is needed to study dually diagnosed patients on variables such as gender, trauma history, polysubstance use versus alcohol use alone, and the presence or absence of antisocial personality disorder.

CONCLUSIONS

The landmark NESARC has not only confirmed that mood disorders and substance use disorders are prevalent among American adults today, but also that their rates of co-occurrence are clinically significant. The traditional separation of treatment approaches and facilities for mood disorders versus alcohol and other substance use disorders is inadequate to meet the treatment needs of the large numbers of patients with problems in both areas. Furthermore, even when both types of disorders are acknowledged and addressed in a given patient, the notion of "primary versus secondary" disorder may also miss the mark, because mood disorders and substance use disorder tend to exacerbate each other in a vicious cycle. Thus, treatment for such comorbidity needs to be comprehensive to maximize the chances of success.

CT is demonstrably efficacious as a treatment for depression, but only a relatively sparse body of work supports its use in the treatment of substance use disorders. Nonetheless, evidence that CT is more effective than alternative treatments for substance use disorders, specifically when the patients are also depressed, demonstrates the promise of CT as a treatment for "dual-diagnosis" patients.

To adapt CT to the treatment of comorbid mood and substance use disorders, therapists need to keep the following factors in mind. First, a good case conceptualization and a well-established therapeutic alliance are essential to address the sensitive area of alcohol and other substance use. Second, it will likely take therapeutic finesse to engage patients in a therapeutic agenda that places the substance use problem on a par with the depressive disorder. One way of achieving this is to encourage patients to collect data on their use of alcohol and other drugs as part of their ongoing self-monitoring homework. Third, ongoing assessment is vital, because patients' alcohol and other drug-using status can change rapidly, perhaps interfering with treatment itself and increasing the risk of suicidality. Fourth, the risk of premature dropout from therapy is high and must be addressed assertively and preemptively, if possible. Finally, as the case study illustrated, CT can work in a complementary fashion with other treatment approaches, such as medications, group therapy, family therapy, and 12SF. CT can effectively modify the faulty beliefs that may needlessly pit one treatment approach against the other.

REFERENCES

Alcoholics Anonymous. (1976). *Alcoholics Anonymous: The story of how many thousands of men and women have recovered from alcoholism* (3rd ed.). New York: Author.

Alverson, H., Alverson, M., & Drake, R. E. (2001). Social patterns of substance-use among people with dual diagnoses. *Mental Health Services Research, 3,* 3–14.

American Psychiatric Association (1994). *Diagnostic and statistical manual of mental disorders* (4th ed.). Washington, DC: Author.

Anton, R. F., Moak, D. H., Waid, L. R., Latham, P. K., Malcolm, R. J., & Dias, J. K. (1999). Naltrexone and cognitive behavioral therapy for the treatment of outpatient alcoholics: Results of a placebo-controlled trial. *American Journal of Psychiatry, 156,* 1758–1764.

Beck, A. T., Steer, R. A., & Garbin, M. G. (1988). Psychometric properties of the Beck Depression Inventory: Twenty-five years of evaluation. *Clinical Psychology Review, 8,* 77–100.

Beck, A. T., Wright, F. D., Newman, C. F., & Liese, B. S. (1993). *Cognitive therapy of substance abuse.* New York: Guilford Press.

Beck, J. S. (1995). *Cognitive therapy: Basics and beyond.* New York: Guilford Press.

Brown, R. A., Evans, D. M., Miller, I. W., Burgess, E. S., & Mueller, T. I. (1997). Cognitive-behavioral treatment for depression in alcoholism. *Journal of Consulting and Clinical Psychology, 65,* 715–726.

Brown, R. A., Monti, P. M., Myers, M. G., Martin, R. A., Rivinus, T., Dubreuil, M. E., et al. (1998). Depression among cocaine abusers in treatment: Relation to cocaine and alcohol use and treatment outcome. *American Journal of Psychiatry, 155,* 220–225.

Carroll, K. M. (2004). Behavioral therapies for co-occuring substance use and mood disorders. *Biological Psychiatry, 56*(10), 778–784.

Carroll, K. M., Nich, C., Ball, S. A., McCance, E., & Rounsaville, B. J. (1998). Treatment of cocaine and alcohol dependence with psychotherapy and disulfiram. *Addiction, 93,* 713–728.

Carroll, K. M., Rounsaville, B. J., Nich, C., Gordon, L. T., Wirtz, P. W., & Gawin, F. H. (1994). Psychotherapy and pharmacotherapy for ambulatory cocaine abusers: Delayed emergence of psychotherapy effects. *Archives of General Psychiatry, 51*, 989–997.

Cornelius, J. R., Salloum, I. M., Mezzich, J., Cornelius, M. D., Fabreago, H., Ehler, J. G., et al. (1995). Disproportionate suicidality in patients with comorbid major depression and alcoholism. *Psychopharmacology Bulletin, 34*, 117–121.

Dixon, L., McNary, S., & Lehman, A. (1995). Substance abuse and family relationships of persons with severe mental illness. *American Journal of Psychiatry, 148*, 224–230.

Evans, K., & Sullivan, M. J. (2001). *Dual diagnosis: Counseling the mentally ill substance abuser* (2nd ed.). New York: Guilford Press.

Fichter, M. M., Glynn, S. M., Weyer, S., Liberman, R. P., & Frick, U. (1997). Family climate and expressed emotion in the course of alcoholism. *Family Process, 36*, 203–221.

First, M. B., Spitzer, R. L., Gibbon, M., & Williams, J. B. W. (1995). *Structured Clinical Interview for DSM-IV Axis I Disorder with Psychotic Screen.* New York: Psychiatric Institute.

Grant, B. F., Stinson, F. S., Dawson, D. A., Chou, P., Dufour, M. C., Compton, W., et al. (2004). Prevalence and co-occurrence of substance use disorders and independent mood and anxiety disorders: Results from the National Epidemiologic Survey on Alcohol and Related Conditions. *Archives of General Psychiatry, 61*, 807–816.

Marlatt, G. A. (Ed.). (1998). *Harm reduction: Pragmatic strategies for managing high-risk behaviors.* New York: Guilford Press.

Marlatt, G. A., & Gordon, J. R. (Eds.). (1985). *Relapse prevention: Maintenance strategies in the treatment of addictive behaviors.* New York: Guilford Press.

Maude-Griffin, P. M., Hohenstein, J. M., Humfleet, G. L., Reilly, P. M., Tusel, D. J., & Hall, S. M. (1998). Superior efficacy of cognitive-behavioral therapy for urban crack cocaine abusers: Main and matching effects. *Journal of Consulting and Clinical Psychology, 66*(5), 832–837.

McLellan, A. T., Kushner, H., Metzger, D., Peters, R., Smith, I., Grissom, G., et al. (1992). The fifth edition of the Addiction Severity Index. *Journal of Substance Abuse Treatment, 9*, 199–213.

Moore, R. G., & Garland, A. (2003). *Cognitive therapy for chronic and persistent depression.* Chichester, UK: Wiley.

Morgenstern, J., LaBouvie, E., McCrady, B. S., Kahler, C. W., & Frey, R. M. (1997). Affiliation with Alcoholics Anonymous: A study of its therapeutic effects and mechanisms of action. *Journal of Consulting and Clinical Psychology, 65*, 768–777.

Mueser, K. T., Drake, R. E., & Wallach, M. A. (1998). Dual diagnosis: A review of etiological theories. *Addictive Behaviors, 23*(6), 717–734.

Mueser, K. T., & Glynn, S. M. (1999). *Behavioral family therapy for psychiatric disorders* (2nd ed.). Oakland, CA: New Harbinger.

Mueser, K. T., Noordsby, D. L., Drake, R. E., & Fox, L. (2003). *Integrated treatment for dual disorders: A guide to effective practice.* New York: Guilford Press.

Newman, C. F. (2004). Substance abuse. In R. L. Leahy (Ed.), *New Advances in cognitive therapy* (pp. 206–227). New York: Guilford Press.

Nishith, P., Mueser, K. T., Srsic, C. S., & Beck, A. T. (1997). Differential response to cognitive therapy in parolees with primary and secondary substance use disorders. *Journal of Nervous and Mental Disease, 185*(12), 763–766.

O'Brien, C. P., Charney, D. S., Lewis, L., Cornish, J. W., Post, R. M., Woody, G. E., et al. (2004). Priority actions to improve the care of persons with co-occurring substance abuse and other mental disorders: A call to action. *Biological Psychiatry, 56*(10), 703–713.

Ouimette, P. C., Finney, J. W., & Moos, R. H. (1997). Twelve-step and cognitive-behavioral treatment for substance abuse: A comparison of treatment effectiveness. *Journal of Consulting and Clinical Psychology, 65,* 230–240.

Petrakis, I. L., Poling, J., Levinson, C., Nich, C., Carroll, C., & Rounsaville, B. J. (2005). Naltrexone and disulfiram in patients with alcohol dependence and comorbid psychiatric disorders. *Biological Psychiatry, 57*(10), 1128–1137.

Prochaska, J. O., DiClemente, C. C., & Norcross, J. C. (1992). In search of how people change: Applications of addictive behaviors. *American Psychologist, 47,* 1102–1114.

Ramsey, S. E., Brown, R. A., Stuart, G. L., Burgess, E. S., & Miller, I. W. (2002). Cognitive variables in alcohol dependent patients with elevated depressive symptoms: Changes and predictive utility as a function of treatment. *Substance Abuse, 23*(3), 171–182.

Ramsey, S. E., Kahler, C. W., Read, J. P., Stuart, G. L., & Brown, R. A. (2004). Discriminating between substance-induced and independent depressive episodes in alcohol dependent patients. *Journal of Studies on Alcohol, 65*(5), 672–676.

Rosenberg, S. D., Drake, R. E., Wolford, G. L., Mueser, K. T., Oxman, T. E., Vidaver, R. M., et al. (1998). The Dartmouth Assessment of Lifestyle Instrument (DALI): A substance use disorder screen for people with severe mental illness. *American Journal of Psychiatry, 155,* 232–238.

Rounsaville, B. J. (2004). Treatment of cocaine dependence and depression. *Biological Psychiatry, 56*(10), 803–809.

Saunders, J. B., Aasland, O. G., Babor, T. F., De La Fuente, J. R., & Grant, M. (1993). Development of the Alcohol Use Disorders Identification Test (AUDIT): WHO Collaborative Project on Early Detection of Persons with Harmful Alcohol Consumption II. *Addiction, 88,* 791–804.

Siqueland, L., Crits-Christoph, P., Gallop, R., Barber, J. P., Griffin, M. L., Thase, M. E., et al. (2002). Retention in psychosocial treatment of cocaine dependence: Predictors and impact on outcome. *American Journal on Addictions, 11*(1), 24–40.

Trimpey, J. (1996). *Rational Recovery: The new cure for substance addiction.* New York: Pocket Books.

11

PERSONALITY DISORDERS

Arthur Freeman
Gwen E. Rock

Among the greatest myths in the process of assessment is that clinicians will typically find patients who fall neatly into the categories set forth in the nosology of the fourth text revised edition of the *Diagnostic and Statistical Manual of Mental Disorders* (DSM-IV-TR; American Psychiatric Association, 2000). What is far more typical is that the individual being assessed has co-occurring disorders, in addition to the "main problem." These co-occurring conditions may or may not rise to the level of a diagnosable disorder, or they may simply present several confusing and confounding factors. Probably one of the best examples occurs when depression is comorbid with any of the personality disorders. It is in fact unusual for a patient to seek treatment solely for a personality disorder (PD). They more typically come to treatment with complaints of depression or anxiety. It is when the clinician begins to collect life-history data that the picture (or reality) of the Axis II disorder may emerge. Often, patients seeking treatment come to therapy in an attempt to quell or control the more noticeable and common Axis I problems. They may be unaware of the more pervasive and persistent problems that are coded on Axis II. In fact, PDs, while not "visible" upon referral, may not come to light until the individual is well into the treatment process.

Each comorbid PD has its own separate panoply of traits and characteristics. The co-occurring Axis II disorders or complications may amplify
depressive or anxious symptoms. This chapter describes the problems in
assessment, diagnosis, presentation, and treatment PDs that co-occur with
depression.

COMORBIDITY OF DEPRESSION AND PDs

Patients diagnosed with PDs are likely to experience Axis I disorders/symp-
toms, typically Axis I presentations of mood, anxiety, and substance-related
disorders (Robinson, 2003). Comorbid conditions can impede therapeutic
interventions focused on treating either Axis I or Axis II disorders by complicating the symptom picture. Patients may present with "symptom profu-
sion," wherein they appear to have multiple problems and multiple diagnoses. For example, in the National Institute of Mental Health (NIMH) study
on the co-occurrence of PDs among depressed patients, 74% of the patients
diagnosed with major depression also had PDs (Shea et al., 1990).

Comorbidity of depression and personality disorders in the adult population is gaining interest among clinicians (Farmer & Nelson-Gray, 1990;
Ruegg & Frances, 1995). A number of studies have found that depression
often co-occurs with Axis II disorders among adult patients in mental health
clinics (e.g., Marin, Kocsis, Frances, & Klerman, 1993; Pepper, Klein, Anderson, Riso, Ouimette, & Lizardi, 1995; Pfohl, Stangl, & Zimmerman, 1984;
Sanderson, Wetzler, Beck, & Betz, 1992; Zimmerman, Pfohl, Coryell,
Corenthal, & Stangl, 1991). The depression that is most often noted is a
diagnosis of major depressive disorder (MDD). It is essential in this discussion to address the issue of integrating dysthymia into the diagnostic picture.
Many patients have "double depression," in which they experience a major
depressive episode superimposed upon a history of dysthymia. These
patients may be helped to deal with the depression, which then allows them
to return to their more pervasive and persistent dysthymic style. The high
prevalence rates of depression and comorbid conditions lead one to consider
revisiting the possibility of reclassifying dysthymia as a PD instead of a mood
disorder that is identified as depressive PD (DPD; American Psychiatric
Association, 2000, pp. 788–789). Although these disorders have differing
diagnostic criteria, in creativity either in combining both or in creating a
separate diagnosis might be reasonable options. As DSM-IV-TR states, "It
remains controversial whether the distinction between depressive personality disorder and Dysthymic Disorder is useful" (American Psychiatric Asso-

ciation, 2000, p. 788). Perhaps, the chronic, low-grade depressive symptoms that are a part of the dysthymic-pattern PD might be better viewed as a disorder that is not co-occurring, but rather a pervasive and persistent style that must be viewed as a separate entity.

ASSESSMENT OF COMORBID PDs

The assessment process for evaluating PDs has four key elements. The first is assessment through formal and/or structured assessment and testing. The second involves the assessment of what we call "soft-signs" for assessing PDs. The third involves the therapist's familiarity with and understanding of the criteria sets of the DSM. Also important is to be aware of the research on the treatment of each disorder. Finally, the clinician must have the knowledge and ability to understand and conceptualize the impact of a PD (or multiple disorders) on Axis I problems.

Formal Assessment of PD

The psychological community has several measures to assess for PDs; however, not all measures provide accurate information that can be therapeutically relevant for the patient with co-occurring disorders. Beck, Freeman, Davis, and Associates (2004) suggest a number of measures.

The most practical assessment tools for therapists are self-report questionnaires, because they tend to capture more information about the patient. The Millon Clinical Multiaxial Inventory–III (MCMI-III; Millon, Millon, & Davis, 1994) and the Personality Diagnostic Questionnaire—Revised (PDQ-R; Hyler & Rieder, 1987) assess personality disorders as they relate to DSM-IV-TR. The Personality Belief Questionnaire (PBQ; Beck & Beck, 1991) and the Schema Questionnaire (SQ; Young & Brown, 1994) focus more on the cognitive aspects typically associated with patients with PDs.

Another category of assessment tools is the structured and nonstructured clinical interviews. The following structured interviews have shown good reliability and validity, and continue to be widely used: Structured Clinical Interview for DSM-IV (SCID-II; First, Spitzer, Gibbon, & Williams, 1995), the Personality Disorder Examination—Revised (PDE-R; Loranger, Susman, Oldham, & Russakoff, 1987), and the Structured Interview for DSM-IV Personality Disorders (SIDP-R; Pfohl, Blum, Zimmerman, & Stangl, 1989).

The use of nonstructured interviews that are not prompted by a series of predetermined questions can be useful in assessing PDs. However, they require that the therapist have knowledge and expertise of not only DSM-IV-TR criteria but also DSM-IV-TR prevalence and comorbidity data (American Psychiatric Association, 2000). Clinical experience is a must for the therapist to derive enough of information from the subject to ascertain an accurate clinical picture of the patient to determine the presence of a PD (Beck et al., 2004). The interview must involve questions about the "pervasiveness, persistence, and level of impairment" of the problems, then finally questions about belief systems, thoughts, assumptions, and behaviors (Beck, Freeman, Davis, & Associates, 2004).

A useful screening tool is the Freeman Quick Score (FQS; 2006). This scale identifies the existence of a PD, but does not specify the disorder. The specific disorder is then screened with any of the previously mentioned scales for specificity.

Soft Signs Suggesting the Need for the Assessment of PDs

Beck, Freeman, Davis, and Associates (2004) and Fusco and Freeman (2004) provide the following clinical clues or heuristic signs that might suggest comorbid Axis II problems or disorders:

1. *The chronicity of behavior patterns by self-report or reports from significant others.* The therapist collects data that suggest the presenting pattern has been in place for a significant amount of time—for example, "Oh, I have done that since I was a kid," or "He has always been that way."

2. *The patient has had several attempts at therapy.* The patient's history includes a number of therapists and/or long periods of therapy—for example, for example, "I've seen therapists going back to 1968."

3. *Therapy is usually crisis oriented.* The therapy process is oriented more to the *crisis du jour* than to development of specific problem solving-skills or a problem-solving pattern—for example, "I couldn't wait to get here. Listen to what's happened to me this week."

4. *The patient is noncompliant with current or previous treatment regimen.* The patient misses appointments, arrives late, or fails to do homework—for example, "Why should I have to do this? It is so much bull_____t."

5. *The patient has poor monitoring skills.* He/she seems unable or reluctant to self-monitor and/or unable to monitor the reactions of others—for example, "I wasn't aware that they were upset. How was I supposed to know that?"

6. *The patient seems to be unaware of the impact of his/her words and behaviors on others.* The patient acts in a manner and/or says things that get him/her into trouble—for example, "They overreacted. They shouldn't be that upset. I just commented on her family."

7. *The patient's behavior is rigid and compulsive.* The person maintains a pattern of behavior that appears impermeable to incoming data—for example, "This is how I have always done it."

8. *The patient is resistant to change.* The individual keeps using unsuccessful behaviors even after years of failure in their use—for example, "Why should I be the one that has to change?"

9. *The patient is other-blaming.* He/she blames others rather than assuming personal responsibility for his/her actions—for example, "If they were willing to allow me the slack to do it my way, then the problems would be over."

Issues in the Assessment of PDs

The therapists who suspects that a patient has a PD should such corroborating data. Several variables can warrant an invalid self-report of PDs, so that deriving additional information about the patient from informants can be useful. These informants may be individuals close to the patient (perhaps a spouse, partner, family member, etc.) that can either substantiate or deny information derived from the patient. An outside informant's participation in the assessment process enhances the richness of the clinical picture by providing clues not readily seen by the patient or the therapist. For example, DSM-IV-TR requires that a history of conduct disorder be part of the clinical history when assigning a diagnosis of antisocial PD (ASPD; American Psychiatric Association, 2000, p. 706). Given that lying is one of the criteria for ASPD, why should the clinician believe the patient's report of his/her one adolescent history? The patient may want to impress the therapist with what a tough fellow he was as an adolescent ("Yeah, I was once tough bastard. I ran away 10 times and killed small animals"). Or the patient may want to appear far less chronic ("Me? No. I never had trouble as an adolescent").

The therapist should be familiar with research on the treatment of PDs. In addition, he/she should have a clear understanding of the nature of PDs and how they affect daily functioning. Furthermore, the therapist must be keenly aware of the mild, moderate, and severe manifestations of the disorders. Last, the therapist must recognize the prevalence of co-occurring disorders and discern between Axis I and Axis II disorders (Freeman, Pretzer, Fleming, & Simon, 2004).

IMPACT OF PDs ON THE TREATMENT OF DEPRESSION

The therapist who identifies the patient as having a PD in addition to the presenting depression has several choices. First, he/she can treat the depression and never deal with the Axis II problem. This might involve pharmacotherapy, psychotherapy, or a combination of both. Second, the therapist may decide that he/she needs to deal with the PD rather quickly, inasmuch as the Axis II disorder is stimulating and fueling the depression. Third, the depression may be the initial target of therapy, in that the therapist decides that the depression is exacerbating the PD symptoms. In most cases, however, the Axis I and Axis II disorders are bidirectionally stimulating, so that the Axis I disorder—in this case, the depression—exacerbates the Axis II disorder. In turn, the Axis II disorder fuels the depression. What occurs is a continuous loop, with each axis stimulating the other, with a net result in a loss of adaptation. The clinician is then left asking him/herself where to intervene in this loop.

In all cases, the depression needs to be the primary focus of the therapy for several reasons. First, depression is most likely what has brought the patient to therapy. Second, it is the subject of the initial therapy contract. Third, the depression may yield more easily than the PD to pharmacotherapeutic interventions. Fourth, most clinicians have more skill at treating depression than they have in treating PDs. Fifth, for the patient, relief of the depression lifting may be a satisfactory therapeutic outcome. Finally, as noted earlier, the easing of the depression in terms of depth, duration, or frequency may have a salutary effect on the Axis II disorder(s). A second factor to consider is that the treatment of the depression can be a skills-building area in which the patient gains skills that he/she may then apply to the more complex and difficult PD symptoms.

The presence of comorbid conditions greatly impacts and complicates the psychotherapy process, in that separate and unique characteristics of each disorder must be accounted for at every point in the therapeutic process. PDs negatively impact the overall appearance and manifestation of co-occurring depression and/or anxiety (Daley et al., 1999). Additionally, several studies have indicated that the presence of comorbid conditions significantly diminishes treatment effects (reviewed in Beck et al., 2004).

Patients with PDs typically do not believe they have interpersonal problems with others; instead, they blame problematic situations on others. These patients more likely believe that the difficulties that they experience both inter- and intrapersonally stem from their being victimized by others or by the "system." It is less likely that they are prepared or willing to assume personal responsibility for their difficulties, inasmuch as the behaviors noted in the PD diagnostic criteria sets are ego-syntonic for these individuals. There are, however, some patients with PDs who are aware of their problematic behaviors; however, they lack the skills and/or the motivation to cope effectively or to change behaviors. Given the aforementioned characteristics of depressed patients with comorbid PDs, it is understandable how such behaviors impede most therapeutic interventions, particularly when PDs are not identified or addressed. Assessing and conceptualizing problems become extremely fragmented, and the ability to establish a working alliance becomes increasingly difficult; as a result, treatment plan goals are not successfully set or ultimately met.

COGNITIVE THERAPY FOR DEPRESSION IN PATIENTS WITH COMORBID PDs

Once some of the symptoms of depression have been relieved, the therapeutic focus switches to core schemas about self and life, which tend to trigger problems and depressive symptoms (Young, Weinberger, & Beck, 2001). Educating the patient about schemas is pertinent in this phase, for instance, explaining that schemas are rules by which people live and how they make sense of the world. Next, it is important for the patient reflectively to explore and identify personal schemas. Through the identification process, "CT [cognitive therapy] aims at counteracting the effects of schemas and replacing dysfunctional techniques and methods with new approaches, making the patient less vulnerable to future depressions" (Young, Weinberger, & Beck, 2001, p. 278).

Once the core and active schemas have been identified, the corollary schema can be investigated and tested. For example, the schema might be, "The world is a dangerous place," and the corollary schema might be, "The most dangerous thing in the world are relationships. Relationships can injure you," or "Avoid relationships." The decision can then be made as to the therapeutic interventions. Schemas can be constructed, reconstructed, modified, reinterpreted, or camouflaged. If the individual has no schema for dealing with a particular experience, the schema may have to be built or constructed within the therapy (e.g., a patient is aggressive but has no schema for assertive behavior). Rules for being assertive may have to be constructed within the therapeutic collaboration.

Reconstructing schemas is akin to urban renewal. The individual's present schematic structure is not working well. The structure can be deconstructed and a more flexible and useful structure may be put in its place. For example, if the schema is "Men are always dangerous," the reconstructed schema might be "Men are not always dangerous." Schematic modification involves keeping much of the schema yet changing small parts of it to better accommodate new experience (e.g., " Men are *often* dangerous"). In schematic reinterpretation, the individual maintains the schema but finds new and more adaptive uses and applications of it. For example, if the schema is, "I am special and should be noticed," then the reinterpretation might be, "I will become a teacher (actor, politician) and always be on stage." Finally, in schematic camouflage, individuals learn to mask or hide certain schemas that they recognize as being asocial, undesirable, or destructive to self or others. For example, someone with the schema, "If no one is there to see me break the law, then it is OK," might never break the law if he/she were always being watched. Prisoners who merit time off from the imposed sentence for good behavior in prison might not fare well outside of a highly controlled environment.

Relapse prevention is key to the second phase of treatment. The patient continues in an active role identifying problem areas, hypothesizing solutions, and following through with homework assignments. In this phase, the therapist's role changes more to that of a consultant discussing problems and potential solutions, practicing solutions, and discussing the effects of homework assignments. As the patient becomes more comfortable with self and homework assignments, the number of sessions decreases until therapy is eventually completed (Young et al., 2001).

Adaptation/Modification of "Standard" CT for Depression

According to J. S. Beck (1995), modifying "standard" CT for PDs involves using the therapeutic relationship as a means to improve overall current level of functioning. The term often applied to this clinical phenomenon is "therapeutic alliance." We divide the alliance into two parts, the *therapeutic bond* and the *therapeutic relationship*. The choice of using one or the other depends on the goals of the treatment, the disorder being treated, and the personal style of the patient. There may exist a bond but not an alliance. For example, the therapeutic bond (relationship) that works best with younger children may make older children suspicious. Patients with high levels of anxiety may need more relationship or contact. However, the bond alone is not sufficient for change. In working with more ego-syntonic issues such as those inherent in PDs, there may be far greater value in the therapeutic alliance, which requires that there be an agreement or contract on the goals, tasks, and focus of therapy.

Disseminating Information to Patients

A patient seeking services has the right to know his/her diagnosis. Careful dissemination of evaluation results may help both to structure the beginning of the therapeutic alliance and to provide relief to the patient regarding unanswered questions. Sharing evaluation results and diagnoses in a thoughtful manner is essential and may instill hope in the therapeutic process. Patient education regarding the disorder and its implications, chronicity, and treatability, as well as the treatment plan and patient participation is extremely important (Freeman & Fusco, 2005). The patient must be told that PDs, like most other disorders, may not always be cured; however, PDs can be treated to help the individual to live a healthier, more adaptive, and fulfilling life. Finally, it is imperative to emphasize that appropriate patient participation is the key ingredient in therapeutic success. Once the patient understands his/her diagnosis, the work begins with treatment planning and identification of specific interventions to help the patient develop the skills to live effectively with the diagnosed PD. The contract for the working alliance can then be negotiated.

SPECIFIC PDs AND CT FOR DEPRESSION

In conceptualizing issues of comorbidity, it is important to decipher how the co-occurrence of specific PDs impacts depression. To simplify this process the following PDs are categorized in clusters, as presented in DSM-IV-TR (American Psychiatric Association, 2000). Interestingly, the clusters themselves present complicating factors associated with both the co-occurrence of depression and treatment outcomes. Below we briefly describe how each co-occurring PD compounds the assessment and treatment of depression. Each section also includes specific suggestions for modifying CT for depression with the co-occurring PD.

Cluster A

Patients diagnosed with Cluster A disorders are least likely to benefit from therapeutic interventions based upon their behavioral styles, which often involve greater isolation and higher levels of what might be termed "eccentric" behavior. Therapy to them might seem very threatening and be interpreted as an invasion of privacy (Beck et al., 2004; Magnavita, 1997; Millon, 1999; Millon & Davis, 2000).

Schizoid PD and Schizotypal PD

There is little evidence of co-occurring Axis I disorders among patients diagnosed with schizoid PD (SPD), because most of these patients display few emotions and prefer few, if any, interpersonal relationships (Beck et al., 2004; Magnavita, 1997; Millon, 1999; Millon & Davis, 2000). Much of the behavioral and cognitive pattern of the individual with SPD parallels that of depression. They have a "profound defect in the ability to form social relationships and an underresponsiveness to all forms of stimulation" (Millon, 1999, p. 283). Furthermore, Millon states, "They tend to choose interests and vocations that will allow them to maintain their social detachment" (p. 283). The significant difference is that for the individual with SPD, the pattern is a way of life, whereas for the depressed patient, it is an interruption in life.

> Dan, age 68, met the criteria for SPD but came to therapy having self-labeled himself as "depressed." He had sought therapy over the past 40 years for periods ranging from 6 months to 7 years. Dan claimed that the therapy helped him, but he was unable to describe what help he gained in the therapy(s). Over the years he had taken a broad range of antidepressants with no effect. One therapist labeled him as having "untreatable depression." It was clear that Dan's personality problems were the core of his view of his own depression. When his most recent therapist asked Dan whether he had ever heard the term "schizoid," Dan said that he had not. The treatment question was whether this approach would be helpful or open a can of worms. Could Dan's depression possibly be addressed without addressing the schizoid personality pattern? The therapist decided that it would be useful to open this particular can of worms. He shared the DSM criteria with Dan and discussed the nature of personality styles and disorders. Dan sat with DSM-IV-TR on his lap and read and reread the entry. He responded, "That's me. That is surely me. So all of these years it wasn't my fault that I couldn't get rid of my depression. They [previous therapists] were treating my broken leg by trying to put a cast on my arm." Dan could identify the problems he wanted to deal with by differentiating between the depression and SPD.

Similar to SPD, the inability to relate to others and the interpersonal problems associated with schizotypal PD (SchPD) contribute to overall depressive symptoms (Beck et al., 2004; Magnavita, 1997; Millon & Davis, 2000). The SchPD pattern, which is the most eccentric of the group, can often mask the depression, whereas the depression can exacerbate the eccentricity of the individual with SchPD. The depressive has what might be termed a "minor thought disorder," wherein the individual misinterprets his/her reality. For example, the individual may strongly believe, "Nobody likes me," regardless of data to the contrary. The individual with SchPD may have ideas of reference relating to the motives, actions, or thoughts of others.

Paranoid PD

The patient with paranoid PD (PPD) is similar to both the patient with SPD and to that with SchPD. Depression is common among paranoid patients, as they tend to have low self-esteem and use fear responses and behaviors as a means to cover up depression (Millon & Davis, 2000). As a means of coping with their fears, patients with PPD typically isolate themselves when they feel shame and humiliation. These perceptions then contribute to the overall depressive state and the depressive-like pattern (Beck et al., 2004; Magnavita, 1997; Millon, 1999; Millon & Davis, 2000). The members of this diagnostic group rarely choose to seek therapy, inasmuch as they have strongly held beliefs regarding the untrustworthiness of others. The very idea of unburdening themselves to another person is antithetical to their deepest core beliefs. They are often referred by family members, or by an employer within the context of an employee assistance program.

> Lester Jensen was referred for five "counseling" sessions because of his "constant down mood and problems getting along with his coworkers." He had worked in the same drafting room at an architectural firm for the past 7 years. There were six other men who worked in the room. Mr. Jensen insisted on being addressed formally by his coworkers and stated that he was "not friends with any of the people at work." He sat with his drafting table facing the wall, so that he would not have to see the other men. "I know that they talk about me. They make fun of me. They steal my ideas, so I tell them off on a regular basis." He also was clear that he would not be self-disclosing with the therapist, as he knew that the therapist was going to tell the managers at his firm everything that was said in the sessions. The therapist took the tack that there were ways that Mr. Jensen could get these people off of his back, so that he could have his privacy. The therapist used the five sessions to outline specific behaviors that Mr. Jensen could perform that might have the effect of keeping others at bay and maintaining his privacy (and safety), without injuring his position at work.

Cluster B

Patients with Cluster B disorders have as their major shared style a pattern of high arousal. When their arousal needs are not met, they often become frustrated, angry, and disappointed, which then manifest as depression or depressive-like symptoms. We may term this depressive reaction as "deprivation depression." When they have their arousal needs met, they do not experience the same disappointment and subsequent depressive reaction. An alternative reaction is the more commonly described frustration–aggression hypothesis. If they do not receive the arousal that they believe that they need, they may become aggressive, either verbally or behaviorally, to create the needed arousal.

Patients diagnosed with Cluster B disorders have more of a chance for change than do patients in the Cluster A category (Magnavita, 1997). Although therapeutic growth is slow at times, change can and does happen, generally over a longer period of time. Interestingly enough, the therapeutic challenge lies in the complexity of Cluster B disorders, because patients with each disorder seem to respond differently to treatment interventions (Magnavita, 1997). When others do not meet their needs, demands, or expectations, individuals with Cluster B disorders may feel empty, cheated, misunderstood, or depressed. When their needs are met, they may temporarily feel good, but when that feeling wanes, they are back to needing another "fix" of attention or arousal.

Histrionic PD

People with histrionic PD (HPD) typically experience symptoms of low-grade depression as opposed to major depressive episodes (Millon & Davis, 2000). Generally speaking, individuals with HPD experience difficulty in relationships and typically feel empty and bored, but conceal their negative feelings with dramatic outbursts/behaviors in an attempt to divert the spectator's attention. Most times individuals with HPD do not seek therapy; however, when they do, it is for immediate relief from typical Axis I disorders (Beck et al., 2004; Millon, 1999; Millon & Davis, 2000).

> Angela dressed very carefully for her date with her new beau, Fred. They were going to a party at Fred's boss's home, and Angela was determined to be a "knockout." Fred worked as an associate at a prestigious and conservative law firm. Angela knew that he was being considered as a partner. She knew that she could help him in his quest for a partnership by how she would look. She described her dress as very revealing, but "if you've got it, flaunt it." She stated that her intent was

to "dazzle them," which would positively impact on Fred's goal. When Fred came to pick her up, his first question was, "Is *that* what you are wearing?" The answer was all too obvious. Yes, it was what she planned to wear, and it caused Fred great concern. He then asked if she could wear a shawl to "cover herself." Angela reacted, in her words, "as if he had hit me with a club." She brought a shawl spent the evening in a corner. She described the other women at the party as "unattractive, dowdy, drab, gross, and matronly." She could not understand why Fred would not want her to "liven the place up." She decided that there was something wrong with Fred if he wanted to be a law partner in such a conservative law firm. She felt "down, way down." When Fred did not call for another date, then refused to meet with her to discuss their relationship, Angela reported being "crushed." It was as if he ran her over with a truck, had a plane crash onto the truck, and then blew it all up."

dramatic respond

Antisocial PD

Many patients with ASPD experience depression related to issues of rejection, abandonment, or remorse for past actions (Beck et al., 2004; Millon, 1999; Millon & Davis, 2000). Most times the depression manifests itself in hopelessness and triviality, in that patients with ASPD experience consequences of their actions and believe that there is no hope for change for the future. Depression becomes cyclical, in that the patient with ASPD is not able to see a way out. The perpetual cycle is manifested in the actions of the antisocial personality, followed by depression, which may spur on more antisocial activities. Depression co-occurring with ASPD perpetuates the cycle, which makes it difficult to motivate patients to change.

Ken, age 24, was interviewed in a county jail. He had been arrested for drug possession with intent to sell. The first part of the interview was filled with his bravado that he would beat the charge. After all, it was a small amount of drugs, it was only his second arrest, there were larger dealers, and he had a good lawyer who could beat the system. Based on all of these factors, Ken stated that he would easily be acquitted. He then shifted to justification and rationalization. After all, he claimed, "There are many places in the world where drug possession and sales are legal," and he would not have been bothered. His next strategy in the interview was to be challenging and angry. Who did these people think they were, messing with him? When asked about the possibility of his going to jail and not being able to be with his girlfriend and their two children, ages 2 and 3, Ken spoke of his children and the possibility of being in jail for 5–7 years. He became sad and a far more depressed affect emerged. The depressive reaction was not simply a passing sadness, but a far more pervasive sorrow that he would likely be separated from his girlfriend and their children.

Borderline PD

Borderline PD (BPD), the most commonly diagnosed personality disorder, affects about 3% of the population, and is mostly comprised of women (Robinson, 2003). However, for cultural reasons, men with BPD characteristics and traits are most likely to be diagnosed with ASPD. Depression is usually seen as a comorbid disorder among patients diagnosed with BPD. According to Akiskal (1981), depression is so commonly associated with BPD that it is difficult to distinguish whether it is a lifestyle consequence or rather more genetically based. Typically, issues of depression center on the patient's low self-esteem, feelings of inadequacy, helplessness, and marked difficulties in maintaining appropriate and long-term relationships. Many times patients with BPD seek therapy due to relationship difficulties and the negative consequences of failed relationships attempts or the interpersonal feelings generated by them (Fusco & Freeman, 2004; Millon & Davis, 2000).

> Carrie, age 36, sought therapy because of what she described as her chronic depression. She had been married three times for periods of 1, 4, and 6 years, respectively. Each marriage ended in divorce and was accompanied by Carrie's expressions of anger. She accused her husbands of cheating in their hearts when they looked at other women in a mall, on television, or in a magazine. She would walk behind her husband in a mall, so that she could see who he was looking at. Carries used each and every charge and denial as further evidence that she would soon be abandoned. The fact that each marriage had ended substantiated her view. In all three marriages, she and her spouse went for couple therapy. In every case, Carrie believed that the therapist was siding with her husband when he/she pointed out anything that Carrie was doing to help to create the problem. Carrie saw no outcome other than spending the rest of her life alone. This was enough to create an ongoing depressive mood.

Narcissistic PD

Patients diagnosed with narcissistic PD (NPD) typically are resistant to therapeutic interventions because of the characteristics and traits associated with their PD (Beck et al., 2003; Millon & Davis, 2000). They often end up in power struggles with the therapist to prove that they are indeed special. Their pattern is, however, more a low-grade depression, or a series of depressive episodes, as opposed to major depressive episodes. Basically, patients with NPD tend to use their defense mechanisms and distorted thinking as a means to resist treatment needs or attempts, complicating the process of treating symptoms of comorbid depression. Usually the strain of repeated attempts at presenting a false, presumptuous demeanor and failing to reap the benefits eventually takes its toll on the individual with NPD, perhaps contributing to low-grade depression, usually hidden from others and based on fear, anger, and envy (Beck et al., 2004; Millon & Davis, 2000).

> Shelly, a 45-year-old accountant, came to therapy at the demand of his wife. She was concerned by his behavior over the years and had recently become more concerned inasmuch as she saw their two sons emulating Shelly's pattern. Shelly sought to regale the therapist with stories of his accounting legerdemain: how he had cheated the IRS out of millions of dollars over the years, and how his clients were so dumb that he could cheat them, too. Each "victory" would help Shelly soar, but soon afterward he fell to earth. Therapy focused on helping him get more of what he wanted (the highs) without the depressive crashes.

Cluster C

Patients diagnosed with any of the Cluster C PDs have the best outcomes for therapy, particularly when compared to individuals with Cluster A or Cluster B disorders (Magnavita, 1997). Typically, patients with Cluster C disorders experience high levels of anxiety and fear, and have difficulty expressing emotions. Based upon this premise, patients in this cluster experience more impairment as they seek treatment services to fix Axis I disorders, such as depression and anxiety; therefore, patients in this cluster are more motivated to change behaviors, feelings, and cognitions to relieve symptom distress (Magnavita, 1997).

Avoidant PD

Depression co-occurring with avoidant PD (APD) is very common, because avoidant persons isolate themselves as means of protecting their well-being, yet desire human interaction (Millon & Davis, 2000). Avoidant individuals are different than Cluster A personalities, in that they desire human interaction, but fear potential rejection, embarrassment, criticism and subsequent depression. Oftentimes, these fears make the avoidant appear introverted or shy. The push–pull effect of pushing people away, but then wishing for their company can take a toll on the avoidant's life. Depression symptoms manifest in the patient's self-imposed social, cognitive, and emotional isolation. Eventually, depressive symptoms are generated and presented as full-blown depressive episodes or as low-level, but enduring patterns of depression (Beck et al., 2004; Millon & Davis, 2000).

> Robin, age 27, came to treatment with her self-diagnosed problems of avoidant personality, dependent personality, social anxiety, and major depression—all diagnoses she obtained from various websites. At one website for avoidant/social anxiety disorders, a person in the chatroom "guaranteed" that these were Robin's disorders. Robin had been in psychotherapy for several years for the treatment of her anxiety. What emerged rather quickly in the current therapy was that Robin was far more narcissistic than anxious, and that being in the center of everyone's radar was her major goal. The more anxious she was, the more attentive her husband, parents, friends, and coworkers, all of whom she had previously alerted to her needs.

Dependent PD

There is overwhelming evidence that patients diagnosed with dependent PD (DPD) often have comorbid depression. In fact, most research attempts to determine whether depression can be distinguished as separate from DPD (Beck et al., 2003; Millon, 2000). Depressive issues generally center on perceived hopelessness and helplessness, thereby contributing to the difficulty of treating this particular population. Usually patients with DPD have negative reactions to normal adverse situations contributing to the therapeutic difficulties. Poor motivation and lack of coping skills tend to complicate the treatment process; causing the patient to be more dependent on outside resources and to feel less competent.

> Sally, age 38, came to therapy because she was overwhelmed by her work. A first-grade teacher, she was "weeks behind" on grading student test papers. Sally reported that her dining room table was covered with these spelling and arithmetic tests. When asked why she had so much trouble in grading papers, Sally reported that she could not use an answer key; therefore, she graded each question on each paper individually. When asked why she could not use an answer key, Sally stated that if there was a misprint on a single test paper and she used an answer key, she would be in danger of grading a correct answer as incorrect, and the student would "suffer" a lower grade. Sally reported that one of her childhood fantasies was that while she was in the bath-

tub a shark would come out of the drain and devour her. Sally could bathe only if her mother sat in the bathroom. This continued until Sally was 12 years old.

Obsessive–Compulsive PD

Depression is often a co-occurring disorder among patients diagnosed with obsessive–compulsive PD (OCPD) (Millon & Davis, 2000). The general pessimistic and negative attitudes about self, others, and life that contribute to issues of depression suggest that perhaps this is a lifestyle choice. For instance, some patients with OCPD use depression as a form of self-punishment, perpetuating the cycle of obsessive–compulsive behaviors. The depression maintains their need to engage cognitively, behaviorally, and emotionally in obsessive–compulsive rituals to find ultimate relief that, consequentially, is never fully achieved. Thus, patients continue the perpetual cycle of attempting to find relief, like a dog chasing its tail. The earlier case of Sally illustrates quite clearly both DPD and OCPD.

CASE ILLUSTRATION

Background Information

Ann was a 35-year-old, divorced, lesbian, living in a rather rural community in Kansas. She was the oldest of three children. Her recollection was of a rather turbulent childhood. Her parents separated and divorced when she was approximately 7 years old. Ann reported great dislike of her father and has had no contact with him. She said that her biological father was a "scam artist and con man." After her parents' separation and subsequent divorce, Ann's mother frequently left her children unattended to go out with friends and boyfriends. Many times, Ann and her siblings stayed home alone, waited in cars while their mother was in a bar, or stayed with friends or family members. Ann reported that her mother used alcohol frequently, and that many men had come to the house for approximately 5–7 years. Eventually, Ann's mother "settled down" and married her current husband of 20 years.

Ann's self-report was of poor quality, because she had difficulty remembering many events in her childhood. She did report that it was chaotic being shifted from home to home, wondering when, or if, her mother would ever come home. At times there was evidence of parental neglect and abuse, in that Ann became the primary caretaker of her siblings and herself, making sure that they all had food, were clean, and did their homework. In Ann's teenage years, evidence of impulsive behaviors began cropping up. Although she did not remember any sexual or physical abuse, Ann had an early onset of sexual activity and promiscuity, mostly with males. She reported feeling confused about her sexuality, but suppressing it, because it "wasn't right." Shortly after high school, Ann married an acquaintance while working at a local hospital. The marriage lasted 1½ years, because Ann was unhappy and began socializing with "different" friends. In addition, she reported that she was "running around" instead of staying home with her husband. Eventually, sexual dissatisfaction and relational difficulties associated with Ann's not being home contributed to the decline of the marriage.

While Ann was married, she became involved with a lesbian softball team (i.e., different friends) in an adjacent town. It was through this team that Ann met acquaintances and began participating in lesbian affairs. During this period, frequent "partying" involved various drugs and alcohol. Ann felt that her alcohol, marijuana, and cocaine use had escalated and become problematic. During this time period, Ann was arrested for DWI (driving while intoxicated) and assault; she spent the night in jail. In an attempt to establish some normalcy, Ann moved to Pennsylvania, where she enrolled in a junior college and completed an associates in arts degree, with a major in social services over a 3-year period. The extended time was because Ann worked at the college while attending classes.

While working at the college, Ann engaged in an affair with a college professor that lasted for approximately 1 year, at which point she ended the affair. She was later introduced to "Tom," the father of her 14-year-old son. While Ann dated Tom, she was still involved with her lesbian friends and lovers. She became pregnant and decided to move in with Tom to build a normal lifestyle for their unborn child. For 7 of the 9 years that she lived with Tom there was little communication and no sexual contact. Ann reported being disgusted with Tom, which further repelled her from having sexual relations with men. When she divorced Tom, he asked for and received custody of Brian, age 9. Ann had visitation rights but rarely exercised them, because she felt bad for "surrendering" her son so easily.

Ann had had three jobs in the past 2 years. She reported that because she had difficulty getting along with anyone at her jobs, she had either quit or failed to return to each job. During the past year she had engaged in treatment services for depression and anxiety issues related to her job.

Ann came for therapy while on sick leave from her job. She reported that she could no longer handle the stress of her job or the people at the job site. She was employed as a prison guard in an all-male facility. After a verbal altercation with her supervisor and a failed relationship with a male prison guard, Ann began experiencing panic attacks and an overall depressed mood. She reported that the anxiety also stemmed from prisoners harassing her, but at no time was she physically assaulted. The local psychiatrist Ann was seeing prescribed several anxiolytic drugs, as well as several different antidepressants. However, even after frequent medication changes, nothing seems to be working. The doctor suggested that perhaps enlisting the help of a therapist might complement the medication regimen.

Assessment

When assessing Ann, the therapist found past evidence of suicidal ideation, fears of abandonment, maintenance of self-destructive relationships, disrupted education, legal difficulties, and substance abuse. Her reported major problems areas were (1) depression, (2) low self-esteem, (3) relationship difficulties, (4) vocational difficulties, (5) periodic suicidal thoughts, (6) estrangement from her son, and (7) lack of friends. At intake, her score on the Beck Depression Inventory (BDI) was 42. The Beck Hopelessness Scale (BHS, Beck, 1993), and Scale of Suicidal Ideation (SSI, Beck, 1991) were also administered. Ann's scores on both measures fell in the low-to-moderate range.

Treatment

In establishing the problem list with Ann, the therapist asked Ann to relate a critical incident to illustrate each of the problem areas (Fusco & Freeman, 2004). This allowed the therapist to gain clarity into each of the problem areas as perceived by Ann. For example, when Ann saw her son playing softball in a local school yard, she wanted to move closer to see him (and, presumably, to have him see her), but she stayed in her car and watched him from a distance. This epitomized Ann's behavior—distant and shielded, but still yearning for contact.

The initial focus of treatment was Ann's depression and suicidal thinking. Using traditional CT, the therapist introduced her to the concepts of automatic thoughts, schemas, and cognitive distortions. Ann caught on quickly and read several books on CT, including *Feeling Good* (Burns, 1980) and *Woulda, Coulda, Shoulda* (Freeman & DeWolf, 1989). She was introduced to the three-column technique, and after 6 weeks, Ann's BDI score had dropped to 28. Ann's cores on the BHS and SSI were also lower.

Ann was then asked to switch to a more schematic focus rather than the symptomatic focus used early in the therapy. Ann was agreeable to that, and was able to identify quite clearly the active and operative schemas in her life. Once these were identified, the "subparts" of the schemas could then be elucidated and used in the therapy. For example, Ann believed that "people cannot be trusted." Subparts of this included, "Men cannot be trusted," "People in positions of authority cannot be trusted," "One must always be on the lookout for potential injury," and "People will injure you if they can." With Ann's agreement, the therapist decided that the active schema could best be modified rather than totally reconstructed. The next phase of the therapy focused on the elicited schemas and how they could best be modified to allow Ann maximum flexibility.

Problems

Problems in therapy came from three areas: Ann, her environment, and her pathology. Although her depressive episodes were less frequent and lasted a shorter time, whenever Ann became depressed, she was unable to cope. At these points, therapy shifted back to the "basics" or to Ann looking at her self-talk, how she was perceiving life experiences, and what meaning these events had for her.

A particular sensitive area was Ann's wish to see and to spend time with her son. Because this would involve the risk of speaking to Tom, then contacting Brian, Ann's negative predictions were catastrophic and global. By dissecting her fear, Ann was able to take a structured, stepwise approach to effecting a change.

Conclusions

Ann was seen for 3 years of weekly sessions. Therapy was terminated when the therapist moved out of state. Ann chose to take a "vacation" from therapy and after 6 months resumed therapy with another therapist.

SPECIAL CONSIDERATIONS

Clearly, this chapter points to the prevalence of depression among patients with PDs. It is evident the depression is very pervasive among most patients with PDs, causing difficulty in accurate diagnoses and subsequent treatment planning. The modification of standard CT provides an example of overcoming the complications of depression with comorbid conditions. Perhaps another approach is to examine depression as a separate issue, out of the mood disorder category and into the personality disorder category. Two examples of this are revisiting dysthymia as a personality disorder and DPD.

Delineating the differences, the relationship, and the substance of DPD and dysthymic disorder is very much like reading a political paper on the merits of one candidate over another. Many studies can be quoted (Ryder & Bagby, 1999; Widiger, Mangine, Corbitt, Ellis, & Thomas, 1995; Bradley, Shedler, & Westen, 2006). Representatives of each side speak eloquently of the advantages of their position. The bottom line, however, is that there is no clear-cut winner. A common theme is the significant overlap between DPD and dysthymia (Bradley et al., 2006). A second theme is that the DPD diagnostic group has ramifications for the trajectory of depressive symptoms in patients with dysthymic disorder and MDD.

It is important to note that the scope of DPD can be characterized by several features of other PDs, leading to specific variants. Millon and Davis (2000) propose and differentiate five variants of DPD. Specifically, the five variants are ill-humored depressive, voguish depressive, self-derogating depressive, morbid depressive, and restive depressive. Typically, the ill-humored depressive tends to exhibit negativistic features, whereas the voguish depressive exhibits histrionic and narcissistic features. On the other hand, the self-derogating depressive exhibits dependent features, whereas the morbid depressive exhibits masochistic features. Finally, the restive depressive experiences avoidant features. Millon and Davis's variants of DPD encompass practically all possibilities of features with which patients with PD may present. Categorizing patients specifically helps the therapist to decipher interventions and techniques that best meet their needs.

REVIEW OF EFFICACY RESEARCH

The treatment of patients with PDs is hampered by the lack of a broad empirical base. The most well-explored disorder is BPD, with special emphasis on self-harm and parasuicidal behavior (Davidson et al., 2006; Weinberg, Gunderson, Hennen, & Cutter, 2006) Self-harm is a clear, targeted therapeutic goal. Attempts to mount similar studies for other PDs are hindered by the very nature of the disorders. For example, how does one go about obtaining a group of patients with NPD or HPD? Advertising or seeking referrals from inpatient units, or from acute care facilities, is not feasible.

Until the field develops a recruitment and screening program for the other PDs, we are unable to support empirically the cognitive-behavioral treatment for disorders other than BPD. We will be in the same bind that plagued the early psychoanalysts: Treating those patients who sought treatment, then extrapolating their clinical findings and insights to all persons—a problem that remains in some quarters even today.

CONCLUSIONS

Patients with PDs as part of the clinical picture are challenging, resistant, and often difficult to treat. They generally require more resources in terms of time, energy, and support systems, as well as longer duration of therapy than other patients. Therapist reactions to these patients range from empathy to hostility, from fondness to aversion, and the many feelings in between. PDs, by definition, are inflexible, pervasive, stable, and enduring, and lead to clinically significant distress or impairment in functioning (American Psychiatric Association, 2000).

Individuals with PDs are typically unaware of the extent of their disorder, despite the sometimes overwhelming effects of their behaviors on themselves and on those around them. In fact, PDs are considered ego-syntonic to the individual; that is, patients' patterns of thinking, feeling, and relating seem comfortable and familiar to them. When the diagnostic picture is complicated by a comorbid depression, whether MDD, dysthymia, or a DPD, treatment is equally confused and complicated.

This chapter has focused on these comorbid disorders and a discussion of how the basic cognitive-behavioral therapy (CBT) model may be adapted for persons with these chronic, severe, and often disabling disorders. Our goal has been to provide clinicians with guidelines in understanding, applying, and conceptualizing these disorders, and in to preparing appropriate treatment planning measures for patients. We discussed several aspects of therapy, with definitions and highlights regarding various issues that may arise when working with these patients. Finally, we offered a number of case examples to illustrate the disorders and the treatment.

Empirical support for the treatment of PDs is sparse, with the exception of BPD. Ideally, as we obtain better recruitment strategies, other PDs can be studied.

Finally, the depression that is often the referral focus, and the first focus of treatment, is central. For this disorder, CBT has many interventions. It is the adaptation of "standard" CBT that makes it effective for treating the comorbid disorders.

REFERENCES

Akiskal, H. S. (1981). Subaffective disorders: Dysthymic, cyclothymic and bipolar II disorders in the "borderline realm." *Psychiatric Clinics of North America, 4,* 25–46.

American Psychiatric Association. (2000). *Diagnostic and statistical manual of mental disorder test revision* (4th ed., text rev.). Washington, DC: Author.

Beck, A. T. (1993). Cognitive therapy: Past, present, and future. *Journal of Consulting and Clinical Psychology, 6,* 194–198.

Beck, A. T., & Beck, J. S. (1991). *The personality belief questionnaire (PBQ).* Bala Cynwyd, PA: Beck Institute for Cognitive Therapy and Research.

Beck, A. T., Freeman, A., Davis, D., & Associates. (2004). *Cognitive therapy of personality disorders* (2nd ed.). New York: Guilford Press.

Beck, J. S. (1995). *Cognitive therapy: Basics and beyond.* New York: Guilford Press.

Bradley, R., Shedler, J., & Westen, D. (2006). Is the appendix a useful appendage?: An empirical examination of depressive, passive aggressive (negativistic), sadistic, and self-defeating personality disorders. *Journal of Personality Disorders, 20,* 524–541.

Burns, D. (1980). *Feeling good.* New York: Morrow.

Daley, S., Hammen, C., Burge, D., Davilia, J., Paley, B., Lindberg, N., et al. (1999). Depression and Axis II symptomatology in an adolescent community sample: Concurrent and longitudinal associations. *Journal of Personality Disorders, 13*(1), 47–60.

Davidson, K., Narrie, J., Tyrer, P., Gumley, et al. (2006). The efficacy of cognitive behavior therapy for borderline personality disorder: Results from the Boscott trial. *Journal of Personality Disorders, 20,* 466–482.

Farmer, R., & Nelson-Gray, R. (1990). Personality disorders and depression: Hypothetical relations, empirical findings, and methodological considerations. *Clinical Psychology Review, 10,* 453–476.

First, M., Spitzer, R., Gibbon, M., & Williams, J. (1995). The Structured Clinical Interview for DSM-III-R Personality Disorders (SCID-II): Part I. Description. *Journal of Personality Disorders, 9,* 83–91.

Freeman, A. (2006). *Freeman Quick Score for Personality Disorders.* Fort Wayne, IN: Freeman Institute.

Freeman, A., & DeWolf, R. (1989). *Woulda, coulda, shoulda.* New York: Morrow.

Freeman, A., Pretzer, J., Fleming, B., & Simon, K. M. (2004). *Clinical applications of cognitive therapy* (2nd ed.). New York: Kluwer.

Fusco, G., & Freeman, A. (2004). *Borderline personality disorder: A patient's guide to taking control.* New York: Norton.

Fusco, G., & Freeman, A. (2004). *Borderline personality disorder: A therapist's manual.* New York: Norton.

Hyler, S., & Rieder, R. (1987). *PDQ-R: Personality Diagnostic Questionnaire—Revised.* New York: New York State Psychiatric Institute.

Loranger, A., Susman, V., Oldham, J., & Russakoff, L. (1987). The personality disorder examination: A preliminary report. *Journal of Personality Disorders, 1,* 1–13.

Magnavita, J. (1997). *Restructuring personality disorders.* New York: Guilford Press.

Marin, D., Kocsis, J., Frances, A., & Klerman, G. (1993). Personality disorders in dysthymia. *Journal of Personality Disorders, 7,* 223–231.

Millon, T. (1999). *Personality-guided therapy.* New York: Wiley.

Millon, T., & Davis, R. (2000). *Personality disorders in modern life.* New York: Wiley.

Millon, T., Millon, C., & Davis, R. (1994). *Millon Clinical Multiaxial Inventory–III (MCMI-III).* Minneapolis: National Computer Systems.

Pepper, C., Klein, D., Anderson, R., Riso, L., Ouimette, P., & Lizardi, H. (1995). DSM-III-R Axis II comorbidity in dysthymia and major depression. *American Journal of Psychiatry, 152,* 239–247.

Pfohl, B., Blum, N., Zimmerman, M., & Stangl, D. (1989). *Structured Interview for DSM-III-R Personality (SIDP-R).* Iowa City: University of Iowa, Department of Psychiatry.

Pfohl, B., Stangl, D., & Zimmerman, M. (1984). The implications of DSM-III personality disorders for patients with major depression. *Journal of Affective Disorders, 7,* 309–318.

Robinson, D. (2003). *The personality disorders explained* (2nd ed). Port Huron, MI: Rapid Psychler Press.

Ruegg, R., & Frances, A. (1995). New research in personality disorders. *Journal of Personality Disorders, 9,* 1–48.

Ryder, A. G., & Bagby, R. M. (1999). Diagnostic viability of dependent personality disorder. *Journal of Personality Disorders, 13,* 99–117.

Sanderson, W., Wetzler, S., Beck, A., & Betz, F. (1992). Prevalence or personality disorders in patients with major depression and dysthymia. *Psychiatry Research, 42,* 93–99.

Shea, M., Pilkonis, P., Beckham, E., Collins, J. F., Elkin, L., Sotsky, S., et al. (1990). Personality disorders and treatment outcome in the NIMH Treatment of Depression Collaborative Research Program. *American Journal of Psychiatry, 147,* 711–718.

Weinberg, I., Gunderson, J. G., Hennen, J., & Cutter, C. J. (2006). Manual assisted cognitive treatment for deliberate self-harm in borderline personality disorders patients. *Journal of Personality Disorders, 20,* 482–493.

Widiger, T. A., Mangine, S. M., Corbitt, E. M., Ellis, C. G., & Thomas, G. V. (1995). *Personality Disorder Interview–IV.* Odessa, FL: Personality Assessment Resources.

Wright, J. (2003). Cognitive-behavior therapy for chronic depression. *Psychiatric Annals, 33*(12), 777–786.

Young, J., & Brown, G. (1994). Schema Questionnaire. In J. E. Young (Ed.), *Cognitive therapy for personality disorders: A schema-focused approach* (rev. ed., pp. 63–76). Sarasota, FL: Professional Resource Exchange.

Young, J., Weinberger, A., & Beck, A. (2001). Cognitive therapy for depression. In D. H. Barlow (Ed.), *Clinical handbook of psychological disorders* (pp. 264–308). New York: Guilford Press.

Zimmerman, M., Pfohl, B., Coryell, W., Corenthal, C., & Strangl, D. (1991). Major depression and personality disorder. *Journal of Affective Disorders, 22,* 199–210.

12

BORDERLINE
PERSONALITY DISORDER

Clive J. Robins
C. Virginia Fenwick
Jacqueline E. Donnelly
Jennie Lacy

Many patients with mood disorders also meet criteria for borderline personality disorder (BPD), which significantly complicates treatment of the mood disorder. Aggregating across numerous studies, it appears that criteria for BPD are met by around 10% of outpatients and up to 65% of inpatients with major depressive disorder (MDD), with early-onset MDD associated with about twice the rate of BPD as later-onset MDD (Fava et al., 1996). Estimates of BPD prevalence are similar in dysthymic disorder and bipolar disorders. These reported co-occurrence rates may be inflated, however, by the fact that individuals are more likely to endorse PD criteria when depressed than when in remission (e.g., Hirschfeld et al., 1983). Among depressed patients, co-occurring BPD is associated with a greater number of major depressive episodes, symptom severity of current depressive episode, early-onset dysthymic disorder, and co-occurrence of MDD and dysthymic disorder (Skodol et al., 1999). Looking at co-occurrence from the opposite direction, McGlashan et al. (2000) reported that for 175 outpatients with

BPD, lifetime rates were 71% for MDD, 17% for dysthymic disorder, 12% for bipolar disorder type I, and 8% for bipolar disorder type II, and other studies have indicated that between 25% and 65% of patients with BPD report a concurrent mood disorder.

SPECIFIC CLINICAL FEATURES OF DEPRESSION ASSOCIATED WITH BPD

Gunderson and Elliott (1985) reviewed early studies that suggest depression in BPD is characterized by loneliness, emptiness, boredom, and feelings of worthlessness and hopelessness, rather than guilt, remorse, and low self-esteem. Suicidal ideation and overt suicidal behaviors are more common among depressed patients who also have Cluster B personality disorders (Shea, Glass, Pilkonis, Watkins, & Docherty, 1987), and McGlashan (1987) reported that depressed patients with BPD were more likely actually to commit suicide during a 15-year follow-up.

MECHANISMS FOR THE CO-OCCURRENCE OF MOOD DISORDERS AND BPD

Although a well-documented relationship exists between BPD and mood disorders, the exact nature of this relationship has been a subject of much speculation and controversy. Farmer and Nelson-Gray (1990) summarized eight hypotheses that have been advanced regarding relations between PDs and depression. Four of these (the *orthogonal, overlapping symptoms, heterogeneity,* and *modification* hypotheses) are primarily descriptive and do not propose a particular mechanism or suggest that no such mechanism exists. Four hypotheses, described below, do propose a causal mechanism to account for co-occurrence.

The *characterological predisposition hypothesis* suggests that individuals with personality disorders engage in maladaptive behaviors that result in stressful life events and difficulties, which in turn increase vulnerability to depression, or that individuals with BPD are susceptible to depression because of a "bad self" or anger turned inward, or "abandonment depression" (Gunderson & Elliott, 1985). There is no direct prospective evidence regarding this hypothesis for BPD, but some maladaptive personality traits, such as dependency, do predict the first onset of major depression (e.g., Hirschfeld et al., 1989).

Conversely, the *complication hypothesis* suggests that depression, particularly chronic or recurrent depression, can lead to the development of PD characteristics, either only during a depressive episode (e.g., increased dependency that may decline again when depression remits) or as a more enduring "scar" effect.

The *attenuation hypothesis* suggests that personality disorders are an attenuated form of mood disorders and have the same causes (e.g., genetics). Akiskal (2004), one of the more prominent proponents of the *attenuation hypothesis* with regard to BPD, notes the high rate of comorbidity with mood disorders, particularly the bipolar spectrum, shared family history, and similarities in sleep electroencephalographic (EEG) and neuroendocrine findings. However, others (e.g., Gunderson & Elliott, 1985; Gunderson & Phillips, 1991) have noted important differences between BPD and mood disorders, and have suggested that co-occurrence is best explained as chance association (the *orthogonal hypothesis*). This question remains the subject of heated debate. Among 16 patients with BPD, 32% reported spontaneous mania or hypomania, and 81% had "soft" signs of bipolarity, such as a bipolar temperament, pharmacological response pattern, or family history of bipolarity (Deltito et al., 2001). Interestingly, in dialectical behavior therapy (DBT, Linehan, 1993a), emotion dysregulation, a cardinal feature of bipolar disorders, is viewed as the core difficulty of persons with BPD, from which the other characteristics largely emerge over time as the individual interacts with an environment that often responds poorly to such dysregulation. Linehan has never suggested that BPD is a bipolar spectrum disorder, but this would not be inconsistent with her model.

Klein and Schwartz (2002) compared the fit between several causal models and data from a 5-year longitudinal study of outpatients with dysthymic disorder. Results suggested that BPD features and depressive symptoms are influenced by partially overlapping processes, consistent with what Farmer and Nelson-Gray (1990) refer to as the "coeffect" hypothesis.

It is likely that several mechanisms contribute to the co-occurrence of BPD and depressive disorders, including shared biological and psychosocial causal influences, the effects of BPD on depression, and the influence of recurrent depression on development of BPD.

IMPACT OF BPD ON OUTCOMES OF DEPRESSIVE DISORDERS

The level of dysfunction and overall prognosis are generally worse for BPD than those for MDD, with high rates of psychiatric inpatient service utilization, self-injury, suicide attempts, and completed suicides. Most patients with

BPD enter treatment for relief from depressive symptoms, yet patients with BPD have poorer outcomes for depression than those without BPD (Mulder, 2002).

Surprisingly, we could locate no reports on the influence of BPD on effects of psychotherapy for depression in a controlled treatment study, only in naturalistic studies. Meyer, Pilkonis, Proietti, Heape, and Egan (2001) reported that BPD features predicted less improvement in depressive symptoms and overall level of functioning over 1 year of treatment (95% received psychotherapy, 65% received medications), whereas other Cluster B and Cluster C disorder features did not. Grilo et al. (2005) found that, among 302 patients with major depression, those with BPD had a lower remission rate (60 vs. 89%) and a longer interval until remission than those without BPD, even when controlling for many parameters of depression course and history. McGlashan (1987) reported that depressed patients with BPD were more likely over a 15-year follow-up to commit suicide, to abuse substances, and to use more psychiatric services. Regarding other measures of functioning, poorer academic and social outcomes have been found over 2–4 years for depressed high school and college students with BPD features (especially affective lability and impulsivity) than for those without such features (e.g., Bagge et al., 2004; Daley, Burge, & Hammen, 2000). What about rates of relapse and recurrence for patients who actually achieve remission from a depressive episode? Ilardi, Craighead, and Evans (1997) found that presence of Cluster B symptoms, but not Cluster A or Cluster C symptoms, predicted shorter periods of remission before relapse/recurrence of depression during a 33- to 84-month follow-up of depressed inpatients. Hart, Craighead, and Craighead (2001) reported similar findings for undergraduates in remission from major depression.

MECHANISMS FOR THE IMPACT OF BPD ON DEPRESSION OUTCOMES

Why does BPD have such adverse impacts on outcomes of depression? Shea, Widiger, and Klein (1992) discussed a number of possibilities, upon which we expand here. One is that depression with BPD may be biologically distinct. No good data directly support this position, although poorer outcomes for biological treatments, at least in uncontrolled studies, are consistent with it.

A second possibility is that, compared to patients with depression only, there are differences in cognitive content and style variables associated with depressed patients with BPD, such as dysfunctional beliefs and biased information-processing mechanisms. For example, Abela, Payne, and Moussaly (2003) found that individuals with both BPD and MDD had more dysfunctional attitudes and hopelessness than those with only MDD. This suggests greater cognitive vulnerability to depression in patients with BPD.

A third factor may be the adverse influence on psychotherapy of BPD behavior patterns, such as being underassertive or aggressive, or fluctuating between the two. Shea et al. (1992) speculated that because cognitive therapy (CT) is "technique-oriented," it might be less adversely affected by the interpersonal deficits patients with BPD than psychotherapies that give a more central role to the therapeutic relationship. In our opinion, this is a mischaracterization of CT, which always requires a well-functioning relationship. The cognitive-behavioral treatments for BPD discussed in this chapter all emphasize the importance of maintaining a strong working alliance.

A fourth factor that may lead to poorer outcomes is the increased incidence of stressful life events in the patient's life, which is at least partially self-generated due to his/her poor interpersonal skills; deficits in tolerating distress; associated impulsive behaviors, such as self-injury or substance abuse; and a tendency to avoid situations that need to be addressed. Helping the patient to deal with frequent situational crises necessarily shifts the focus of therapy away from the development of cognitive and behavioral skill sets that he/she can apply to reduce depressive symptoms and, more generically, to improve quality of life and reduce recurrences.

HOW CONCEPTUALIZATION OF THE RELATIONS BETWEEN DEPRESSION AND BPD INFORMS PSYCHOTHERAPY

In our view, understanding the causal relations between the patient's depression and his/her BPD characteristics has little relevance for how best to sequence psychotherapy, at least cognitive-behavioral therapies. From a behavioral perspective, the concept of discrete disorders, as in DSM-IV, is rarely the most helpful way to conceptualize a patient's problems. Instead, other principles should guide sequencing of therapy, such as first targeting problems that threaten the patient's life or the lives of others (e.g., self-injurious behavior), then problems that undermine treatment (e.g., serious therapy relationship problems), and finally problems that seriously undermine quality of life (e.g., inactivity, depressed mood).

COGNITIVE-BEHAVIORAL CASE FORMULATIONS
AND BPD

The two principal cognitive-behavioral treatment approaches to BPD—CT and DBT—both propose that environmental contexts, biological factors, behavioral skills deficits, dysfunctional cognitive content and styles, and emotional responses all transact with each other and need to be addressed in therapy. However, as one would expect, CT more strongly emphasizes and focuses on cognitions such as dysfunctional attitudes, beliefs, and information-processing styles, whereas DBT more strongly emphasizes biological dysfunction of the emotion regulation system, behavioral skills deficits, and reinforcement contingencies and other environmental influences. We discuss next the relations of some of these factors to BPD.

Sociotropy/Dependency and Autonomy/Self-Criticism

The psychoanalytic theorist Blatt and the cognitive theorist Beck have proposed that highly dependent (Blatt, 1974) or sociotropic (Beck, 1983) individuals have a strong need to develop and maintain close relationships and the approval of others, which leaves them vulnerable to depression following interpersonal losses, rejections, or disruptions, and that highly self-critical (Blatt, 1974) or autonomous (Beck, 1983) individuals have a strong need to meet their own high standards and to avoid being controlled by other people or circumstances, which leaves them vulnerable to depression following perceived failure or lack of control. These two dimensions, and their associated beliefs and behavioral strategies, also may be related to particular personality disorders, including BPD (Beck et al., 1990; Blatt & Shichman, 1983). Unlike most personality disorders, BPD may be characterized by both sociotropic/dependent themes (e.g., fears of abandonment) and autonomous/self-critical themes (e.g., fears of being controlled, core sense of badness).

Empirical studies have found that patients with both BPD and MDD or dysthymia, and those with BPD alone scored higher than patients with pure MDD or dysthymia on both dependency and self-criticism (e.g., Westen et al., 1992) or only on self-criticism (Southwick, Yehuda, & Giller, 1995). In other clinical studies, BPD diagnosis and dimensional scores were related to self-criticism and to autonomy but not to dependency or sociotropy (Ouimette, Klein, Anderson, Riso, & Lizardi, 1994), or were related to both (Morse, Robins, & Gittes-Fox, 2002). Collectively, these studies suggest that sociotropy/dependency and autonomy/self-criticism may be important dimensions for understanding BPD, and that some psychodynamic accounts of BPD have overemphasized dependency concerns (e.g., Blatt & Shichman, 1983; Gunderson & Elliott, 1985), whereas concerns with self-worth and autonomy are at least as prominent, if not more so.

BPD may be characterized by ambivalence and conflict between these two sets of concerns, leading to dramatic shifts in behavioral strategies, such as between being interpersonally mistrustful or distant and being too trusting or intimate. Alternatively, there may be two different subsets of individuals with BPD, with predominantly sociotropic or autonomous concerns. Linehan (1993a) described "attached" patients, who seek closeness and support from the therapist, and "butterfly" patients, who are more distant and likely to drop out or have frequent absences from therapy. Consistent with this, Leihener et al. (2003) reported that, based on a measure of interpersonal problems, inpatients with BPD could be divided into two clusters, stable over 4 months, that they labeled "dependent" (73%) and "autonomous" (27%).

Dysfunctional Attitudes and Beliefs

O'Leary et al. (1991) reported that patients with BPD, with or without major depression, scored higher than controls on a broad measure of dysfunctional attitudes. Cognitive theorists and therapists have described several specific beliefs and attitudes common among individuals with BPD. Beck et al. (1990), suggested that the individual views him/herself as bad, unacceptable, and unlovable, which may be articulated in automatic thoughts such as "I deserve to be hurt," "I must be perfect," and "I need reassurance." Such a patient also views him/herself as weak, powerless, and vulnerable, which may lead to thoughts such as "I can't function on my own" and "I need others around." Finally, he/she views the world as malevolent or dangerous, and experiences thoughts such as "Others are dangerous" and "Others can't be trusted." Such beliefs are proposed to bias information processing through cognitive errors or distortions, such as dichotomous thinking, personalization, and overgeneralization, so that situations and people are perceived as more dangerous or malevolent than they actually are, and so on, and that these perceptions then lead to emotion dysregulation and adoption of behavioral strategies that serve a protective function but can become maladaptive when rigid or extreme. Examples are adoption of perfectionist standards, attempts to elicit reassurance about lovability, idealization and devaluation of others, attempts to avoid emotions, avoidance of control by others, and hypervigilance and lack of trust.

Beck et al. (1990) note that core beliefs of individuals with BPD often are based on a history of trauma or invalidation. Arntz (1994) particularly emphasizes the role of early trauma in giving rise to core beliefs, asserting that "every borderline has experienced chronic traumas in childhood" (p. 422), but he uses the term "trauma" in a broad sense that includes, for example, emotional unavailability of parents and conflict between parents. Such trauma is proposed to lead to developmental stagnation and, consequently, continuation of cognitive processing more typical of children, such as dichotomous thinking. Arntz suggests that "unprocessed trauma" is the primary cause of the emotional reactivity seen in BPD, and a history of being punished for emotional experience and expression leads to other common BPD characteristics, such as emotional reactivity, self-invalidation, and appearing more competent than one feels. However, empirical data suggest that far from all patients with BPD have experienced trauma, even adopting the broader definition used by Arntz.

Arntz, Dietzel, and Dreessen (1999) developed the Personality Disorder Beliefs Questionnaire (PDBQ) which includes 20 assumptions that are thought to characterize each personality disorder. Examples include "I will always be alone," "If others get to know me, they will find me rejectable and will not be able to love me," "I need to have complete control over my feelings otherwise things go completely wrong," "I am an evil person and I need to be punished for it," and "My feelings and opinions are unfounded." According to Arntz et al. the BPD assumptions most strongly differentiated the BPD patients from Cluster C patients and normal controls, compared with the assumptions proposed for patients with five other personality disorders. Arntz, Dreessen, Schouten, and Weertman (2004) found that six of the original 20 BPD assumptions discriminated BPD patients from five other personality disorders. These items are characterized by themes of (1) loneliness, (2) unlovability, (3) rejection/abandonment, and (4) viewing oneself as bad and in need of punishment. Beck's research group developed the Personality Belief Questionnaire (PBQ), which comprises beliefs proposed to be associated with each PD except BPD. Butler, Brown, Beck, and Grisham (2002) found that patients with BPD were best differentiated from patients with other PDs by 14 PBQ items from the Dependent, Paranoid, Avoidant, and Histrionic scales that reflect themes of dependency, helplessness, distrust, fears of rejection, abandonment, loss of emotional control, and attention seeking.

Cognitive Styles and Information-Processing Biases

Certain cognitive processes and information-processing biases, some of which are shared with depression, may also characterize BPD. An explanatory style of attributing negative events to internal, specific, and global causes, for example, has long been known to be associated with, and theorized to be a cause of, depression. Yet this style is even more strongly related to BPD (Rose, Abramson, Hodulik, Halberstadt, & Leff, 1994). Arntz, Appels, and Sieswerda (2000) reported that patients with BPD showed more interference on an emotional Stroop task than did normal controls, indicating that more of their attention was drawn to emotional content. They also made more extreme positive and negative evaluations of personalities in film clips with emotional themes than did normal controls or patients with Cluster C disorders (Veen & Arntz, 2000), empirically demonstrating dichotomous or extreme thinking. Another example of an information-processing bias in BPD is that parasuicidal (suicidal and/or self-injurious) patients lack positive expectations for the future, and those with BPD have even lower expectations than other parasuicidal patients (MacLeod et al., 2004).

Problem-Solving Skills

Patients with BPD frequently have problem-solving deficits, at least in particular domains. Kehrer and Linehan (1996) reported that, among BPD patients, inappropriate interpersonal and emotional problem-solving strategies (both suicidal and nonsuicidal) on a standardized test predicted parasuicidal behavior during the next 4–8 months.

DBT's Biosocial Theory of BPD

DBT organizes the nine DSM-IV criteria for BPD into five broad areas of dysregulation that clarify what skills the patient needs to learn and practice (Linehan, 1993a). These are (1) emotion dysregulation (labile affect and undercontrol/overexpression of anger), (2) relationship dysregulation (stormy, chaotic relationships and fears of abandonment), (3) self-dysregulation (lack of sense of identity, emptiness), (4) behavior dysregulation (suicidal and self-injurious behaviors, and other impulsive behaviors), and (5) cognitive dysregulation (transient stress-related paranoia, dissociative, or quasi-psychotic symptoms).

The development and maintenance of BPD behaviors are viewed as resulting from a transaction between a biological component, dysfunction of the emotion regulation system, and a social–environmental component, an invalidating environment (Linehan, 1993a). BPD may involve a dysfunction of parts of the central nervous system involved in regulation of emotions. There is evidence for genetic influences on emotion dysregulation and on BPD, and early life trauma can have enduring structural effects on the developing limbic system, which is central to emotion regulation. DBT proposes that individuals with BPD are biologically vulnerable to experiencing emotions more intensely than the average person, and have difficulty modulating their intensity.

In an invalidating environment, the individual's communications about his/her private experiences are frequently met with responses that suggest they are invalid, faulty, or inappropriate, or that they oversimplify the ease of solving the problem. Consequently, the individual may come to self-invalidate and not learn how to label accurately, communicate about, or regulate emotions. Communications of negative emotions may be ignored or punished, but extreme communications may be taken more seriously, so the individual learns to inhibit emotional expression or to respond to distress with extreme behaviors.

Over time, as the individual's behavior becomes more extreme in attempts to regulate emotion or to communicate, he/she is likely increasingly to experience invalidation from the environment, including the mental health system, and in response the sensitive individual is likely to feel even more emotionally vulnerable. Thus, in this transactional model, the individual and those in his/her interpersonal environment continuously influence one another. The individual comes to experience frequent and pervasive emotion dysregulation and has poor emotion regulation skills, often relying on ultimately maladaptive coping behaviors. The intense expression of emotions or associated extreme behaviors typically adversely affect relationships, schooling and careers, and are viewed in DBT as largely giving rise to the other symptom criteria involving dysregulation of relationships, sense of self, and cognition. Difficulty in regulating emotion makes it more difficult to develop skills in interpersonal relationships, as well as in tolerating distress; therefore, all three sets of skills are explicitly taught and practiced in DBT (Linehan, 1993b).

Sharing the Case Formulation with the Patient

Practitioners of all forms of CBT share with the patient, typically during the first few sessions, their conceptualization of his/her difficulties. With BPD, some clinicians may be reluctant to discuss the diagnosis or case conceptualization, because patients quickly learn that many clinicians view this diagnosis negatively and resist accepting the label. However, we believe that this knowledge is important insofar as there is somewhat effective treatment, and that the diagnosis can be discussed in a destigmatizing way. One of us (C. J. R.) often simply has the patient read the DSM-IV criteria and asks whether each area is a problem for him/her, then states that rather than focusing on diagnosis, he instead tries to help people with the specific behaviors and

emotional responses they want to change. Discussing the roles that biological predisposition and early development may have played in the formation
of these current patterns and being asked to provide examples for the therapist are often experienced positively by patients and allows them to be less
self-invalidating.

ASSESSMENT AND DIAGNOSIS OF BPD
IN PATIENTS WITH MOOD DISORDERS

Signs Suggesting Need for BPD Assessment

Repeated suicide attempts or other self-injurious behaviors, and strong
urges to engage in those behaviors, are probably the most obvious and frequently used cues to assess for the possibility of BPD in a patient with a
mood disorder. Although these behaviors are certainly not specific to BPD,
they should lead to consideration of that diagnosis. The other two indicators
that we most strongly emphasize, because they are almost universal among
patients with BPD are (1) strong emotional lability in reaction to events; and
(2) excessive concerns about rejection and abandonment, which often show
up in the therapeutic relationship. Anger overexpression, although noted as a
criterion in DSM-IV, is no more related to BPD than are other emotions,
and because it certainly is not specific to BPD, it is not a strong indicator.

Measures for Assessing BPD in Clinical Practice

Patients score higher on measures of personality pathology when depressed
than when in remission (e.g., Hirschfeld et al., 1983), so the clinician who
needs to plan treatment for the depressed patient and suspects BPD or any
other PD should proceed with assessment knowing that there may be an
overendorsement of PD characteristics.

Structured diagnostic interviews for Axis II disorders, essential in most
clinical research, are too time-consuming and require more training than is
practical for most clinicians. Fortunately, a number of screening questionnaires give an approximate idea of whether a patient meets criteria for BPD,
and can then be followed up with more rigorous assessment if desired. In
the first author's (C. J. R.) own clinical practice, all new patients are routinely administered the screening questionnaire for the Structured Clinical
Interview for DSM-IV Axis II Personality Disorders (SCID-II; First, Gibbon, Spitzer, Williams, & Benjamin, 1996). If the Patients who endorse
questions related to five or more DSM-IV criteria for BPD are then administered the BPD section of the SCID-II interview itself. Another commonly

used questionnaire is the Personality Diagnostic Questionnaire-Revised (PDQ-R; Hyler, Oldham, Kellman, & Doidge, 1992). Information from such measures should be combined with that from collateral sources and the clinician's own behavioral observations.

TREATMENT OF DEPRESSION CO-OCCURRING WITH BORDERLINE PERSONALITY DISORDER

Cognitive Therapy

Layden, Newman, Freeman, and Morse (1993) presented the first extended guide to conducting CT for BPD. Treatment is multifaceted, but focuses on helping patients to identify early maladaptive schemas, core unconditional beliefs about the self and the world, and the behavior patterns seen as driven by those schemas, and to work on changing the schemas. Layden et al. suggest that of 15 early maladaptive schemas (EMSs) identified by Young (1990), those most commonly present in BPD are unlovability, incompetence, mistrust, abandonment, emotional deprivation, lack of individuation, and dependency, and that these schemas often conflict with one another, such as dependency and mistrust. In our own experience, many patients with BPD also score high on most of Young's other EMSs, such as fear of losing control, vulnerability to harm, unrelenting standards, guilt/punishment, and social undesirability. They propose that it is important for the clinician to also know the Ericksonian stage of development when the schema was acquired, which largely determines which schemas are most affected; through which perceptual channels; and at what Piagetian level of cognitive processing, which determines the types of cognitive distortions manifested.

In addition to use of all standard CT strategies in treating BPD, special emphasis is given to establishing and maintaining a good therapeutic relationship, crisis intervention strategies, and schema-focused interventions. The most problematic schemas are identified by noting the presenting problem, the types of crises that occur, developmental history, and common automatic thoughts. Schema-focused interventions include completion of worksheets on evidence that contradicts or reframes old core beliefs, use of imagery of trauma from the patient's childhood, and introduction of the adult self to modify the outcome, in addition to other uses of imagery and sensations, and behavioral tests. Layden et al. (1993), Young (1990), and other CT authors (e.g., Beck et al., 1990) discuss stages of treatment; others who treat BPD, from behavioral to psychodynamic experts, appear to agree on similar stage notions. Arntz (1994) suggests that treatment for the patient with BPD involves the following five stages:

1. Construction of a working relationship, which requires therapist patience; avoidance of intimacy, confrontation, or lack of clarity; allowing the patient some control; observing one's own limits; and admitting errors.
2. Symptom management, through functional analysis and patient practice of alternative behaviors.
3. Correction of thinking errors, such as dichotomous thinking, personalizing, and catastrophizing.
4. Trauma processing and schema change through graduated exposure, cognitive restructuring, and psychodrama.
5. Termination, which needs to be particularly well planned and gradual, and to involve booster sessions.

DBT: Some Contrasts with CT and Possibilities for Integration

In comparison with other treatment approaches, CT and DBT share many important features, both being forms of cognitive-behavioral therapy. Both recognize the need for cognitive change, exposure to feared situations, skills training, and attention to reinforcers. Nonetheless, some differences between approaches, at least in emphasis, are worth noting. CT emphasizes developmental experiences as determinants of schema development and other key cognitive processes viewed as underlying BPD, whereas DBT proposes a biosocial model in which such developmental experiences transact with biologically based emotional vulnerability. DBT does not include the construct of schema; instead it involves patterns of cognitive behaviors (thoughts) and is generally a more behavioral, less cognitive treatment. Structurally, DBT explicitly includes four treatment modes—individual psychotherapy, group skills training, telephone consultation, and a therapists consultation team, whereas CT involves individual therapy and may include telephone consultation. This may in part be a function of the need created by the severity level of the patients treated in Linehan's programs. DBT emphasizes more and provides more detailed treatment guidelines for self-injurious behaviors. Deliberate management of reinforcement contingencies, particularly use of the therapeutic relationship contingently, is emphasized more in DBT, and there is probably a higher threshold for hospitalization. Dialectical principles and strategies are more explicitly emphasized in DBT, though in many ways CT certainly addresses similar dialectics, such as acceptance and validation versus change and problem solving. Teaching mindfulness practices as acceptance skills to patients with BPD is fairly unique to DBT and possibly an important component (Robins, 2002).

One of the challenges in working with a patient with BPD is the sheer number of problems with which he/she often presents and the fact that the problem viewed as most urgent by the patient and/or therapist often changes from session to session. A loss of focus and continuity can easily result. This is addressed in DBT in part by establishing a clear list of therapy targets and arranging these in a hierarchical order of priority that depends on their severity and impact on functioning in the long-term rather than on a short-term sense of urgency. Patients who have severe behavioral dyscontrol, such as repeated self-injury, hospitalizations, or severe eating disorder or substance abuse, are considered to have the highest level of severity and to require Stage 1 treatment, in which the primary focus is simply on getting those behaviors under control. Within Stage 1, the highest priority is given not only to life-threatening behaviors, including suicide attempts, but also to any deliberate self-injury, regardless of intent or severity, as well as to major changes in suicidal ideation and behaviors related to harming others. Whenever one of these behaviors has occurred since the last therapy session, understanding that incident and problem-solving about it for the future become the primary focus of the session. The second highest priority is therapy-interfering behavior, because insufficient attention to this can lead the therapist to lose motivation to work with the patient or to the patient dropping out of treatment prematurely. The third priority target category in Stage 1 is severe quality-of-life–interfering behaviors, such as serious substance abuse or other mental health problems that, if not addressed, make a life of reasonable quality almost impossible.

Stage 2 focuses on some of the sources of the patient's misery, which he/she is likely to continue experiencing even after behaviors are more under control. This might include exposing the patient to trauma-related cues and other trauma-focused work, and helping the patient to become more willing and able to tolerate experiencing the full range of emotions that he/she may have been avoiding and escaping from through self-injurious or other problem behaviors. The most important thing is that the therapist not embark on this until there is evidence that the patient is sufficiently equipped to handle the strong emotions it may elicit, without resorting to extreme behaviors. If the patient no longer has serious difficulties with severe behavioral dyscontrol or posttraumatic stress disorder–related phenomena, the therapist can proceed to Stage 3, in which the goal is to help the person solve the ordinary problems in living that bring most people to psychotherapy, such as relationship difficulties, low self-esteem, dysthymia, and so on. To complete the continuum from extreme mental ill health to optimal mental health, Linehan has recently added a Stage 4 to her treatment model, in which the goal is to help the individual to have a greater capacity for joy and freedom.

In this stage model, because severe disabling depression is usually viewed as a severe quality-of-life problem, it is a focus during Stage 1, if the patient has no life-threatening or recent therapy-interfering behavior that takes precedence. A lower level of depression that does not seriously interfere with a person's ability to work or to be in relationship with others, however, is usually viewed as a target for Stage 3 treatment.

In our treatment program, we treat patients with BPD in Stage 1 using a standard DBT model. Stage 2 treatment draws primarily on protocols for treating the effects of trauma, such as prolonged exposure or cognitive processing therapy. In this model, cognitive styles and patterns, though never ignored, are less a focus in Stage 1 than is typical in CT, in part because of the theoretical perspective that distorted cognition often is a result rather than a cause of intense emotions, so that it is more useful to focus on development of behavior skills for regulating emotions. In addition, many patients with BPD experience a focus on distorted cognition, particularly early in treatment, as invalidating; therefore, they reject it and may reject treatment. By Stage 2, and particularly Stage 3, it is often far more useful to use standard CT forms, exercises, and so on, none of which are incompatible with continuing DBT.

If one does not have access to all the modes of treatment of a DBT program, there may be ways that elements of DBT can usefully be incorporated into a CT-oriented individual therapy. Following the previous sequence of treatment stages and target hierarchy is strongly recommended. Problem behaviors that occur can be subjected to detailed, moment-by-moment behavioral analysis to help both therapist and patient develop insight into the situations that are likely to occasion such behavior—the person's thoughts, emotions, urges, and behaviors in response to the situation—and the consequences that may influence the behavior through reinforcement or punishment. This can lead to useful ideas about changing several behaviors in the future. A focus on skills building is essential in our view. Although patients with BPD often have deficits in motivation to engage in skillful behavior, because of fear, hopelessness, reinforcement contingencies, or other factors, it is easy to underestimate the extent to which these patients simply do not have more skillful means in their repertoires. Although a consistent focus on skills training is difficult in individual therapy when crises often occur (hence, the rationale for skills-training group), it is at times possible to teach whatever skill is needed for a current situation, and Linehan's (1993b) skills training manual is a helpful resource. The emphasis in DBT on looking for and highlighting what is valid in a patient's responses can easily be incorporated into CT, as those writing about CT for BPD have done.

We recommend that, particularly early in treatment, the approach to thoughts be different than that in standard CT. Rather than encouraging a patient to evaluate the validity of his/her thinking, it is often more helpful simply to point out repeatedly that the patient's thought or belief is just a thought or belief, not a fact, and to help him/her to develop a stance of observing thoughts as sensations or external objects of perception, as in mindfulness-based cognitive therapy (MBCT; Segal, Williams, & Teasdale, 2002). Mindfulness exercises can be helpful tools for decentering from cognition in this way.

Pharmacotherapy

Although depressed patients with BPD usually have poorer responses to medications than those without BPD, randomized trials suggest that three classes of medications (classic and "atypical" antipsychotics, all types of antidepressants, and mood stabilizers) may be helpful for at least some patients with BPD. It is not uncommon to encounter patients with BPD who are on four or five psychotropic medications, and to be unsure which, if any, medication is helping, and which may be leading to more symptoms or side effects. In an attempt to avoid such polypharmacy and base choice of medications on close observation of patient response, Soloff (2000) has published an algorithm for successive medication trials in the form of a Decision Tree based on symptoms and response. No single class of medications is superior to the others or is recommended as the standard of care or even drug of first choice. Rather, initial choice of medication is best determined by which particular symptoms are currently most prominent—antipsychotics for cognitive dysregulation or extreme anxiety, antidepressants or mood stabilizers for mood dysregulation, and mood stabilizers for anger problems or impulsive behaviors. Favorable results for benzodiazepines have been reported in only one, older trial, and these medications have the serious drawback of potentially leading to disinhibition of behavior, the last thing one would want in an impulsive patient.

CASE ILLUSTRATION

Presenting Problems and Background

C. N., a 25-year-old woman who worked in science research, had lived until her late childhood in a country with a culture very different from that in the United States. She was treated for 1 year with the DBT model by C. V. F.,

supervised by C. J. R. This followed 1 year of treatment by the same therapist with a more psychodynamic supervisor. Her presenting problems
included dysthymia and substance abuse. She was referred for DBT after an
overdose on a mixture of unprescribed pharmaceutical drugs (sedative–
hypnotic abuse) and street drugs (cocaine) that required hospitalization. C.
N. denied actively wanting to die, endorsing instead the desire to sleep and
escape life. She also had problems with her primary support group given
that her domestic partner was an alcoholic and a drug dealer. All of her
friends and acquaintances were drug users.

Diagnoses

At the time of referral, C. N. endorsed the following DSM-IV symptoms of
dysthymia: hypersomnia, low energy and fatigue, low self-esteem, poor concentration, and feelings of hopelessness, in addition to depressed mood for
most of the day for more days than not for 5 years. She met seven of nine
criteria for BPD (five or more are required for diagnosis) at the time of
referral: frantic efforts to avoid real or imagined abandonment; a pattern of
unstable and intense interpersonal relationships (with mother, sisters, boyfriend); potentially self-damaging impulsivity (substance abuse, spending,
reckless driving); recurrent suicidal attempts, gestures, or threats; affective
instability due to marked reactivity of mood; chronic feelings of emptiness;
and inappropriate, intense anger that is difficult to regulate. She endorsed
several symptoms of sedative–hypnotic abuse: recurrent use resulting in failure to fulfill major role obligations at work and with family; recurrent use in
physically hazardous situations (while driving); and continued use despite
persistent fights with her boyfriend regarding her substance use.

Case Conceptualization

Relevant Developmental History

C. N. reported that in 1 year during middle childhood, her father died and a
family member sexually abused her. She felt blamed by her family for
encouraging the rape. Reactions to the sudden loss of her father were not
processed, and she was not permitted to mention him ever again. She
reported a lifelong history of both physical and emotional abuse from her
mother and a family that often referred to her as "crazy" and "ill" due to her
frequent emotional outbursts. She also reported several incidents of date
rape during her late adolescence and early adulthood.

Self-Injurious Behaviors

C. N. had had a history of self-injurious drug use since her early teens. Her most common form of deliberate self-injury involved abusing large quantities of sedatives, which she obtained from her boyfriend. She engaged in risky drug use approximately once a month, usually with the desire to become numb. On occasion, she engaged in cutting her hand and hitting her leg with a pole. Other risky behaviors included reckless driving, sleeping overnight in a parking lot in a dangerous part of town, and walking alone along a highway late at night. All of these behaviors were considered intentionally or potentially self-injurious, and their reduction was the primary target of treatment in Stage 1.

Stage of Treatment and Target Hierarchy

Given that C. N. exhibited severe behavioral dysregulation, she was considered to be in treatment Stage 1. The primary targets, in descending order, were her self-injurious and risky behaviors, urges to engage in these behaviors, and suicidal ideation. The next level of targets included her lateness, missing sessions due to substance use, and noncompletion of the diary card. The third targeted area was behaviors that compromised her quality of life, such as anger, depression/misery, and lack of social support outside of a community of drug users. Treatment targets were tracked on her diary card.

Sample Behavioral Analysis

A representative chain analysis of events surrounding C. N.'s self-injury is as follows: Her mother made a demand with which C. N. did not want to comply and about which she then felt guilty. She then argued with her boyfriend, while he was drunk, about his failure to meet her needs and about his alcohol use. Because her boyfriend did not exhibit any reaction, C. N. first felt hurt, unacknowledged, and powerless, then intense rage. She was physically violent toward her boyfriend (punching his face, slamming his head into the ground, kicking him, purposely breaking his eyeglasses), and he did not fight back. She then felt intense guilt and told herself that she was just like her physically abusive mother. C. N. then took sedatives to escape her feelings of guilt. As a consequence, she then stayed in bed and missed several days of work due to fatigue and depression associated with drug use. Another consequence was that her boyfriend then spent time with her cleaning up and repairing objects in the house.

Treatment Strategies for Each Class of Targets

Decreasing Self-Injurious Behaviors

Several strategies were implemented to address parasuicidal drug use. C. N. attended a DBT skills training group to learn to tolerate her intense guilt and rage. Problem-solving chain analyses like the one outlined earlier were used in individual therapy to identify points at which various coping skills could be employed. These were primarily from the Distress Tolerance and Emotion Regulation modules. For example, C. N. found that leaving the situation and engaging in intense exercise and holding ice in her hand were both strategies that reduced her rage, as did writing down her feelings. To regulate lower levels of emotion, she found that a mindful focus on her breathing, knitting, watching television, and telling herself, "Let it go," were all successful distractors and ways of calming herself, at least temporarily. She also agreed to dispose of her stash of pills to avoid ease of access in a crisis.

Treatment also involved generating a list of statements to challenge the automatic thoughts "I'm a loser," and "I'm just like my mother," which often directly preceded self-injury according to C. N.'s chain analyses.

C. N. also reported that her drug use was often motivated by her desire to hurt herself to make her boyfriend feel bad and thereby punish him. Therefore, individual therapy also focused on C. N.'s use of the assertiveness skills she was learning in the Interpersonal Effectiveness module of the DBT skills group, to express better her needs and her feelings of disappointment or anger when these were not met. Cognitive restructuring work also focused on whether hurting her boyfriend actually led to any substantive positive outcomes for her, even if it might have felt satisfying momentarily, or whether, as in the previous example, it simply resulted in C. N. feeling bad about herself and further damaging the relationship.

Decreasing Therapy-Interfering Behaviors

As C. N.'s self-injurious behavior decreased, the therapeutic target became reduction of her therapy-interfering behaviors of lateness and noncompliance with completing the diary card. She was frequently very late for therapy sessions. She revealed that she was also habitually late for work. Further examination revealed that whereas she budgeted her time quite effectively, she demonstrated an inability to say "no" to others' requests that she help them. Therefore, the interpersonal effectiveness skills she was learning in the group were employed to reduce this deficit. These same skills were applied to the many situations in which C. N. received unwanted sexual attention or contact. Over time, she became quite skillful at saying "no" to unreasonable demands of others. Learning to set appropriate limits also served to reduce conflict and to regulate emotion associated with her family's demands of her.

Regarding completion of the diary card, C. N. remained noncompliant for several months. When asked why she had not completed it, C. N. stated that she had forgotten, or that she had left it at home. She also wanted to avoid thinking about her problematic anger and substance use due to shame associated with this behavior. When the therapist requested that she complete the diary card in session, C. N. did so. The therapist highlighted that because session time was taken up with completion of diary card, there was not time to attend to many quality-of-life–related items on the agenda for the session. On occasions when C. N. did complete the diary card beforehand, the therapist reinforced this behavior with praise and by allotted that time to discussion of items on C. N.'s agenda. Whereas C. N. continued to complete the diary card in session sometimes, incidences of daily completion of the diary card increased.

Decreasing Quality-of-Life–Interfering Behaviors

As her self-injurious and therapy-interfering behaviors gradually decreased, more therapy time could be devoted to C. N.'s serious quality-of-life–interfering behaviors. A major one was her total involvement in the drug community. She was strongly encouraged to build a friendship network outside of this subculture to support her commitment not to abuse drugs. Interpersonal effectiveness skills were employed to assist her in asking acquaintances to socialize with her. In addition, a typical day involved going to work, exercising, eating dinner, and going to bed. C. N. often commented that she dreaded each day and looked forward to nothing. In keeping with the overarching treatment goal of building a life worth living, she was strongly encouraged to engage in daily pleasant activities and to be mindful of any positive emotions they occasioned, just in that moment, without worrying about whether she deserved it, whether it was going to last, and so forth (i.e., combining a traditional CT strategy with the use of mindfulness skills she learned in the DBT group). In addition, C. N. decided to adopt a pet, which gave her much joy and a feeling of mastery in taking good care of it.

C. N. also often became overwhelmed and dropped all of her responsibilities, missing work and therapy sessions as a result of severe emotional dysregulation and associated depression. Treatment involved encouraging her to focus on endurance by being kind to herself and planning minibreaks throughout the day in order to avoid burnout. The skill of opposite action (discussed in the Emotion Regulation module), in this case, behavioral activation, a skill commonly used in cognitive-behavioral therapy for depression, helped combat C. N.'s feelings of inertia, lethargy, and hopelessness when she felt depressed and compelled to stay in bed all day.

Outcomes

C. N. had marked decreases in self-injurious behaviors (overdosing, cutting, and hitting herself); moderate increases in attendance and timeliness for therapy and completion of self-monitoring forms; moderate increases in work attendance, interpersonal assertiveness, and involvement in hobbies; and moderate decreases in drug and alcohol use, self-blame and guilt, anger, and depressive symptoms. Progress across the year of treatment was far from linear, however. C. N. experienced several relapses in which she overdosed, engaged in other self-injury, or was physically violent toward her boyfriend. Indeed, arguments with and physical violence toward her boyfriend continued relatively unchanged. There were several discussions about the wisdom of continuing in what was clearly a very problematic relationship, especially because her boyfriend continued to sell drugs. On one level, C. N. was aware that it was a huge problem, but she remained very ambivalent and not ready to end the relationship. Also, therapy-interfering behaviors, no-shows and lateness, increased around the time of therapist transfer. The plan was for her to transfer to another trainee therapist, but unfortunately she chose not to follow through with that plan. In general, the therapist and supervisor felt that C. N. had made significant progress during 1 year of treatment, that she likely would have made further progress after perhaps a rocky period with a new therapist, and that it was unfortunate that she chose not to continue.

REVIEW OF EFFICACY RESEARCH

Cognitive Therapy

Descriptions of CT for BPD have been available for many years (e.g., Arntz, 1994; Freeman & Fusco, 2004; Layden et al., 1993; Beck et al., 1990), but the first systematic outcome study of CT for BPD, an open, uncontrolled trial, was published only fairly recently (Brown, Newman, Charlesworth, Crits-Christoph, & Beck, 2004). In that study, CT was provided once weekly for 50 weeks, with up to 12 additional sessions to be used as needed during the 1-year period, to 32 patients with BPD (28 women, 4 men), with either recent self-injurious behavior (66%) or some nonzero level of suicidal ideation. Treatment emphasized helping patients to identify and modify mal-

adaptive beliefs and, because of the common problems in therapeutic relationships and unstable, chaotic lifestyles of many patients with BPD, also
incorporated specific alliance-building strategies and behavioral skills building (which make it more similar to DBT than most previous accounts of
CT for BPD or other PDs). Patients showed significant decreases over the
course of treatment on all measures collected, including suicidal ideation,
hopelessness, depression, and number of BPD criteria they met. Although
there are still no randomized controlled trials of CT for BPD, this uncontrolled trial certainly provides promising data that warrant such a trial.

Dialectical Behavior Therapy

Linehan, Armstrong, Suarez, Allmon, and Heard (1991) reported the first
randomized controlled trial (RCT) of DBT. Since then, DBT has generated
by far the greatest number of studies of any psychosocial treatment for BPD
(reviewed by Robins & Chapman, 2004). In addition to a number of
uncontrolled studies, there are now four RCTs of standard DBT for BPD, as
well as two RCTs of adaptations of DBT for BPD or suicidal behavior; two
RCTs of an adaptation of DBT for patients with BPD and comorbid substance abuse; and two nonrandomized but controlled trials of adaptations of
DBT, one for suicidal adolescents and one for inpatients with BPD. There
have also been two RCTs of DBT adaptations for eating disorders (binge-
eating disorder and bulimia) and two RCTs of adaptations for older adult
depressed patients, with or without comorbid personality disorders. In all, 11
RCTs of standard DBT, or close adaptations of it, have all reported beneficial effects.

CONCLUSIONS

BPD co-occurs quite commonly with depressive disorders. We reviewed
several proposed explanations for this co-occurrence and concluded that
several mechanisms might be operative. The presence of BPD usually complicates the treatment of depressive disorders with CT, as well as other treatments, and is associated with a poorer long-term outcome of depression.
Understanding the mechanisms that maintain the pattern of behaviors
referred to as BPD and focusing treatment strategies on those mechanisms
are essential for a good clinical outcome. Several theoretical constructs from
the CT model, including specific dysfunctional attitudes and beliefs, cognitive processing styles, and information-processing biases, have been shown to
be associated with BPD. We also described the biosocial theory of BPD,

which is a foundation of DBT though space has precluded discussion of emerging supportive evidence regarding emotional sensitivity and experiences of invalidation. We have discussed several self-report questionnaires that screen for and assess features of BPD, adaptations of standard CT specific for BPD, and some principal features of the DBT model and how they might be integrated into CT. Emerging evidence that indicates DBT, and possibly CT, have efficacy in greatly decreasing the severity of several problems associated with BPD, including depression. We have illustrated the use of these principles and strategies in a case example.

REFERENCES

Abela, J. R. Z., Payne, A. V. L., & Moussaly, N. (2003). Cognitive vulnerability to depression in individuals with borderline personality disorder. *Journal of Personality Disorders, 17,* 319–329.

Akiskal, H. S. (2004). Demystifying borderline personality: Critique of the concept and unorthodox reflections on its natural kinship with the bipolar spectrum. *Acta Psychiatrica Scandinavica, 110,* 401–407.

Arntz, A. (1994). Treatment of borderline personality disorder: A challenge for cognitive-behavioural therapy. *Behaviour Research and Therapy, 32,* 419–430.

Arntz, A., Appels, C., & Sieswerda, S. (2000). Hypervigilance in borderline disorder: A test with the emotional stroop paradigm. *Journal of Personality Disorders, 14,* 366–373.

Arntz, A., Dietzel, R., & Dreessen, L. (1999). Assumptions in borderline personality disorder: Specificity, stability and relationship with etiological factors. *Behaviour Research and Therapy, 37,* 545–557.

Arntz, A., Dreessen, L., Schouten, E., & Weertman, A. (2004). Beliefs in personality disorders: A test with the Personality Disorder Belief Questionnaire. *Behaviour Research and Therapy, 42,* 1215–1225.

Bagge, C., Nickell, A., Stepp, S., Durrett, C., Jackson, K., & Trull, T. J. (2004). Borderline personality disorder features predict negative outcomes 2 years later. *Journal of Abnormal Psychology, 113,* 279–288.

Beck, A. T. (1983). Cognitive therapy of depression: New perspectives. In P. J. Clayton & J. E. Barrett (Eds.), *Treatment of depression: Old controversies and new approaches* (pp. 265–290). New York: Raven Press.

Beck, A. T., Freeman, A., Pretzer, J., Davis, D. D., Fleming, B., Ottaviani, R., et al. (1990). *Cognitive therapy of personality disorders.* New York: Guilford Press.

Blatt, S. J. (1974). Levels of object representation in anaclitic and introjective depression. *Psychoanalytic Study of the Child, 27,* 107–157.

Blatt, S. J., & Shichman, S. (1983). Two primary configurations of psychopathology. *Psychoanalysis and Contemporary Thought, 6,* 187–254.

Brown, G. K., Newman, C. F., Charlesworth, S. E., Crits-Christoph, P., & Beck, A. T.

(2004). An open clinical trial of cognitive therapy for borderline personality disorder. *Journal of Personality Disorders, 18,* 257–271.

Butler, A. C., Brown, G. K., Beck, A. T., & Grisham, J. R. (2002). Assessment of dysfunctional beliefs in borderline personality disorder. *Behaviour Research and Therapy, 40,* 1231–1240.

Daley, S. E., Burge, D., & Hammen, C. (2000). Borderline personality disorder symptoms as predictors of four-year romantic relationship dysfunction in young women: Addressing the issue of specificity. *Journal of Abnormal Psychology, 109,* 451–460.

Deltito, J., Martin, L., Riefkohl, J., Austria, B., Kissilenko, A., Corless, P., et al. (2001). Preliminary communication: Do patients with borderline personality disorder belong to the bipolar spectrum? *Journal of Affective Disorders, 67,* 221–228.

Farmer, R., & Nelson-Gray, R. O. (1990). Personality disorders and depression: Hypothetical relations, empirical findings, and methodological considerations. *Clinical Psychology Review, 10,* 453–476.

Fava, M., Alpert, J. E., Borus, J. S., Nierenberg, A. A., Pava, J. A., & Rosenbaum, J. F. (1996). Patterns of personality disorder comorbidity in early-onset vs. late-onset major depression. *American Journal of Psychiatry, 153,* 1308–1312.

First, M. B., Gibbon, M., Spitzer, R. L., Williams, J. B. W., & Benjamin, L. (1996). *User's guide for the Structured Clinical Interview for DSM-IV Axis II Personality Disorders (SCID-II).* New York: Biometrics Research Department, New York State Psychiatric Institute.

Freeman, A., & Fusco, G. M. (2004). *Borderline personality disorder: A therapist's guide to taking control.* New York: Norton.

Grilo, C. M., Sanislow, C. A., Shea, M. T., Skodol, A. E., Stout, R. L., Gunderson, J. G., et al. (2005). Two-year prospective naturalistic study of remission from major depressive disorder as a function of personality disorder comorbidity. *Journal of Consulting and Clinical Psychology, 73,* 78–85.

Gunderson, J. G., & Elliott, G. R. (1985). The interface between borderline personality disorder and affective disorder. *American Journal of Psychiatry, 142,* 277–288.

Gunderson, J. G., & Phillips, K. A. (1991). A current view of the interface between borderline personality disorder and depression. *American Journal of Psychiatry, 148,* 967–975.

Hart, A. B., Craighead, W. E., & Craighead, L. W. (2001). Predicting recurrence of major depressive disorder in young adults: A prospective study. *Journal of Abnormal Psychology, 110,* 633–643.

Hirschfeld, R. M. A., Klerman, G. L., Clayton, P. J., Keller, M. B., McDonald-Scott, M. A., & Larkin, B. H. (1983). Assessing personality: Effects of the depressive state on trait measurement. *American Journal of Psychiatry, 140,* 695–699.

Hirschfeld, R. M. A., Klerman, G. L., Lavori, P., Keller, M. B., Griffith, P., & Coryell, W. (1989). Premorbid personality assessment of first onset of major depression. *Archives of General Psychiatry, 46,* 345–350.

Hyler, S. E., Oldham, J. M., Kellman, H. D., & Doidge, N. (1992). Validity of the Personality Diagnostic Questionnaire—Revised: A replication in an outpatient sample. *Comprehensive Psychiatry, 33,* 73–77.

Ilardi, S. S., Craighead, W. E., & Evans, D. D. (1997). Modeling relapse in unipolar depression: The effects of dysfunctional cognitions and personality disorders. *Journal of Consulting and Clinical Psychology, 65,* 381–391.

Kehrer, C. A., & Linehan, M. M. (1996). Interpersonal and emotional problem solving skills and parasuicide among women with borderline personality disorder. *Journal of Personality Disorders, 10,* 153–163.

Klein, D. N., & Schwartz, J. E. (2002). The relation between depressive symptoms and borderline personality disorder features over time in dysthymic disorder. *Journal of Personality Disorders, 16,* 523–535.

Layden, M. A., Newman, C. F., Freeman, A., & Morse, S. B. (1993). *Cognitive therapy of borderline personality disorder.* Needham Heights, MA: Allyn & Bacon.

Leihener, F., Wagner, A., Haaf, B., Schmidt, C., Lieb, K., Stieglitz, R., & Bohus, M. (2003). Subtype differentiation of patients with borderline personality disorder using a circumplex model of interpersonal behavior. *Journal of Nervous and Mental Disease, 191,* 248–254.

Linehan, M. M. (1993a). *Cognitive-behavioral treatment of borderline personality disorder.* New York: Guilford Press.

Linehan, M. M. (1993b). *Skills training manual for treating borderline personality disorder.* New York: Guilford Press.

Linehan, M. M., Armstrong, H. E., Suarez, A., Allmon, D., & Heard, H. L. (1991). Cognitive-behavioral treatment of chronically suicidal borderline patients. *Archives of General Psychiatry, 48,* 1060–1064.

MacLeod, A. K., Tata, P., Tyrer, P., Schmidt, U., Davidson, K., & Thompson, S. (2004). Personality disorder and future-directed thinking in parasuicide. *Journal of Personality Disorders, 18,* 459–466.

McGlashan, T. H. (1987). Borderline personality disorder and unipolar affective disorder: Long-term effects of comorbidity. *Journal of Nervous and Mental Disease, 175,* 467–473.

McGlashan, T. H., Grilo, C. M., Skodol, A. E., Gunderson, J. G., Shea, M. T., Morey, L. C., et al. (2000). The collaborative longitudinal personality disorders study: Baseline Axis I/II and II/II diagnostic co-occurrence. *Acta Psychiatrica Scandinavica, 102,* 256–264.

Meyer, B., Pilkonis, P. A., Proietti, J. M., Heape, C. L., & Egan, M. (2001). Attachment styles and personality disorders as predictors of symptom course. *Journal of Personality Disorders, 15,* 371–389.

Morse, J. Q., Robins, C. J., & Gittes-Fox, M. (2002). Sociotropy, autonomy, and personality disorder criteria in psychiatric patients. *Journal of Personality Disorders, 16,* 549–560.

Mulder, R. T. (2002). Personality pathology and treatment outcome in major depression: A review. *American Journal of Psychiatry, 159,* 359–371.

O'Leary, K. M., Cowdry, R. W., Gardner, D. L., Leibenluft, E., Lucas, P. B., & De

Jong-Meyer, R. (1991). Dysfunctional attitudes in borderline personality disorder. *Journal of Personality Disorders, 5,* 233–242.

Ouimette, P. C., Klein, D. N., Anderson, R., Riso, L. P., & Lizardi, H. (1994). Relationship of sociotropy/autonomy and dependency/self-criticism to DSM-III-R personality disorders. *Journal of Abnormal Psychology, 103,* 743–749.

Robins, C. J. (2002). Zen principles and mindfulness practice in dialectical behavior therapy. *Cognitive and Behavioral Practice, 9,* 50–57.

Robins, C. J., & Chapman, A. L. (2004). Dialectical behavior therapy: current status, recent developments, and future directions. *Journal of Personality Disorders, 18,* 73–89.

Rose, D. T., Abramson, L. Y., Hodulik, C. J., Halberstadt, L., & Leff, G. (1994). Heterogeneity of cognitive style among depressed inpatients. *Journal of Abnormal Psychology, 103,* 419–429.

Segal, Z. V., Williams, J. M. G., & Teasdale, J. D. (2002). *Mindfulness-based cognitive therapy for depression.* New York: Guilford Press.

Shea, M. T., Glass, D. R., Pilkonis, P. A., Watkins, J., & Docherty, J. P. (1987). Frequency and implications of personality disorders in a sample of depressed outpatients. *Journal of Personality Disorders, 1,* 27–42.

Shea, M. T., Widiger, T. A., & Klein, M. H. (1992). Comorbidity of personality disorders and depression: Implications for treatment. *Journal of Consulting and Clinical Psychology, 60,* 857–868.

Skodol, A. E., Stout, R. L., McGlashan, T. H., Grilo, C. M., Gunderson, J. G., Shea, M. T., et al. (1999). Co-occurrence of mood and personality disorders: A report from the Collaborative Longitudinal Personality Disorders Study (CLPS). *Depression and Anxiety, 10,* 175–182.

Soloff, P. H. (2000). Psychopharmacology of borderline personality disorder. *Psychiatric Clinics of North America, 23,* 169–192.

Southwick, S. M., Yehuda, R., & Giller, E. L. (1995). Psychological dimensions of depression in borderline personality disorder. *American Journal of Psychiatry, 152,* 789–791.

Veen, G., & Arntz, A. (2000). Multidimensional dichotomous thinking characterizes borderline personality disorder. *Cognitive Therapy and Research, 24,* 23–45.

Westen, D., Moses, M. J., Silk, K. R., Lohr, N. E., Cohen, R., & Segal, H. (1992). Quality of depressive experience in borderline personality disorder and major depression: When depression is not just depression. *Journal of Personality Disorders, 6,* 382–393.

Young, J. E. (1990). *Cognitive therapy for personality disorders: A schema focused approach.* Sarasota, FL: Professional Resource Exchange.

13

MEDICAL CONDITIONS

Kenneth E. Freedland
Robert M. Carney
Judith A. Skala

Controlled treatment trials have shown that cognitive therapy (CT) is efficacious for a wide range of problems, but medically ill patients have been
excluded from many of these studies. Consequently, less is known about CT
for problems such as depression, stress, or anxiety in medically ill patients than
in healthy individuals. This is starting to change as a number of research groups
are testing cognitive-behavioral interventions for these problems in a variety
of medical patient populations. Researchers have also been working on
cognitive-behavioral interventions for problems that are specific to medically
ill patients, such as difficulties in coping with frightening or painful symptoms.
This chapter focuses primarily on CT for depression in various medical conditions, but it extends to the treatment of related problems as well.

RESEARCH ON THE COMORBIDITY OF DEPRESSION
AND MEDICAL ILLNESS

Epidemiology

There is a well-established association between chronic medical illness and
depression in the general population. In one study, for example, the 6-
month prevalence of affective disorder was 6% in medically well individuals,

9% in respondents with a chronic medical illness, and 12% in those who were being treated for a medical condition (Wells, Golding, & Burnam, 1988).

A recent review concluded that disability is the only significant health-related risk factor for depression in individuals age 50 years or older. Some studies find that poor health status and the onset of a new medical illness predict the onset of depression, but other studies do not (Cole & Dendukuri, 2003). This suggests that the disabling effects of chronic medical illnesses are more reliably depressogenic than are other aspects of these conditions. There is also a robust association between physical inactivity and depression, regardless of health status (Goodwin, 2003). These findings provide valuable clues as to which health-related problems are likely to be fruitful targets of treatment in CT for depression in medically ill patients.

Many studies have examined comorbid depression in patients with specific chronic medical illnesses. Prevalence estimates are consistently higher when depression is defined by self-report questionnaires rather than by structured interviews and diagnostic criteria. The estimated prevalence of major depression also varies within and between medical illnesses. Studies of various cardiac patient populations consistently find that about 15–20% of patients meet the DSM-IV criteria for a major depressive episode (Rudisch & Nemeroff, 2003), but very different prevalence estimates have been found in some subgroups. In patients with congestive heart failure (CHF), the prevalence ranges from 2% in older adult patients with mild CHF to 67% in younger patients with severe CHF (Freedland et al., 2003). Although depression is common in patients with cancer, the prevalence of major depression varies widely among different types of cancer (Massie, 2004). This literature has been summarized in a number of recent review articles (e.g., Anderson, Freedland, Clouse, & Lustman, 2001; Evans et al., 2005; Massie, 2004; Rudisch & Nemeroff, 2003).

Severity of illness is a complex construct, and there are multiple ways to measure it. Furthermore, many patients have more than one illness, so no measure of the severity of any single condition captures the total burden of medical illness. Across conditions, the severity of depression correlates more strongly with measures of the clinical or functional severity of illness than with physiological indicators. For example, the number of diseased coronary arteries is a very weak correlate of depression in patients with coronary heart disease (CHD), but the severity of functional limitations and of symptoms such as angina are strong correlates (Spertus, McDonell, Woodman, & Fihn, 2000; Sullivan, La Croix, Russo, & Walker, 2001). Here again, it is evident that the most depressogenic aspects of chronic medical illnesses tend to be the ones that adversely affect how the patient feels and functions in daily life, as opposed to physiological factors that may be more important determinants of the patient's prognosis or of the treatability of the medical condition.

Much of the current interest in comorbid depression revolves around the discovery that it has prognostic importance in certain medical illnesses, especially in heart disease. Depression predicts cardiac morbidity and mortality in patients with stable CHD (Carney et al., 1988), a recent acute myocardial infarction (MI; Frasure-Smith, Lesperance, & Talajic, 1993), recent coronary artery bypass surgery (Connerney, Shapiro, McLaughlin, Bagiella, & Sloan, 2001), and CHF (Freedland et al., 1991). There is also considerable interest in the prognostic importance of depression in other major illnesses, such as diabetes and cancer (Evans et al., 2005). Depression is associated with poor glycemic control and an increased risk of serious complications in patients with diabetes (De Groot, Anderson, Freedland, Clouse, & Lustman, 2001; Lustman et al., 2000). There is very limited evidence linking depression to the incidence of cancer (Penninx et al., 1998), but it may be a risk factor for mortality in patients who already have cancer (e.g., Herrmann et al., 1998). Little is known about whether treatment of depression can improve the medical outcomes of any of these conditions.

CONCEPTUALIZATION OF COMORBID MEDICAL CONDITIONS

Co-Occurrence of Depression and Medical Illness

It is often assumed that if a patient is depressed after a serious medical event, then the depression must be *due* to the medical event. In many cases, however, the patient was already depressed when the event occurred and/or had a prior history of depressive episodes. For example, 44% of patients who met the criteria for major depression after being diagnosed with CHD had had a prior major depressive episode (Freedland, Carney, Lustman, Rich, & Jaffe, 1992). This is not surprising, in that the incidence of depression rises sharply in adolescence and early adulthood (Kessler et al., 2003), many years before the usual onset of most chronic illnesses. CHD, for example, usually appears after age 50 in men and age 60 in women (American Heart Association, 2004).

Depression may also precede major medical events, such as stroke, because it is a risk factor for them (Larson, Owens, Ford, & Eaton, 2001). Conversely, stroke patients are also at high risk for depression (Whyte & Mulsant, 2002). Patients can also become depressed before, during, or after a major medical event for reasons having little or nothing to do with the medical illness.

It is important to assess the course of the patient's depression and compare it to the course of his/her medical illness, and to determine whether this is the latest in a series of recurrent depressive episodes or the patient's first. A major medical event, such as the diagnosis of cancer, can precipitate a depressive episode even in patients who have never been depressed before, but such salient stressors can overshadow equally important diatheses. Cerebrovascular disease, for example, may have an etiological role in late-onset depression, even when the depression seems to have been precipitated by an unrelated medical event (Krishnan, Hays, & Blazer, 1997). Although the efficacy of CT for vascular depression has not been studied, it would be surprising if it were as efficacious for vascular depression as it is for the more common forms of depression that affect younger individuals. Clinical trials of antidepressants for patients with vascular depression have found these patients do not respond as well as other depressed patients (Kales, Maixner, & Mellow, 2005). Thus, it is not safe to assume that CT is necessarily be easier to administer or more efficacious for medical patients who are having their first depressive episode than for those who have struggled for years with chronic or recurrent depression.

Medical Illness as a Target of Treatment

Other chapters have considered whether to treat comorbid conditions sequentially or concurrently. This is a clearly pivotal question for CT with patients who have multiple psychiatric conditions, but is it relevant to the treatment of comorbid depression in medical illness? Depressed medical patients, too, can have multiple psychiatric and psychosocial problems (Bankier, Januzzi, & Littman, 2004). For example, if depression is the reason for referral of a patient with CHF, he/she may also have clinically significant anxiety. Thus, sequencing of treatments for multiple psychiatric conditions may be necessary in the context of medical illness.

Most cognitive therapists who work with medically ill patients are mental health professionals with no medical training and no license to treat medical illnesses. Those who *do* have medical training usually limit their practice to the treatment of psychiatric problems and leave the treatment of medical comorbidities to other specialists or primary care physicians. This does not mean, however, that cognitive therapists play no role whatsoever in their patients' medical care. To the contrary, therapists often recognize untreated medical problems and are instrumental in bringing them to the attention of patients' physicians. They help patients with both medical problem solving and decision making, and with the assertiveness and communication skills needed to interact with health care providers, third-party payers, employers, and assistance agencies. Also, the targets of treatment in CT for depression in medical patients often include health behavior problems such as smoking, lack of exercise, or medication nonadherence. Thus, therapists often play an important role in their patients' medical care.

CT has the potential to produce *adverse* medical consequences in some cases. For example, a patient may feel discouraged and isolated after an acute MI because he has stopped joining his friends on the golf course. Behavioral activation might be used to encourage him to get back out on the tee, but this could be a risky activity under the circumstances. Behavioral activation is an essential component of CT for depressed medical patients, but consultation with the patient's physician is necessary if there is any question about the safety of an activation plan.

CT could have unintended consequences by increasing the overall burden of health care. Weekly visits with a cognitive therapist might make it difficult for patients to keep up with other aspects of their health care, such as frequent visits to physicians and adherence to multiple medication regimens. This was observed in a trial of CT for depression in patients with diabetes (Lustman, Griffith, Freedland, Kissel, & Clouse, 1998b). The participants were randomly assigned to 10 weeks of CT or to a control group. Participation in CT helped to improve patients' glycemic control in the long run, but it decreased their adherence to the diabetes self-care regimen in the short run (Lustman, Freedman, Griffith, & Clouse, 1998a). Thus, medical patients with complex, demanding treatment regimens may have difficulty in adhering simultaneously to CT and to self-care for medical illness. It may be possible to mitigate this by integrating CT into a broader interdisciplinary care plan.

CT might also produce unintended adverse effects by being *intrusive*, particularly for medical patients who are recruited or referred rather than self-referred. When a patient has been recruited for a trial of CT for depression or referred for clinical CT services, it is advisable to assess whether the patient acknowledges feeling distressed, and whether he/she welcomes treatment and sees it as potentially beneficial rather than as intrusive.

Conceptualization

Medical illness and medical care can enter into cognitive-behavioral case conceptualization in a number of ways. For example, symptom and disease attributions can help to inform case conceptualization. It is important to determine whether patients attribute depression or anxiety symptoms to their medical illness, and whether they attribute their medical illness to stress, depression, anxiety, or other problems (Day, Freedland, & Carney, 2005; Freedland, 2005).

In developing a case conceptualization, it is important to consider the extent to which the patient is distressed about the consequences or implications of his/her illness, rather than about the illness per se. Dysfunctional Thought Records reveal that many patients spend little time ruminating about their medical condition but frequently have distressing thoughts about its consequences or implications. For example, a patient may experience less distress about her cancer than about the belief that she is to blame for it. A patient may have few automatic thoughts about his recent heart attack, yet be overwhelmed with concerns about being unable to return to his former lifestyle, or with guilt about letting his family down by not taking better care of himself. When patients dwell on recent medical events, therapists can expect these events to dominate collaborative agenda setting during the first few sessions. However, many patients are eager to leave their medical crises behind and move on with their lives. In such cases, it is not helpful to emphasize the medical event in the case conceptualization or treatment plan.

Whether the relationship between the patient's medical and psychological problems is a central focus of therapy or only a peripheral issue varies from case to case. An individual may be identified as a "cancer patient" or a "heart patient," yet be depressed about something distantly related, if related at all, to the medical illness. One patient, for example, had been hospitalized repeatedly for heart and lung disorders. She had been ill for 10 years and was coping very well with her medical problems, but she was distressed about her grandson's drug abuse and about her daughter's irresponsibility as a parent. It would have been counterproductive, at best, to make this patient's medical problems the centerpiece of the case conceptualization. This is in contrast to other cases, in which medical problems are responsible for much of the patient's distress.

Depressed patients' medical illnesses should be considered from a developmental lifespan perspective. Core beliefs, intermediate cognitions, and compensatory strategies begin to develop early in life, at a stage when the chronic illnesses of middle- and old-age are just remote abstractions. When medical illness strikes, it often does so unexpectedly, in ways that violate the patient's beliefs. It is hard to adjust to a serious medical illness if one believes, for example, "Other people can get sick, but not me." It is also hard to adjust to illnesses that strike at a younger age than their victims have any reason to expect. One of our patients developed severe CHF in his early 30s, not long

312   CT FOR COMORBID DEPRESSION

after the birth of his first child. He expressed a profound sense of shock and existential betrayal at having been stricken with "something that only happens to old people" and that would prevent him from being the father and husband he had always wanted to be. In some cases, however, medical illnesses do not violate core beliefs, but instead confirm and activate them. The onset of cancer, for example, might reinforce a patient's long-held belief that "I'm defective" or that "I've been doomed from the start."

Medical illnesses can also disrupt compensatory strategies that were more or less successful during the healthier years of the patient's life. An individual with a core belief of unlovability, for example, might compensate for it with a very active social life. If the emergence of a chronic illness prevents her from maintaining her social activities, she may have no alternative strategies with which to defend herself against feeling unwanted.

A developmental lifespan perspective is also helpful in conceptualizing the psychosocial effects of medical illnesses that affect younger individuals. For example, a recent study examined the efficacy of CT for depression in patients with epilepsy. The participants were young adults whose epilepsy deprived them of opportunities to gain independence, to pursue a career, to develop an adult social network, or to find a partner. The depressogenic problems that confronted them were the opposite of those experienced by many older individuals, who enjoyed decades of good health and independence before developing a chronic medical illness.

ASSESSMENT OF COMORBID MEDICAL CONDITIONS

In contrast to comorbidities such as panic or personality disorder, cognitive therapists do not have a direct role in evaluating medical comorbidities. They should review the patient's medical history and current medications nevertheless, and evaluate whether the presenting problems may be due, at least in part, to side effects of medications, or to the neuropsychiatric effects of a medical condition. Cognitive therapists should also assess psychosocial issues related to the patient's medical condition, such as functional impairment, the interpersonal impact of the illness, and health-related quality of life. Numerous assessment instruments have been developed for these purposes, but only some of them have been used in conjunction with CT for medical patients. For example, the Depression Interview and Structured Hamilton (DISH), a semistructured interview for assessing depression in medically ill patients (Davidson et al., 2006; Freedland et al., 2002), was developed for the multicenter Enhancing Recovery in Coronary Heart Disease (ENRICHD) clinical trial and has since been used in a number of other studies.

A variety of questionnaires have been used to assess causal attributions about specific medical illnesses, such as heart disease. The Illness Perception Questionnaire (IPQ; Weinman, Petrie, Moss-Morris, & Horne, 1996), which has been used in a number of recent studies, evaluates the extent to which the patient believes that emotional distress in the form of stress, anxiety, depression, and so forth, has contributed to the onset or progression of his/her medical illness. Therapists can use this information to determine whether to emphasize the potential health benefits of overcoming depression, coping with stress, and so forth, when inducting the patient into CT and working to maintain his/her motivation to participate fully in treatment.

The 36-item Short-Form Health Survey (SF-36), a widely used measure of health-related quality of life (Stewart et al., 1989), assesses the perceived impact of medical problems on activities, role functioning, and emotional well-being. Therapists can use it to determine whether the patient's medical problems are a significant source of distress and impairment. It yields physical and mental factor scores. CT can have differential effects on these scores, particularly with patients whose physical health status is declining over time. Treatment for depression can help them maintain or improve the mental component of their quality of life, even while the physical component is deteriorating.

ADAPTATION OF STANDARD CT IN THE TREATMENT OF DEPRESSION IN MEDICALLY ILL PATIENTS

There are more similarities than differences between standard CT and cognitive-behavioral interventions for depressed medical patients. Some of the differences stem from the fact that many of these patients are referred by their physician, urged by their spouse to see a therapist, or recruited for participation in a clinical trial. Their demographic profile tends to differ from that of depressed but otherwise healthy patients who seek CT on their own initiative. Although some chronic illnesses are prevalent among young adults, most of the major chronic illnesses are more common among middle-aged and older individuals. Consequently, patients with conditions such as arthritis or heart disease who are referred for CT are older on average than the majority of patients who are seen in more typical cognitive-behavioral practices.

It is not uncommon for medical patients to feel insulted, humiliated, or angry when their physician refers them to a mental health professional, or to arrive at the therapist's doorstep with erroneous ideas about the purpose and process of therapy. This is an especially important consideration for older patients, those with no prior history of psychiatric problems and no prior contacts with mental health professionals, and individuals who are wary of being mistreated by health care professionals. These considerations place a premium on the process of inducting the patient into therapy and on establishing a *collaborative* therapeutic relationship.

When working with seriously medically ill patients, there is often a greater emphasis on the *utility* of distressing cognitions than on their *validity*. Medical illnesses often create a daunting cascade of financial, occupational, interpersonal, and practical problems. It is counterproductive, for example, to discuss "catastrophizing" with patients who are facing genuine personal catastrophes. It is better to address the utility of distressing thoughts about these problems, to provide ample emotional support, and to help with problem solving.

However, dysfunctional cognitions are neither off-limits nor irrelevant in CT for depressed medically ill patients, who often have the same kinds of depressogenic cognitions about self, world, and future that are common among healthier depressed patients (Beck, Rush, Shaw, & Emery, 1979). Depressogenic and anxiogenic cognitions about medical illness and its consequences are also common. Because health-related dysfunctional cognitions are not explicitly included in the Dysfunctional Attitudes Scale (DAS; Burns, 1980; Weissman & Beck, 1978), we recently developed a 20-item supplement to the DAS to assess ones that are often reported by chronically ill patients. The Dysfunctional Attitudes about Health supplementary scale includes items such as "It's unfair for me to have health problems," "People will resent it if they have to take care of me," and "Because of my illness, I'm not the same person I used to be." It is useful for assessing self-blame for the medical illness, unfounded fears about its interpersonal consequences, and other health-related dysfunctional cognitions. The entire scale is included in Skala, Freedland, and Carney (2005).

Some health-related cognitions are distressing not because they reflect cognitive distortions, but because they are *misconceptions* about illness or treatment. For example, it is not unusual for patients with CHD to hold the mistaken belief that every episode of angina is a small heart attack that causes permanent damage. This stems from a misunderstanding about angina rather than from a cognitive distortion such as catastrophizing. Patients who hold this distressing misconception tend to avoid physical activity and exercise, which contravenes the recommendations that they were probably given by their cardiologist or cardiac rehabilitation specialist (Furze, Bull, Lewin, & Thompson, 2003). Although these misconceptions constitute a different kind of cognitive error than the ones that are emphasized in standard CT, they can be modified by a combination of health education and cognitive-behavioral techniques (Lewin et al., 2002).

One of the most important adaptations of CT is in how it is delivered to medically ill patients. Some patients are able to come in for weekly therapy outpatient sessions, and doing so may be a component of their behavioral activation plan. Others, however, cannot, or will not, participate in frequent clinic visits for reasons such as being too ill, disabled, weak, or fatigued; lack of transportation; scheduling conflicts with work or with other clinic visits, treatments, rehabilitation programs, or support groups; or an appraisal that frequent clinic visits for CT are not worth the time or effort. The latter does not necessarily indicate a lack of motivation or interest in treatment. It may instead represent a rational cost–benefit analysis, if medical illness and medical care are severely disrupting the patient's daily life.

Many medically ill patients who cannot, or will not, participate in weekly clinic visits can still benefit from CT if their therapists are willing to reach out to them. In the ENRICHD trial, for example, therapists often conducted sessions at the patient's home or at bedside if the patient had been rehospitalized. Many sessions were also conducted via telephone. Telephone-based therapy has been used in several recent cognitive-behavioral trials with generally favorable results (Bastien, Morin, Ouelette, Blais, & Bouchard, 2004; Blumenthal et al., 2006; Mohr et al., 2000; Simon, Ludman, Tutty, Operskalski, & Von, 2004).

Timing and duration of treatment are also important considerations in adapting CT to the needs of medically ill patients. Aside from limitations imposed by third-party payers or other practical constraints, the duration of CT is usually determined by considerations such as the severity and chronicity of depression, the presence of psychiatric comorbidities, and the complexity of the patient's psychosocial problems. When working with medical patients, the course of the medical illness also has to be taken into account. For example, many survivors of a acute MI are too ill to tolerate CT immediately after their hospitalization, at least not in the usual hour-long, weekly or biweekly format. Consequently, it may be necessary to start with brief, supportive contacts and to postpone intensive therapy until the patient is ready. Other medical problems can follow distinctly different trajectories. For example, CHF is a progressive illness with a poor long-term prognosis. Patients with CHF typically experience a decline over time in their health status and physical functioning, so patients with comorbid depression often require 6 months or more of CT to reach complete remission of depression.

It may not be possible to conduct a typical "linear" course of CT for depression in seriously medically ill patients; it may be necessary to intervene in a series of bouts instead. Patients may require more frequent sessions during particularly stressful phases of their illness and less frequent sessions during more favorable periods. It may be necessary to interrupt intensive therapy for weeks or months at a time during rehospitalizations or other medical crises, and to resort to brief, supportive contacts. Furthermore, patients may have different needs and different treatment goals after an acute medical event, major surgery, and so forth, than they did before.

Thus, the nature and course of the patient's medical condition can affect the timing and duration of CT for depression. *Flexibility* and *individual tailoring of treatment* are essential in delivering CT to these patients. Treatment protocols that are too rigidly standardized cannot accommodate the complexity of CT for depression in the context of major medical illnesses.

CASE ILLUSTRATION

R. D., a 54-year-old African American woman identified as depressed by a nurse at her cardiac surgeon's office, reported low mood, crying, irritability, fatigue, poor concentration, disrupted sleep, and suicidal thoughts. At her initial visit, R. D. was diagnosed with major depression. She reported loss of interest for nearly 2 years and long-standing problems with low self-esteem. Most of her symptoms had been present for at least 2 months. Her Beck Depression Inventory (BDI) score was 28 and her Beck Anxiety Inventory (BAI) score was 24. On the SF-36, she described her health as poor, getting worse, and limiting her in all but basic self-care activities. She was randomly assigned to the CT arm of a trial of treatment for depression after coronary bypass surgery.

R. D.'s initial clinical evaluation revealed that she had been divorced for 7 years after a long marriage. She had lost a sibling in an accident a few months earlier and reported thinking, "Why wasn't it me? I'm sick and lonely, and I can't accomplish anything anymore." She had been on disability for 5 years after doing clerical work for 17 years at a firm where her reliability and competence had been well recognized. Her early years included financial hardships and a debilitating childhood accident from which she fully recovered over a period of years without medical care. She recalled that other children rejected her because of her disability.

R. D. had several major medical problems, including diabetes with severe complications. Despite the severity of her illness, her husband had accused her of faking symptoms to get out of doing housework. She had had coronary artery bypass graft (CABG) surgery about 10 years earlier and a second CABG operation 10 months prior to enrollment in the study. She stated that her first CABG surgery was not at all like her second experience, in that her recovery from the latter seemed slow and incomplete. Other health problems included hypertension and asthma. R. D. was on 14 different daily medications. After discussing the pros and cons with her therapist, she asked her physician to prescribe an antidepressant; escitalopram (10 mg per day) was added to her regimen. R. D. reported one prior episode of depression during her fourth pregnancy. She sought counseling at the time and described it as "helpful."

At the beginning of CT, she appeared very tired. She produced a one-item problem list, "my health problems," but she talked mostly about other concerns, particularly feelings of shame about her depression. R. D.'s problem list was revised to include her depression and her thoughts about it. Because of her fatigue, she was given a light CT homework assignment.

She completed her homework and read Beck's *Coping with Depression* booklet. When R. D. reported that she was not doing anything that she enjoyed anymore, she was asked to try doing some needlework, one of her favorite activities. Time-based pacing with frequent rest was introduced as a way for R. D. to accomplish her chores without experiencing severe fatigue. At the next session, R. D. reported that her children questioned her rest breaks in the middle of doing chores; this made her realize that she had accepted unfair blame for her illnesses and for the breakup of her marriage. When asked to explain these beliefs, she realized that the facts did not support them. Her mood brightened considerably when she discussed this. She began to recognize her self-blaming thoughts and to dispute them. With her therapist's assistance, she also developed a set of coping cards for situations in which believes she was being unfairly blamed.

Testing her thoughts and disputing worries became the cornerstone of therapy for the next several sessions. Several stressful events occurred during this period and were opportunities R. D. to practice new coping skills. By the fourth week of therapy, she was readily identifying and challenging her automatic thoughts, and her BDI score had dropped to 16. During a frightening health crisis, she used her homework forms to test her thoughts, but she did not achieve the results she had come to expect. She called her therapist, and they collaboratively reviewed her thinking about the situation and developed a new coping card.

At her sixth session, R. D.'s problem list was reevaluated. She believed that others did not understand her diabetes–related symptoms. She felt alone with her health problems and was uncomfortable about asking others for help. She developed a set of responses to her distressing automatic thoughts about these issues, and wrote them on her coping cards. Her social network was also examined, and strategies were developed to improve her social functioning. Problem-solving strategies included returning to her church and associating with others who accepted depression as an illness rather than a weakness or lack of faith; calling the American Diabetes Association to inquire about joining a support group; and obtaining educational materials about diabetes for her children to read. She was also given homework assignments to borrow household items from a neighbor, and to decline to offer help when someone called her about a problem that could realistically be solved, or at least tolerated, without her assistance. At her eighth session, R. D.'s BDI score was 10 and her BAI score was 13.

During the next phase of the intervention, R. D.'s cognitive conceptualization was discussed at length and regularly reviewed. After examining several situations, along with her automatic thoughts, emotions, and behaviors, and considering the contributions of her early years to her current thinking, the therapist suggested that R. D. seemed to hold core beliefs about being defective and unlovable. She affirmed this, as well as her long-standing intermediate belief that she would be acceptable to others only if she did all she could for them, while hiding her own pain. She also confirmed that she had relied on the compensatory strategies of pushing herself to do all she could for others, while ignoring her limitations, then isolating herself from others to avoid having to say "no" and to escape the harsh judgments that she expected. Her response to this intervention was to state that she had no reason to continue on the same path, especially since she believed that changing her thoughts and behaviors was helping her.

Although R. D. was slow to make contact with the American Diabetes Association, she had taken the initial steps. She had borrowed a kitchen item from her neighbor, and she had attended some church services. At Session 10, her BDI score was 7 and her BAI was 8. A relapse prevention plan was collaboratively formulated. At R. D.'s 11th and final session, her BDI score was 5 and her BAI was 7. Dysfunctional attitudes and the use of various techniques to overcome depression were assessed at the beginning and end of therapy. The changes in both of these areas were reviewed. She was given a copy of her questionnaires to review in case of relapse.

At her follow-up assessments, R. D. continued to do remarkable well. She had joined a support group and had found ways to remain active despite her need for rest. Her BDI score was below 3, and all of her other scores remained at a much-improved level. During a phone call after she had completed the study, R. D. shared some of her thoughts about the process. She reported that she had not wanted to start therapy because it seemed too exhausting, and she had secretly hoped that her therapist would give up and leave her alone. She had wondered why "these white women wanted to bother with her" even though she had "so little to offer anyone." R. D. said that the fact that someone who genuinely cared about her kept showing up made all the difference, and that after the third or fourth week, she had decided that she could trust her therapist.

R. D.'s case reflects not only the challenge of overcoming racial and other demographic barriers to a trusting relationship with a therapist, but also one of the chief difficulties of working with medically ill patients. In many cases, these patients are tired and overwhelmed, and they have exhausted their personal resources. Many patients who need help are unable to come to a clinic for therapy visits. Consequently, they remain "under the radar screen" of the health care system and are underserved. Cognitive therapists may be able to help their depressed, medically ill patients to overcome some of these barriers via phone contacts, as well as home visits, as long as they are feasible for the therapist and welcomed by the patient.

REVIEW OF EFFICACY RESEARCH

Heart Disease

ENRICHD was a large, multicenter, randomized trial of treatment for depression and low perceived social support after acute MI. Participants were randomly assigned to receive up to 6 months of individual CT or usual care. The CT protocol has been described elsewhere (ENRICHD Investigators, 2001). Patients who were either severely depressed or nonresponsive to CT were also given sertraline. There were statistically significant but modest between-group differences in depression and social support at 6 months. There was no difference in the primary medical endpoint, reinfarction-free survival (Berkman et al., 2003).

A few small studies have tested cognitive-behavioral interventions for depression in cardiac patients. In an uncontrolled trial, Carney et al. (2000) treated depressed outpatients with stable CHD with up to 16 sessions of individual CT. In patients who were mildly depressed, BDI scores dropped from 15 ± 4 to 5 ± 4; in severely depressed patients, the scores dropped from 28 ± 7 to 10 ± 7. Other trials are in progress, including studies at our center of CT for depression after heart surgery and for depression in patients with CHF.

Other Medical Conditions

CT has been tested in other medically ill patient populations, with outcomes such as improved adjustment to illness, increased ability to cope with stress, and better health-related quality of life. Few studies have tested the efficacy of CT for comorbid depression in a defined medical illness. For example, the Lustman et al. (1998b) study described earlier is so far the only published trial of CT for depression in patients with diabetes.

Most of the clinical trials published so far have been small, single-site studies, and only some have demonstrated favorable outcomes. In one study, for example, stroke patients were randomly assigned to 10 sessions of CT, an attention control intervention, or usual care. No significant differences were found on posttreatment measures of depression, functional status, or satisfaction with care (Lincoln & Flannaghan, 2003). Sharpe et al. (2001) randomly assigned patients with arthritis to eight sessions of CT or to usual care. The CT group scored significantly lower on the Hospital Anxiety and Depression Scale (HADS) at 6 months. In contrast, Parker et al. (2003) reported that a combination of CT and antidepressants for depression in patients with arthritis was not more efficacious than antidepressants alone.

Given et al. (2004) randomly assigned patients with malignant tumors who were undergoing chemotherapy to a 10 sessions of CT or to usual care. Severely depressed patients derived greater benefit from CT than those who were mildly depressed. In contrast, Trask, Paterson, Griffith, Riba, and Schwartz (2003) randomized patients with malignant melanoma to four sessions of CT or to a control group. There were no significant differences in emotional distress on the posttreatment outcome assessments.

Mohr et al. (2000, 2001) conducted a series of small treatment trials for depression in patients with multiple sclerosis. In one study, patients were randomly assigned to 8 weeks of telephone-administered CT or to usual care. Posttreatment scores on the Profile of Mood States Depression subscale were significantly lower in the CT group than the control group (Mohr et al., 2000). In another study, patients were randomly assigned to 16 weeks of CT, supportive–expressive group therapy, or sertraline. Patients who had received CT or sertraline were significantly less depressed at the posttreatment assessment than those who had received supportive therapy (Mohr et al., 2001).

Finally, in a large, randomized trial, Simon et al. (2004), compared telephone-administered CT combined with case management, case management alone, and usual care for primary care patients who were starting antidepressant therapy. Depression outcomes were significantly better in the CT plus case management group than in the usual care group.

CONCLUSIONS

CT has considerable potential as a treatment for depression and related problems in patients with chronic medical illnesses. For most illnesses, however, there is not yet enough evidence from rigorous clinical trials to claim that CT is a safe and efficacious treatment for comorbid depression. It will take years to amass the evidence needed to determine whether CT can truly be called an empirically supported therapy for comorbid depression in patients with chronic medical conditions. For now, clinicians who seek evidence to support the use of CT with medically ill patients have relatively little to draw upon except for ENRICHD, a handful of small comorbid depression trials in various medical populations, and CT trials conducted in generally healthy but depressed patient populations, such as the recent trial by DeRubeis et al. (2005). Several relevant studies are currently in progress, and there is good reason to hope that a number of high-quality trials will be published over the next decade.

ACKNOWLEDGMENT

We wish to thank Iris Csik, MSW, LCSW, for her comments and suggestions.

REFERENCES

American Heart Association. (2004). *Heart disease and stroke statistics—2005 update.* Dallas, TX: American Heart Association.

Anderson, R. J., Freedland, K. E., Clouse, R. E., & Lustman, P. J. (2001). The prevalence of comorbid depression in adults with diabetes: A meta-analysis. *Diabetes Care, 24,* 1069–1078.

Bankier, B., Januzzi, J. L., & Littman, A. B. (2004). The high prevalence of multiple psychiatric disorders in stable outpatients with coronary heart disease. *Psychosomatic Medicine, 66,* 645–650.

Bastien, C. H., Morin, C. M., Ouellet, M. C., Blais, F. C., & Bouchard, S. (2004). Cognitive-behavioral therapy for insomnia: Comparison of individual therapy, group therapy, and telephone consultations. *Journal of Consulting and Clinical Psychology, 72,* 653–659.

Beck, A. T., Rush, A. J., Shaw, B. F., & Emery, G. (1979). *Cognitive therapy of depression.* New York: Guilford Press.

Berkman, L. F., Blumenthal, J., Burg, M., Carney, R. M., Catellier, D., Cowan, M. J., et al. (2003). Effects of treating depression and low perceived social support on clinical events after myocardial infarction: The Enhancing Recovery in Coronary Heart Disease Patients (ENRICHD) randomized trial. *Journal of the American Medical Association, 289,* 3106–3116.

Blumenthal, J. A., Babyak, M. A., Keefe, F. J., Davis, R. D., Lacaille, R. A., Carney, R. M., et al. (2006). Telephone-based coping skills training for patients awaiting lung transplantation. *Journal of Consulting and Clinical Psychology, 74,* 535–544.

Burns, D. D. (1980). *Feeling good: The new mood therapy* (1st ed.). New York: Morrow.

Carney, R. M., Freedland, K. E., Stein, P. K., Skala, J. A., Hoffman, P., & Jaffe, A. S. (2000). Change in heart rate and heart rate variability during treatment for depression in patients with coronary heart disease. *Psychosomatic Medicine, 62,* 639–647.

Carney, R. M., Rich, M. W., Freedland, K. E., Saini, J., teVelde, A., Simeone, C., et al. (1988). Major depressive disorder predicts cardiac events in patients with coronary artery disease. *Psychosomatic Medicine, 50,* 627–633.

Cole, M. G., & Dendukuri, N. (2003). Risk factors for depression among elderly community subjects: A systematic review and meta-analysis. *American Journal of Psychiatry, 160,* 1147–1156.

Connerney, I., Shapiro, P. A., McLaughlin, J. S., Bagiella, E., & Sloan, R. P. (2001). Relation between depression after coronary artery bypass surgery and 12-month outcome: A prospective study. *Lancet, 358,* 1766–1771.

Davidson, K. W., Kupfer, D. J., Bigger, J. T., Califf, R. M., Carney, R. M., Coyne, J. C., et al. (2006). Assessment and treatment of depression in patients with cardiovascular disease: National Heart, Lung, and Blood Institute Working Group Report. *Psychosomatic Medicine, 68,* 645–650.

Day, R. C., Freedland, K. E., & Carney, R. M. (2005). Effects of anxiety and depression on heart disease attributions. *International Journal of Behavioral Medicine, 12,* 24–29.

DeGroot, M., Anderson, R., Freedland, K. E., Clouse, R. E., & Lustman, P. J. (2001). Association of depression and diabetes complications: A meta-analysis. *Psychosomatic Medicine, 63,* 619–630.

DeRubeis, R. J., Hollon, S. D., Amsterdam, J. D., Shelton, R. C., Young, P. R., Salomon, R. M., et al. (2005). Cognitive therapy vs medications in the treatment of moderate to severe depression. *Archives of General Psychiatry, 62,* 409–416.

ENRICHD Investigators. (2001). Enhancing Recovery in Coronary Heart Disease (ENRICHD) study intervention: Rationale and design. *Psychosomatic Medicine, 63,* 747–755.

Evans, D. L., Charney, D. S., Lewis, L., Golden, R. N., Gorman, J. M., Krishnan, K. R., et al. (2005). Mood disorders in the medically ill: Scientific review and recommendations. *Biological Psychiatry, 58,* 175–189.

Frasure-Smith, N., Lesperance, F., & Talajic, M. (1993). Depression following myocardial infarction: Impact on 6-month survival. *Journal of the American Medical Association, 270,* 1819–1825.

Freedland, K. E. (2005). Heart disease attributions: introduction to the miniseries. *International Journal of Behavioral Medicine, 12,* 21–23.

Freedland, K. E., Carney, R. M., Lustman, P. J., Rich, M. W., & Jaffe, A. S. (1992). Major depression in coronary artery disease patients with vs. without a prior history of depression. *Psychosomatic Medicine, 54,* 416–421.

Freedland, K. E., Carney, R. M., Rich, M. W., Caracciolo, A., Krotenberg, J. A., Smith, L. J., et al. (1991). Depression in elderly patients with congestive heart failure. *Journal of Geriatric Psychiatry, 24,* 59–71.

Freedland, K. E., Rich, M. W., Skala, J. A., Carney, R. M., Davila-Roman, V. G., & Jaffe, A. S. (2003). Prevalence of depression in hospitalized patients with congestive heart failure. *Psychosomatic Medicine, 65,* 119–128.

Freedland, K. E., Skala, J. A., Carney, R. M., Raczynski, J. M., Taylor, C. B., Mendes de Leon, C. F., et al. (2002). The Depression Interview and Structured Hamilton (DISH): Rationale, development, characteristics, and clinical validity. *Psychosomatic Medicine, 64,* 897–905.

Furze, G., Bull, P., Lewin, R. J., & Thompson, D. R. (2003). Development of the York Angina Beliefs Questionnaire. *Journal of Health Psychology, 8,* 307–315.

Given, C., Given, B., Rahbar, M., Jeon, S., McCorkle, R., Cimprich, B., et al. (2004). Does a symptom management intervention affect depression among cancer patients?: Results from a clinical trial. *Psycho-Oncology, 13,* 818–830.

Goodwin, R. D. (2003). Association between physical activity and mental disorders among adults in the United States. *Preventive Medicine, 36,* 698–703.

Herrmann, C., Brand-Driehorst, S., Kaminsky, B., Leibing, E., Staats, H., & Ruger, U. (1998). Diagnostic groups and depressed mood as predictors of 22-month mortality in medical inpatients. *Psychosomatic Medicine, 60,* 570–577.

Kales, H. C., Maixner, D. F., & Mellow, A. M. (2005). Cerebrovascular disease and late-life depression. *American Journal of Geriatric Psychiatry, 13,* 88–98.

Kessler, R. C., Berglund, P., Demler, O., Jin, R., Koretz, D., Merikangas, K. R., et al. (2003). The epidemiology of major depressive disorder: Results from the National Comorbidity Survey Replication (NCS-R). *Journal of the American Medical Association, 289,* 3095–3105.

Krishnan, K. R., Hays, J. C., & Blazer, D. G. (1997). MRI-defined vascular depression. *American Journal of Psychiatry, 154,* 497–501.

Larson, S. L., Owens, P. L., Ford, D., & Eaton, W. (2001). Depressive disorder, dysthymia, and risk of stroke: Thirteen-year follow-up from the Baltimore Epidemiologic Catchment Area study. *Stroke, 32,* 1979–1983.

Lewin, R. J., Furze, G., Robinson, J., Griffith, K., Wiseman, S., Pye, M., et al. (2002). A randomised controlled trial of a self-management plan for patients with newly diagnosed angina. *British Journal of General Practice, 52,* 194–201.

Lincoln, N. B., & Flannaghan, T. (2003). Cognitive behavioral psychotherapy for depression following stroke: A randomized controlled trial. *Stroke, 34,* 111–115.

Lustman, P. J., Anderson, R. J., Freedland, K. E., de Groot, M., Carney, R. M., & Clouse, R. E. (2000). Depression and poor glycemic control: A meta-analytic review of the literature. *Diabetes Care, 23,* 934–942.

Lustman, P. J., Freedland, K. E., Griffith, L. S., & Clouse, R. E. (1998a). Predicting response to cognitive behavior therapy of depression in type 2 diabetes. *General Hospital Psychiatry, 20,* 302–306.

Lustman, P. J., Griffith, L. S., Freedland, K. E., Kissel, S. S., & Clouse, R. E. (1998b). Cognitive behavior therapy for depression in type 2 diabetes mellitus: A randomized, controlled trial. *Annals of Internal Medicine, 129,* 613–621.

Massie, M. J. (2004). Prevalence of depression in patients with cancer. *Journal of the National Cancer Institute Monographs, 32,* 57–71.

Mohr, D. C., Boudewyn, A. C., Goodkin, D. E., Bostrom, A., & Epstein, L. (2001). Comparative outcomes for individual cognitive-behavior therapy, supportive-expressive group psychotherapy, and sertraline for the treatment of depression in multiple sclerosis. *Journal of Consulting and Clinical Psychology, 69,* 942–949.

Mohr, D. C., Likosky, W., Bertagnolli, A., Goodkin, D. E., Van Der, W. J., Dwyer, P., et al. (2000). Telephone-administered cognitive-behavioral therapy for the treatment of depressive symptoms in multiple sclerosis. *Journal of Consulting and Clinical Psychology, 68,* 356–361.

Parker, J. C., Smarr, K. L., Slaughter, J. R., Johnston, S. K., Priesmeyer, M. L., Hanson, K. D., et al. (2003). Management of depression in rheumatoid arthritis: A combined pharmacologic and cognitive-behavioral approach. *Arthritis and Rheumatism, 49,* 766–777.

Penninx, B. W., Guralnik, J. M., Pahor, M., Ferrucci, L., Cerhan, J. R., Wallace, R. B., et al. (1998). Chronically depressed mood and cancer risk in older persons. *Journal of the National Cancer Institute, 90,* 1888–1893.

Rudisch, B., & Nemeroff, C. B. (2003). Epidemiology of comorbid coronary artery disease and depression. *Biological Psychiatry, 54,* 227–240.

Sharpe, L., Sensky, T., Timberlake, N., Ryan, B., Brewin, C. R., & Allard, S. (2001). A blind, randomized, controlled trial of cognitive-behavioural intervention for patients with recent onset rheumatoid arthritis: Preventing psychological and physical morbidity. *Pain, 89,* 275–283.

Simon, G. E., Ludman, E. J., Tutty, S., Operskalski, B., & Von, K. M. (2004). Telephone psychotherapy and telephone care management for primary care patients starting antidepressant treatment: A randomized controlled trial. *Journal of the American Medical Association, 292,* 935–942.

Skala, J. A., Freedland, K. E., & Carney, R. M. (2005). *Heart disease.* Ashland, OH: Hogrefe.

Spertus, J. A., McDonell, M., Woodman, C. L., & Fihn, S. D. (2000). Association between depression and worse disease-specific functional status in outpatients with coronary artery disease. *American Heart Journal, 140,* 105–110.

Stewart, A. L., Greenfield, S., Hays, R. D., Wells, K., Rogers, W. H., Berry, S. D., et al. (1989). Functional status and well-being of patients with chronic conditions: Results from the Medical Outcomes Study. *Journal of the American Medical Association, 262,* 907–913.

Sullivan, M. D., LaCroix, A. Z., Russo, J. E., & Walker, E. A. (2001). Depression and self-reported physical health in patients with coronary disease: Mediating and moderating factors. *Psychosomatic Medicine, 63,* 248–256.

Trask, P. C., Paterson, A. G., Griffith, K. A., Riba, M. B., & Schwartz, J. L. (2003). Cognitive-behavioral intervention for distress in patients with melanoma: Comparison with standard medical care and impact on quality of life. *Cancer, 98,* 854–864.

Weinman, J. A., Petrie, K. J., Moss-Morris, R., & Horne, R. (1996). The Illness Perception Questionnaire: A new method for assessing the cognitive representation of illness. *Psychology and Health, 11,* 114–129.

Weisman, A. N., & Beck, A. T. (1978, November). *Development and validation of the Dysfunctional Attitudes Scale: A preliminary investigation.* Paper presented at the meeting of the Association for the Advancement of Behavior Therapy, Chicago, IL.

Wells, K. B., Golding, J. M., & Burnam, M. A. (1988). Psychiatric disorder in a sample of the general population with and without chronic medical conditions. *American Journal of Psychiatry, 145,* 976–981.

Whyte, E. M., & Mulsant, B. H. (2002). Post stroke depression: Epidemiology, pathophysiology, and biological treatment. *Biological Psychiatry, 52,* 253–264.

14

FAMILY OR
RELATIONSHIP PROBLEMS

Lisa A. Uebelacker
Marjorie E. Weishaar
Ivan W. Miller

Depression and family problems frequently co-occur. In this chapter, we describe an integrated approach that a cognitive therapist may use to conceptualize and manage depression and family problems in adults and older adolescents. Although we do not describe how to conduct full-scale family therapy per se, we do focus on (1) how to conceptualize depression from an integrated cognitive and interpersonal viewpoint; and (2) a menu of interventions that are consistent with cognitive therapy and include the family. These interventions, which range from a one-session family meeting to concurrent family and individual therapy, allow the clinician to develop an integrative case conceptualization and then act on it.

Given the heterogeneity of family structures in the United States today, it is critical not to adhere to a rigid definition of family. Family can include, but is not limited to, partners, parents, children, stepchildren, extended family, neighbors, godparents, ex-partners with joint care for children, or roommates. A broad definition of family may be particularly important when working with certain ethnic or racial groups. For example, when asked to describe their family, some African Americans include "fictive kin," or people who are not related by blood or by marriage, but are considered to be part of the family (Chatters, Taylor, & Jayakody, 1994). Therefore, when working with a depressed patient, we remain open to including a wide variety of people in the conceptualization and treatment of depression and family problems. Although much family work is with spouses or partners, this is only one subset of the many possibilities. For those therapists who are accustomed to working with partners, it is worth noting that many of the principles that apply to working with partners apply to working with the family as a whole.

CO-OCCURRENCE OF DEPRESSION AND FAMILY PROBLEMS

A significant body of research documents the frequent co-occurrence of depression and family problems. An unfortunate limitation of this research is that despite the variety of family structures we described earlier, much of the available research on adults focuses on spouses or partners. We include research on the family as a whole whenever possible.

Major Depression Is Associated with Poor Family Functioning

Epidemiological research suggests that marital distress is associated with significantly increased levels of major depression in men and women (Whisman & Bruce, 1999). Poorer general family functioning also characterizes depressed adults relative to nondepressed control subjects (Friedman et al., 1997). Approximately 69% of the depressed individuals in this study reported significant family problems. Furthermore, poorer marital or family functioning is associated with depression symptoms in different ethnic or racial groups, including Mexican Americans (Vega, Kolody, & Valle, 1988) and African Americans (Brown, Brody, & Stoneman, 2000).

Family Problems Predict Onset, Delayed Recovery, and Relapse of Major Depression

Using a nationally representative sample, Whisman and Bruce (1999) found that people with marital distress were nearly three times more likely to develop a new major depressive episode in the next year than those who did not report marital distress. Humiliating events, such as infidelity or threats of divorce, may leave people particularly vulnerable to major depression (Cano & O'Leary, 2000). These data are supported by retrospective studies in which large portions of depressed individuals reported that marital problems occurred before the onset of their depression (e.g., Kendler, Karkowski, & Prescott, 1999), and that they believed marital problems had a causal role in the onset of the depression (O'Leary, Riso, & Beach, 1990).

Family problems are also associated with a decreased likelihood of recovery from depression (Keitner, Ryan, Miller, & Zlotnick, 1997). "Expressed emotion," which refers to the tendency of family members to be critical, hostile, and overinvolved with a family member with a psychological disorder, also predicts relapse of major depression (Hooley & Teasdale, 1989).

Depression Predicts Increases in Family Problems

In some cases, depression may predict poorer family functioning in the future (Dehle & Weiss, 1998). Individuals with major depression are 1.7 times more likely than those without a psychological disorder to experience a subsequent divorce (Kessler, Walters, & Forthofer, 1998). Indeed, partners report feeling burdened by a depressed spouse's feelings of hopelessness, worrying, and lack of energy (Benazon & Coyne, 2000).

Impact of Family Problems on Cognitive Therapy for Depression

Although one might speculate that the presence of serious family problems decreases the efficacy of cognitive therapy (CT) for depression, there is actually very little research on this topic. Individuals in CT who reported that relationship problems were a cause of their depression (relative to those who did not) were less likely to complete homework and showed a poorer response to treatment (Addis & Jacobson, 1996). Beach and O'Leary (1992) also found that depressed married women with negative marital environments had more residual depression symptoms after CT than after behavioral couple therapy. Finally, depressed women treated with an antidepressant and either CT or supportive therapy were less likely to remit if they had reported having low support from their husband before beginning treatment (Bromberger, Wisner, & Hanusa, 1994). In summary, the small amount of existing evidence suggests that relationship problems may interfere with response to individual CT.

CONCEPTUALIZATION OF COMORBIDITY
OF FAMILY PROBLEMS

For depressed individuals who are experiencing family difficulties, the cognitive therapist may develop an integrative case conceptualization that takes into account family and interpersonal issues, as well as individual cognitions, emotions, and behaviors. A few points about conceptualizations bear mentioning here. As Jacobson and Christensen (1996b) point out, a conceptualization (or formulation) is not a static concept; rather, it evolves and changes over time as new information is introduced. In addition, a conceptualization does not represent the absolute truth; rather, it is a social construction that derives its value from how useful it is for the patient and family members.

An integrative (interpersonal and intrapersonal) conceptualization takes into account the emotions, cognitions, and behaviors of the depressed patient, as well as those of his/her family members. Both self-schemas and interpersonal schemas should be assessed; that is, one must consider how family members view themselves and the world, as well as their relationships with others. Most importantly, what makes the conceptualization truly integrative is an understanding of the transactional patterns that occur between different individuals in the family; that is, how a given individual's thoughts, feelings, and behaviors impact on the thoughts, feelings, and behaviors of other family members, and how other family members have an impact on that individual. How do these cycles serve to maintain or limit depression in the family? Finally, the therapist also needs to consider the impact of external stressful situations on family members.

We believe that, in most cases, conceptualizations are most useful when no one is blamed for depression or for problematic family interactions. Rather, the conceptualization focuses on differences between people (e.g., different expectations), a mismatch between a person and a situation, transactional patterns that may have been functional at one point but are no longer useful, or a stressor that activates an underlying diathesis. Therapy, then focuses not on blame, but on responsibility for or commitment to change.

In some cases, family problems may precipitate depression; in others, the depression may occur first. Many times, family problems and depression have a complex reciprocal impact on each other: as family problems increase, depression worsens, which may in turn lead to more problems within the family. Family problems that may contribute to the cause of depression include (but are not limited to) history of childhood abuse, aggression within the current family, infidelity, conflict, alcohol or drug problems, and caregiving for an ill relative. Changes in family structure, such as a birth or a child leaving for college, are stressors that may also contribute to or maintain depression. Problems that may be a consequence of depression include symptoms of depression that have an impact on other family members, such as sexual problems, criticism, negativity, anger, decreased interest in other family members or inability to fulfill family responsibilities, or poor problem solving. Suicidal thoughts or attempts may precipitate a family crisis, with other family members feeling a host of negative emotions, including anxiety, anger, shock, grief, or guilt. Because it is hard to know how best to cope with depression in a loved one, the way family members react to a depression may also lead to difficulties. For example, family members may become overprotective if a family member is depressed, and shield him/her from activities that may actually be helpful (e.g., social activities). Family members may not have a good understanding of depression, and may blame the depressed individual for depression symptoms. Alternatively, family members may blame themselves or each other if another family member is depressed (e.g., parents may blame each other for a child's problems).

To illustrate, we give a brief example of a cognitive case conceptualiza-tion, then an example of the same case with an integrative cognitive–interpersonal case conceptualization.

Jane presented to a cognitive therapist saying that she had been feeling depressed and tearful since her marriage 6 months earlier. Her problem list included frequent fights with her husband Bill, not having very many female friends, and being dissatisfied with her work as a teacher. Frequent cognitions included "My husband doesn't care about me," "I'll never make more friends," and "Nothing ever goes right for me." Jane had a deep-seated fear of being alone in the world. She reported that she did attempt to discuss her feelings with her husband, but that he was not interested in hearing about how she felt. She described Bill as uncaring, distant, and cold.

After meeting with both Jane and her husband, the cognitive therapist expanded the case conceptualization further by integrating how Jane's and Bill's thoughts and behaviors interacted. She found that each had come into the marriage with different expectations. Jane expected to experience a new level of closeness, above and beyond what she had felt when they were dat-ing. Bill expected things to continue exactly as before, and he continued to spend two nights per week out with friends. Jane was disappointed and started to feel unloved, interpreting her husband's behavior (i.e., being with friends) to mean that he did not care about her. As she became more con-vinced of this interpretation, Jane requested that he spend more time with her. Bill said that he cared a lot for Jane, so he tried to comply, but he did not want to give up his nights with his friends. Jane began to think that the only way she would know Bill cared about her was if he gave up those nights, and she told him so. This felt very threatening to Bill, and he became determined that he could never give up his nights out. Bill clearly expressed the desire to "make his marriage work" even though he was frustrated because he did not know how to improve things. The partners were polarized in a classic "demand–withdraw" pattern (Christensen & Heavey, 1990): The more Jane demanded, the more Bill withdrew from her; conversely, the more he withdrew, the more depressed and anxious she felt, and the more she demanded from him.

ASSESSMENT OF FAMILY PROBLEMS

Because of the centrality of the family in the lives of most individuals, assessment of family problems is part of the overall initial assessment for any individual with depression. If there is an indication that family problems exist, the clinician may want to consider the following instruments to assist with that assessment.

Family Assessment Device

The Family Assessment Device (FAD) is a 60-item self-report questionnaire, with subscales that assess the areas of family functioning outlined in the McMaster model: Problem Solving, Communication, Roles, Behavior Control, Affective Responsiveness, and Affective Involvement. Problem solving refers to a family's ability to solve both instrumental and affective problems. Communication refers to the ability of the family to communicate clearly and directly, and to understand each other. Roles refers to a family's ability to adequately and appropriately complete necessary family functions, including provision of resources (e.g., food, money), completion of household chores, nurturance and support, sexual gratification of a couple, life skills development (e.g., attending school or work), and systems management and maintenance (e.g., leadership and decision making). Behavior Control refers to standard patterns of behavior and rules for behavior within a family. Affective Responsiveness refers to family members' abilities to respond to events or situations with appropriate quality and quantity of feelings. Affective involvement refers to whether family members demonstrate interest in and value the interests or activities of other members of the family. The FAD has good psychometric properties and cutoff scores that discriminate between families rated as healthy and dysfunctional by experts (Miller, Epstein, Bishop, & Keitner, 1985). There is some evidence to demonstrate its reliability and predictive validity in U.S. studies that included multiracial or multiethnic populations (e.g., Corcoran, 2001).

McMaster Structured Interview for Family Functioning

The McMaster Structured Interview for Family Functioning (McSIFF; Bishop, Epstein, Keitner, Miller, & Zlotnick, 1980) is a 90-minute structured interview designed to assess the areas of family functioning in the McMaster model. Clinicians may choose to use this interview (or parts of it) to make sure that they are conducting a comprehensive assessment of family functioning. For example, the interview includes a broad list of family responsibilities (e.g., housecleaning, shopping, preparing meals, child care, providing money) that can be used to understand the basic roles assumed by each family member, as well as whether there is any conflict about those roles.

If a more quantitative assessment is desired, the McSIFF can be scored using the McMaster Clinical Rating System (MCRS; Miller et al., 1994). The MCRS, a 7-item rating scale, includes ratings of each of the six dimensions of the McMaster model, as well as an overall global functioning score. The MCRS has been shown to have good psychometric properties (Hayden et al., 1998; Miller et al., 1994).

Quality of Marriage Index

The Quality of Marriage Index (QMI; Norton, 1983), a brief, 6-item assessment of overall relationship satisfaction, has good psychometric properties (Heyman, Sayers, & Bellack, 1994). Although QMI scores may correlate with FAD scores, the QMI measures *affective* aspects of a relationship (e.g., "I feel like part of a team with my partner"), whereas the FAD is more behaviorally oriented. Because the QMI is so brief, it is easy to use on a regular basis to assess change over time.

Conflict Tactics Scale

The Conflict Tactics Scale (CTS; Straus, 1979) is used to assess the presence of intimate partner physical aggression. It asks about the frequency of various behaviors in the past year, ranging from insulting or swearing at one's partner; pushing, grabbing, or shoving one's partner; to using a knife or gun. Because some individuals do not consider physical aggression to be a problem (even though it occurs in their family), it can be important to ask people directly and privately about the occurrence of physical aggression. The CTS is one means for doing this.

Many more well-validated instruments may be helpful in specific situations. We refer the reader to Sperry (2004) for more information.

APPROACHES TO TREATMENT

There are many options for integrating family interventions into individually based CT for depression. The integrative case conceptualization, as well as pragmatics, guides the choice of family intervention level and the specific strategies used. Options include (1) treating an individual alone; (2) including family members in a few sessions for the purpose of assessment; (3) providing psychoeducation to family members; (4) brief problem solving with family members; (5) including a family member as a therapy "coach"; and (6) conducting full-scale family therapy in addition to (or in lieu of) individual therapy. We describe what may lead a therapist and patient to choose a particular option, what may be accomplished in the context of that option, and any caveats or limitations of that option.

Individual Alone

The first option is to treat the individual alone, even if it is clear that family problems exist. This option might be chosen for pragmatic reasons (i.e., family members cannot or will not attend conjoint therapy). For example, even when a college student has conflict with his/her family of origin, that family may not be local and may therefore not be available to participate in therapy. In other cases, case conceptualization may dictate the choice of seeing an individual alone. For example, when a family member is so cognitively impaired (as in the case of Alzheimer's disease) that conjoint therapy would not be productive, a CT therapist may choose to work solely with an individual to manage the problem (although the therapist may choose to bring in *other* family members as well). In addition, in certain situations, such as in the case of severe family violence, conjoint therapy may be contraindicated (Holtzworth-Munroe et al., 1995).

Individual CT may be used to target depressive symptoms and behaviors that have an impact on the family. Behavioral interventions may focus on increasing the patient's assertiveness and setting limits, decreasing criticism, expression of both positive and negative feelings in a constructive manner, increasing social activities, and completing family-related responsibilities. Cognitive interventions may focus on changing the way an individual interprets his/her family member's behavior, and modifying dysfunctional beliefs about relationships. For example, a depressed individual may have unrealistic expectations, such as "My partner should know what I need without me having to ask" or "Families should never have disagreements" (Uebelacker & Whisman, 2005). Finally, a therapist may want to help individuals weigh the pros and cons of leaving a difficult or dangerous situation, and/or making a plan to do so.

By necessity, individual CT focuses only on changing the thoughts and behaviors of one family member. Therefore, there are limitations on the degree to which it can impact the entire family. If family problems—such as excessive conflict—contributed to the onset of the depression and persist even after the individual is no longer depressed, he/she may be at an elevated risk for relapse. Also, although we do not find it to be the case in general, there are times when positive changes in a patient have adverse effects on the family system. In these situations, a more direct intervention with the entire family may be indicated.

Assessment

The second option is to include family members on a limited basis (i.e., one or two sessions) for assessment purposes. We often call this a "family meeting." This meeting may be the extent of the face-to-face contact with family members, or it may lead to more extensive treatment. Talking with a family member can be helpful with a great number of patients seen in individual therapy; therapists cannot always anticipate what they might learn by inviting a family member in for one meeting. An important goal of such a family meeting should be to help therapist, patient, and family to develop and refine an integrative case conceptualization. Family meetings can be especially helpful if aspects of the patient's presentation are inconsistent or confusing to the therapist.

The therapist might assess three areas: problems and strengths of the identified patient, of the family as a whole, and of one or more family members. First, family members can help the therapist to clarify certain aspects of their understanding of the depressed individual. Talking with a family member may help the therapist to understand to what extent the patient's perceptions of family relationships (or other issues) are distorted vs. to what extent they are based in reality. For example, a patient may complain that his spouse is easily overwhelmed when he talks about his depressed feelings. Including the spouse in an interview may allow the therapist to directly assess whether she is truly overwhelmed by the patient's feelings, or whether the patient is interpreting more ambiguous signals as signs that she is overwhelmed. Family members may also mention a problem to the therapist that the patient has not mentioned, perhaps because he/she does not see it as a problem (e.g., excessive drinking).

Second, if the patient has indicated that there may be significant family problems, or if the therapist has reason to suspect problems, then the therapist may want to meet family members to conduct a brief assessment of family functioning. This increases the therapist's understanding of the context in which the depressed individual experiences certain thoughts and feelings, and allows the therapist to develop further an integrative case conceptualization. We use the McMaster model of family functioning (Ryan, Epstein, Keitner, Miller, & Bishop, 2005), described earlier, as a guide to areas of functioning about which the therapist may want to inquire. Responses to this assessment may lead the therapist to recommend a more extensive family intervention.

Finally, if there is reason to believe that a family member is experiencing an untreated psychological problem (e.g., depression or alcohol abuses), the therapist may inquire about the family member's symptoms. The therapist might begin with a statement: "It's been my experience that when one member of a family is depressed, other family members sometimes feel stressed as well. Do you ever feel stressed? How do you cope with it?" This assessment could lead to recommendations for treatment for the family member.

Psychoeducation

A third option is to provide psychoeducation for families; this may occur in tandem with assessment as a part of a "family meeting." The case conceptualization should guide how the psychoeducation is presented and what aspects are emphasized. Psychoeducation may be helpful for a number of different reasons. First, it may be particularly important when family members are very critical of the patient's behavior. Very critical family members often believe that the patient's negative behavior is controllable, and they may blame the patient for his/her symptoms (Barrowclough & Hooley, 2003). Psychoeducation may help family members to make more benign attributions for their relative's behavior (e.g., "It's not that he is lazy, it is that he is depressed"). This in turn may decrease criticism.

Second, psychoeducation may help family members who are unsure about how best to help their depressed relative. Should they leave him alone? Encourage him to do things? Try to get him to talk to them? The therapist, the depressed individual, and his family members may discuss what types of behaviors on the part of the family members are most helpful. For example, as a group, they may decide that the depressed person needs gentle encouragement to get out of the house, attend social events, exercise, and so forth. They may come to see that their previous strategy (of avoiding the patient when he was depressed and irritable) may have served to maintain the depression. This change in point of view may result not only in increased support for the patient engaging in positive behavior change, but also in increased feelings of efficacy and hopefulness on the part of the family members.

Third, psychoeducation about the process of treatment may also be helpful. Family members may have misconceptions about therapy that interfere with providing necessary emotional and instrumental support to help the patient attend therapy sessions. For example, if family members believe that the patient spends therapy sessions just complaining about them, and that the therapist blames the family members for the patient's problems, they may be less willing to care for children so that the patient may attend his/her session. Another family member may believe that psychotherapy will go on for many years, and be concerned about the potential cost. If family members have an accurate understanding about what treatment involves, they may be more willing to facilitate the patient attending therapy.

In general, "psychoeducation" consists of an explanation of the symptoms of depression, their consequences for family and work functioning, and an explanation of treatment of depression. Therapists may also review potential causes of the patient's depression (always emphasizing the multiple factors that interact, and avoiding any type of approach that may be construed as blaming the family). To target the psychoeducation session to a particular family's needs, the cognitive therapist may begin by inquiring about family members' beliefs and knowledge about depression, about the patient's behavior, about how they should react to the patient, and about therapy and treatment. It is always useful to provide written materials to family members that reinforce the points covered during this session.

One caveat about psychoeducation: Although increased knowledge may help family members to modify negative cognitions about the patient or therapy, it does not guarantee that behavior change will occur. More intensive family therapy may be needed to help family members change established negative behavior patterns.

Brief Problem Solving and Goal Setting

A fourth option is to assist the family with problem solving or goal setting which can be accomplished in the context of a few family meetings. This may be appropriate for some circumscribed family problems, or if the therapist believes that a few, relatively small behavior changes might make a big difference to the depressed individual or to his/her family. For example, a depressed patient who believes "I must take care of everything in the house or else it won't get done" may take on a lot of household responsibilities, but also feel overwhelmed and resentful. This pattern could be explained to the family in a family meeting and family members might brainstorm ways to help the patient, choose to make a list of chores for which each family member is responsible, and set a goal to follow through on that list.

To conduct problem solving, the therapist explains to the family the standard steps of problem solving (e.g., defining a problem, brainstorming possible solutions, discussing the pros and cons of these solutions, deciding upon a solution, and evaluating the solution). The therapist can assist the family in walking through these steps to manage a specific problem. Because this is not full-scale family therapy, the focus is less on learning the process of problem solving (although the process should be explained) and more on solving a particular problem. The limitation of this strategy is that because it is not full-scale therapy, the number and complexity of problems that can be considered are circumscribed.

Family Member as Coach

A fifth option is to include a family member as a "coach" (Emanuels-Zuurveen & Emmelkamp, 1997). In this case, therapy remains focused primarily on the depressed person and not on family problems. Therapists employ standard CT strategies to help the patient manage depression. The coach's role is to attend sessions to provide emotional support to the patient and to serve as a bridge between therapy sessions and the rest of the patient's life. Because the coach is aware of skills that the patient is learning in therapy, he/she will be able to prompt the patient to use them at home. Specific tasks in which a coach may participate include assisting with the choice of activities for behavioral activation, providing support for behavioral activation at home, helping the patient to identify and challenge dysfunctional thoughts at home, or learning other skills (e.g., problem solving) to support the patient in implementing them at home.

It may be particularly helpful for a family member to be engaged as a coach at the early stages of treatment, when depression may interfere with the patient's ability to concentrate, remember, and get mobilized. It is also useful to have a coach if the patient is very avoidant; the coach can remind the patient that his/her worst fears can be confronted or responded to, that earlier predictions of failure or criticism did not pan out, and so forth. In all cases, the patient should want the coach to attend, and the coach should not encourage dependence or be too intrusive.

There are several caveats relative to the use of a partner or family member as a coach. First, it is important that the relationship between the identified patient and the coach be reasonably supportive. If not, the coach may prove to be overly critical, or the patient may not be receptive to his/her comments. In the worst case, the problems between the coach and the patient may interfere with the explicit focus on the patient and his/her problems. Second, the patient must agree that he or she wants to have a family member as a coach. In relationships in which power struggles are frequent, having one person in the role of a coach and the other as a patient may prove to be too great a power imbalance. Third, it is important that the partner or family member not feel overwhelmed by or resentful about the responsibilities of being a coach.

Family Therapy

The final option is to engage family members in conjoint therapy. The therapist may choose this option if assessment has led to a complex case conceptualization that involves serious problems with family interactions. Of course, family members must also be amenable to this type of treatment. A decision to engage in family therapy may not occur until after one or two family meetings with the cognitive therapist.

If a therapist and family agree that family therapy may be helpful, they need to decide whether family therapy should occur in addition to or in lieu of individual therapy for the identified patient. Evidence (reviewed below) suggests that couple therapy—on its own—can be an effective intervention for treating depression. If the case conceptualization suggests that much of the patient's depression is associated with family problems, and the patient has few problematic cognitions or behaviors that are unrelated to family interactions, the family and therapist may choose to do family therapy only. After family therapy is completed, the therapist and patient may evaluate whether further individual therapy is indicated.

If family problems seem to be only a part of the identified patient's problem list, and she has other types of problems as well (e.g., illness, general social skills deficits, etc.), or if the patient seems to demonstrate a pervasive pattern of dysfunctional beliefs about herself, then the combination of CT and family therapy may be indicated. At this point, the therapist and family members need to decide who will conduct the family therapy. There are two options: The individual cognitive therapist may also conduct family therapy, or the cognitive therapist may refer the family to another therapist. The advantage of having one therapist conduct both individual and family therapy is that the therapist and family can further develop an integrative case conceptualization and treatment rationale that is not confusing or contradictory. This conceptualization can then be used to guide both the individual and the conjoint treatment.

However, a therapist may have ethical and other concerns about conducting both individual and family therapy. He/she may be concerned about forming a productive alliance with all family members. If the therapist is seeing one person individually, the rest of the family may believe that the therapist is most closely allied with that particular person. We do not believe that this issue is insurmountable; however, it is important that it be addressed directly with the family, and that all family members be encouraged to voice any concerns that they may have. The therapist needs to ensure that he/she does not inadvertently favor one individual over another. Of course, this concern is not unique to this situation; a family therapist must always be conscious of whether he/she is siding with one particular member of a family.

A second issue is that of confidentiality. We recommend discussing confidentiality at the outset and setting parameters around safety for the patient and other family members. We encourage family members to reveal information that affects the patient's treatment and improves family functioning. Individual sessions may be confidential to allow each participant to disclose information to the therapist that might be important. The therapist can help to identify information that would benefit other family members and encourage the patient to share this information with them. If the patient is not ready to reveal information to others, the therapist can help that person look at the advantages and disadvantages of disclosing the information in family sessions or work on the issues until he/she can disclose them to the family or partner.

For each case, the therapist and family should weigh the pros and cons of whether to have the individual cognitive therapist conduct family therapy. Families' preferences are obviously important. If an outside referral is chosen, close collaboration between the two therapists (with the family's permission) is essential.

Whether a clinician sees family or refers them, family sessions for family therapy should be compatible with the general philosophy and format of CT; that is, family sessions should be problem-focused and present-oriented in family therapy. The therapist strives to have a collaborative relationship with all family members. Conceptualization of family problems focuses on understanding the interactions between cognitions, emotions, and behaviors for each individual, and the impact of each family member on the others. There should be a focus on setting measurable goals and regularly assessing how closely family members are to meet their goals. Family therapy should be time-limited and include other features of CT, such as setting an agenda for each meeting and assigning homework.

We believe that several types of treatments for family problems may be successfully integrated with CT, including cognitive-behavioral couple therapy (Epstein & Baucom, 2002), integrative couples therapy (Jacobson & Christensen, 1996a), and problem-centered systems therapy of the family (Ryan et al., 2005).

General Issues Regarding Inclusion of a Family Member(s) in Treatment

We have discussed several ways to include family members in cognitive-behavioral treatment for depression. A few final issues cut across the various interventions and bear mentioning.

First, whenever multiple family members are involved in a session, even if it is not for formal family therapy, it is useful for the therapist to keep a few principles in mind. It is important to acknowledge that everyone in the room is having different thoughts and reactions, not just the identified patient. All family members need a chance to talk about their reactions and to feel understood. If someone has a lot of reactions, the therapist might ask him/her to write them down to avoid interrupting other people as they talk. Also, in terms of pacing, it is important to move with the slowest person and to check continuously to make sure that everyone understands the information being presented. Finally, it is ideal if the family members finish the session with a common understanding of the problem, or at least agree on ways to manage the problem.

Second, one or two "family meetings" can be useful even if the therapist believes more extensive family intervention is indicated. Some families are wary about the idea of family therapy; however, they may agree to a few family meetings. If the therapist can build a good alliance with family members and help them to have a better understanding of their problems and of what therapy involves, they may be more willing to participate in formal family therapy.

Third, we would like to touch on some of the obstacles to including families in therapy. One obstacle may be the individual therapist's level of skill and comfort in conducting family therapy. More skills and training are needed as one engages in more complex and involved family interventions. We believe that even without a lot of previous experience, most cognitive therapists can conduct a family meeting (perhaps in consultation with a more experienced colleague). Obviously, if the therapist feels that family therapy or a particular family therapy-related issue is outside of his/her scope of expertise, then he/she will need to provide a referral for the family. A second obstacle is family resistance to being part of therapy. The therapist may overcome some resistance by being willing to talk to family members on the phone, explaining what a given session will involve and reassuring the family members that the purpose of the meeting is not to place blame.

CASE ILLUSTRATION

To illustrate further integrative case conceptualizations and family interventions that may be combined with CT, we describe the case of a person in individual CT that included a family meeting. Thomas, a 32-year-old man, lived with Mark, his partner of 5 years. Thomas had recently lost his job, and unable to find another job after looking for a few months, he became depressed and stopped looking. After a few more months of feeling down, he began individual cognitive-behavioral therapy for depression. As part of the initial assessment, he reported that his relationship with his partner Mark was "basically fine, although he's been sort of irritable lately." The therapist explained to Thomas that she liked to have a family meeting with her patients for the purpose of assessment and psychoeducation. Although Thomas was initially resistant to even asking Mark to attend a family meeting—"He's too busy. He'll never want to come"—the therapist helped Thomas to challenge some of the cognitions that prevented him from asking Mark to join them. Eventually, Thomas did ask Mark, and, to his surprise, Mark agreed to come in.

The family meeting began with an assessment. Talking with Mark and Thomas together, the therapist began to piece together the following conceptualization. When Thomas first lost his job, Mark was very accommodating; he did not expect a lot from Thomas, because he knew how terrible Thomas felt. Thomas, who was thinking "I am a failure at everything," relinquished more and more of his responsibilities (e.g., he did not look for a job or do chores at home) as Mark did more and more for him. Thomas's depression did not improve; he stayed home all day and watched TV. Through careful questioning, the therapist learned that Mark was feeling frustrated, but he was reluctant to say anything; he thought, "If I tell Thomas how frustrated I'm feeling, he won't be able to handle it, and he'll get much worse."

Although Thomas was upset to hear that Mark was frustrated, the therapist normalized both men's reactions. She explained to the couple that

Thomas's lack of energy and motivation were common symptoms of depression. She also validated Mark's feeling of frustration about the fact that Thomas had stopped looking for a job or helping around the house. Because depressed individuals often have trouble being activated, she suggested that it might be helpful if Mark asked Thomas to do more around the house, and if they went out together occasionally in the evenings. Because Thomas had begun to learn about the importance of planning both meaningful and pleasant activities in the context of his individual therapy, he agreed that this was important, and that he might be more likely to get things accomplished or to go out if Mark made a direct request of him. The couple left the meeting with a plan to make a list of tasks for which Thomas might take responsibility once again. They also planned to go out to dinner that weekend. In subsequent individual sessions, Thomas reported that he was feeling more active and less depressed, doing more around the house, and that Mark seemed less irritable. The therapist prompted Thomas to continue talking with Mark about what needed to be done around the house, and to make an effort to go out together in the evenings. With the support of both the therapist and Mark, Thomas started looking for a job again and eventually found a job that seemed promising.

REVIEW OF EFFICACY RESEARCH

The literature documenting the effectiveness of integrated individual CT and family approaches to managing depression in adults is small but promising. We provide a brief survey here, in the hope that there will be more research on integrated approaches in the future.

Family Meetings

No research of which we are aware compares CT with one or two family meetings to CT alone. Group Individual Family Therapy for Depression (GIFT; Friedman et al., 2005) involves 10–14 sessions of cognitive-behavioral group therapy, as well as three individual sessions and two family meetings used primarily for assessment and psychoeducation purposes. Data from an open trial of GIFT indicate that the pre- to posttreatment effect size is similar to that seen with other group treatments for depression. Similarly, CT interventions for adolescents have involved a few conjoint family sessions and/or psychoeducation for parents (Treatment for Adolescents with Depression Study [TADS] Team, 2004).

Family Member as Coach

Emanuels-Zuurveen and Emmelkamp (1997) described a therapy that is similar to CT for depression, with the exception that the patient's spouse was included in all sessions. Treatment did not focus on family problems; rather, the focus remained on the depressed person. In a trial that included depressed individuals who were satisfied with their marriages, they found that spouse-aided therapy was equivalent to individual CT in terms of depression outcomes.

Nezu, Nezu, Felgoise, McClure, and Houts (2003) described a problem-solving therapy for distressed breast cancer patients in which a significant other was included in all parts of therapy as a problem-solving coach. The significant other provided social support and feedback to the cancer patient regarding her use of problem-solving skills. Nezu et al. compared problem-solving therapy with a partner as coach to problem-solving therapy alone and a waiting-list control. At the end of treatment, both active treatments were superior to the waiting-list control in terms of reductions in psychological distress. However, at 6-month and 1-year follow-ups, the partner-assisted therapy actually showed better outcomes than the problem-solving therapy alone.

Family Therapy in Lieu of Individual Therapy

Three studies have shown that behavioral couples therapy is an effective treatment for major depression and is comparable to individual CT, at least when the depressed individual also reports having relationship problems (Beach, Fincham, & Katz, 1998). Couple therapy may be particularly helpful when the relationship problems are seen as primary or as causing the depression.

Family Therapy Combined with Individual Therapy

Jacobson, Dobson, Fruzetti, Schmaling, and Salusky (1991) compared behavioral couple therapy, CT, or their combination in depressed (but not necessarily maritally distressed) women. In terms of depression outcomes, they found that the combined treatment performed as well as CT in both maritally distressed and nondistressed women, and that CT was superior to behavioral couple therapy in nondistressed couples. In terms of marital outcomes, there were no significant differences between groups. This was surprising: Jacobson et al. had hypothesized that the combined treatment would be superior to either treatment alone. They have suggested that the reason for the lack of findings was that couples in the combined treatment received suboptimal doses of both behavioral couple therapy and CT (Addis & Jacobson, 1991). Another possibility is that the treatment approach and rationale for the two modalities needed to be more truly integrated.

Finally, Miller et al. (2005) examined the impact of combined treatments on patients with severe major depression. Each patient was randomly assigned to one of four treatment arms: pharmacotherapy alone, pharmacotherapy + CT, pharmacotherapy + family therapy, or pharmacotherapy + CT + family therapy. Depending on their level of cognitive distortions and family dysfunction at baseline, patients were classified as either "matched" or "mismatched" to their particular treatment. For example, assigning a patient with a high level of cognitive distortion but a low level of family dysfunction to pharmacotherapy + family therapy would be considered a "mismatch." These authors reported two findings relevant to the current topic. First, patients who were "matched" to treatment did somewhat better than those who were mismatched. Second, patients in one of the two conditions that included family therapy showed more improvement than those who did not receive family therapy. Although its complicated design tempers conclusive statements about family therapy, this study does provide some evidence that the addition of family therapy to other, individual treatments may improve outcomes in severely depressed individuals. This may be particularly true when they show evidence of family problems.

In summary, the small amount of research on the integration of family interventions with individual CT for depression is promising but not conclusive. However, the basic research documenting a strong association between family functioning and major depression is very compelling. Therefore, we continue to believe that it makes sense theoretically to address family problems directly in conjunction with CT.

CONCLUSIONS

A large amount of evidence suggests that major depression and family functioning are closely linked. Major depression is associated with poorer family functioning in cross-sectional studies; family problems predict onset and course of illness in depression; and depression is linked to subsequent poorer family functioning. In this chapter, we have demonstrated that it is both feasible and useful to formulate an integrative case conceptualization and to include family members in the cognitive-behavioral treatment of depression. We have presented a series of increasingly intensive family interventions that a CT therapist may use, including (1) treating an individual alone, (2) including family members in a few sessions for the purpose of assessment, (3) providing psychoeducation to family members, (4) brief problem solving with family members, (5) including a family member as a therapy "coach," and (6) conducting full-scale family therapy in addition to (or in lieu of) individual therapy. The limited research that is available suggests that including family members in treatment in some way may improve likelihood of success. We hope that this chapter spurs increased interest among both clinicians and researchers in understanding and treating cognitive, behavioral, and interpersonal aspects of depression.

REFERENCES

Addis, M. E., & Jacobson, N. S. (1991). Integration of cognitive therapy and behavioral marital therapy for depression. *Journal of Psychotherapy Integration, 1,* 249–264.

Addis, M. E., & Jacobson, N. S. (1996). Reasons for depression and the process and outcome of cognitive-behavioral psychotherapies. *Journal of Consulting and Clinical Psychology, 64,* 1417–1424.

Barrowclough, C., & Hooley, J. M. (2003). Attributions and expressed emotion: A review. *Clinical Psychology Review, 23,* 849–880.

Beach, S. R., & O'Leary, K. D. (1992). Treating depression in the context of marital discord: Outcome and predictors of response of marital therapy versus cognitive therapy. *Behavior Therapy, 23,* 507–528.

Beach, S. R. H., Fincham, F. D., & Katz, J. (1998). Marital therapy in the treatment of depression: Toward a third generation of therapy and research. *Clinical Psychology Review, 18,* 635–661.

Benazon, N. R., & Coyne, J. C. (2000). Living with a depressed spouse. *Journal of Family Psychology, 14,* 71–79.

Bishop, D., Epstein, N., Keitner, G., Miller, I., & Zlotnick, C. (1980). *The McMaster Structured Interview for Family Functioning.* Providence, RI: Brown University.

Bromberger, J. T., Wisner, K. L., & Hanusa, B. H. (1994). Marital support and remission of treated depression: A prospective pilot study of mothers of infants and toddlers. *Journal of Nervous and Mental Disease, 182*(1), 40–44.

Brown, A. C., Brody, G. H., & Stoneman, Z. (2000). Rural black women and depression: A contextual analysis. *Journal of Marriage and the Family, 62*(1), 187–198.

Cano, A., & O'Leary, K. D. (2000). Infidelity and separations precipitate major depressive episodes and symptoms of nonspecific depression and anxiety. *Journal of Consulting and Clinical Psychology, 68*(5), 774–781.

Chatters, L. M., Taylor, R. J., & Jayakody, R. (1994). Fictive kinship relations in black extended families. *Journal of Comparative Family Studies, 25,* 297–312.

Christensen, A., & Heavey, C. L. (1990). Gender and social structure in the demand/

withdraw pattern of marital conflict. *Journal of Personality and Social Psychology, 59,* 73–81.

Corcoran, J. (2001). Multi-systemic influences on the family functioning of teens attending pregnancy prevention programs. *Child and Adolescent Social Work Journal, 18*(1), 37–49.

Dehle, C., & Weiss, R. (1998). Sex difference in prospective associations between marital quality and depressed mood. *Journal of Marriage and the Family, 60,* 1002–1011.

Emanuels-Zuurveen, L., & Emmelkamp, P. M. (1997). Spouse-aided therapy with depressed patients. *Behavior Modification, 21,* 62–77.

Epstein, N. B., & Baucom, D. H. (2002). *Enhanced cognitive-behavioral therapy for couples: A contextual approach.* Washington, DC: American Psychological Association.

Friedman, M. A., Cardemil, E. V., Uebelacker, L. A., Beevers, C. G., Chestnut, C., & Miller, I. W. (2005). The GIFT program for major depression: Integrating group, individual, and family treatment. *Journal of Psychotherapy Integration, 15,* 147–168.

Friedman, M. A., McDermut, W. H., Solomon, D. A., Ryan, C. E., Keitner, G. I., & Miller, I. W. (1997). Family functioning and mental illness: A comparison of psychiatric and nonclinical families. *Family Process, 36*(4), 357–367.

Hayden, L. C., Schiller, M., Dickstein, S., Seifer, R., Sameroff, S., Miller, I., et al. (1998). Levels of family assessment: I. Family, marital, and parent–child interaction. *Journal of Family Psychology, 12*(1), 7–22.

Heyman, R. E., Sayers, S. L., & Bellack, A. S. (1994). Global marital satisfaction versus marital adjustment: An empirical comparison of three measures. *Journal of Family Psychology, 8,* 432–446.

Holtzworth-Munroe, A., Markman, H., O'Leary, K. D., Neidig, P., Leber, D., Heyman, R. E., et al. (1995). The need for marital violence prevention efforts: A behavioral-cognitive secondary prevention program for engaged and newly married couples. *Applied and Preventive Psychology, 4*(2), 77–88.

Hooley, J. M., & Teasdale, J. D. (1989). Predictors of relapse in unipolar depressives: Expressed emotion, marital distress, and perceived criticism. *Journal of Abnormal Psychology, 98,* 229–235.

Jacobson, N. S., & Christensen, A. (1996a). *Integrative couple therapy: Promoting acceptance and change.* New York: Norton.

Jacobson, N. S., & Christensen, A. (1996b). Studying the effectiveness of psychotherapy: How well can clinical trials do the job? *American Psychologist, 51*(10), 1031–1039.

Jacobson, N. S., Dobson, K., Fruzetti, A. E., Schmaling, K. B., & Salusky, S. (1991). Marital therapy as a treatment for depression. *Journal of Consulting and Clinical Psychology, 59,* 547–557.

Keitner, G. I., Ryan, C. E., Miller, I. W., & Zlotnick, C. (1997). Psychosocial factors and the long-term course of major depression. *Journal of Affective Disorders, 44*(1), 57–67.

Kendler, K. S., Karkowski, L. M., & Prescott, C. A. (1999). Causal relationship between stressful life events and the onset of major depression. *American Journal of Psychiatry, 156*(6), 837–841.

Kessler, R. C., Walters, E. E., & Forthofer, M. S. (1998). The social consequences of psychiatric disorders: III. Probablility of marital stability. *American Journal of Psychiatry, 155,* 1092–1096.

Miller, I. W., Epstein, N. B., Bishop, D. S., & Keitner, G. I. (1985). The McMaster Family Assessment Device: Reliability and validity. *Journal of Marital and Family Therapy, 11*(4), 345–356.

Miller, I. W., Kabacoff, R. I., Epstein, N. B., Bishop, D. S., Keitner, G. I., Baldwin, L. M., et al. (1994). The development of a clinical rating scale for the McMaster Model of Family Functioning. *Family Process, 33*(1), 53–69.

Miller, I. W., Keitner, G. I., Ryan, C. E., Solomon, D. A., Cardemil, E. V., & Beevers, C. G. (2005). Treatment matching in the post-hospital care of depressed inpatients. *American Journal of Psychiatry, 162,* 2131–2138.

Nezu, A. M., Nezu, C. M., Felgoise, S. H., McClure, K. S., & Houts, P. S. (2003). Project Genesis: Assessing the efficacy of problem-solving therapy for distressed adult cancer patients. *Journal of Consulting and Clinical Psychology, 71,* 1036–1048.

Norton, R. (1983). Measuring marital quality: A critical look at the dependent variable. *Journal of Marriage and the Family, 45,* 141–151.

O'Leary, K. D., Riso, L. P., & Beach, S. R. (1990). Attributions about the marital discord/depression link and therapy outcome. *Behavior Therapy, 21,* 413–422.

Ryan, C. E., Epstein, N. B., Keitner, G. I., Miller, I. W., & Bishop, D. S. (2005). *Evaluating and treating families: The McMaster approach.* New York: Brunner/Routledge.

Sperry, L. (2004). *Assessment of couples and families.* New York: Brunner-Routledge.

Straus, M. A. (1979). Measuring intrafamily conflict and violence: The Conflict Tactics Scales. *Journal of Marriage and the Family, 41,* 75–88.

Treatment for Adolescents With Depression Study (TADS) Team. (2004). Fluoxetine, cognitive-behavioral therapy, and their combination for adolescents with depression. *Journal of the American Medical Association, 292,* 807–820.

Uebelacker, L. A., & Whisman, M. A. (2005). Relationship attributions, beliefs, and spouse behaviors among depressed women. *Cognitive Therapy and Research, 29,* 143–154.

Vega, W. A., Kolody, B., & Valle, R. (1988). Marital strain, coping, and depression among Mexican-American women. *Journal of Marriage and the Family, 50*(2), 391–403.

Whisman, M. A., & Bruce, M. L. (1999). Marital distress and incidence of major depressive episode in a community sample. *Journal of Abnormal Psychology, 108,* 674–678.

IV

COGNITIVE THERAPY
FOR DEPRESSION WITH
SPECIAL POPULATIONS

IV

COGNITIVE THERAPY FOR DEPRESSION WITH SPECIAL POPULATIONS

15

ETHNIC MINORITIES

Laura Kohn-Wood
Glenetta Hudson
Erin T. Graham

The Surgeon General's report on mental health (U.S. Department of Health and Human Services, 1999) detailed the efficacy of available treatments for mental disorders in the United States. Cognitive therapy (CT) and cognitive-behavioral therapy (CBT) approaches to the treatment of major mood and anxiety disorders show particularly favorable outcomes in comparison to other psychotherapy and psychopharmacological interventions (for review see the Special Section of the *Journal of Consulting and Clinical Psychology*, February, 1998). However, a major finding from the supplement to the Surgeon General's report on culture, ethnicity and mental health (U.S. Department of Health and Human Services, 2001) was the lack of information regarding treatment outcomes for ethnic/minority populations. Previously, researchers have highlighted the need to include ethnic/minority populations in psychotherapy research and have provided recommendations to increase their inclusion in research trials. Despite these attempts, studies of empirically validated treatment approaches have typically not included ethnic/minority groups; therefore, little is known regarding the diverse applicability of existing interventions, including CT (Hall, 2001).

A related issue is the underutilization of mental health services by ethnic/minority populations (Snowden & Yamada, 2005). Researchers have suggested that numerous instrumental and perceptual barriers preclude therapy involvement for ethnic minorities (U.S. Department of Health and Human Services, 2001). Specifically, underutilization among Latinos has been attributed to inaccessibility, lack of services, and cultural acceptability (Hohmann & Parron, 1996). With few ethnic minorities participating in treatment and little information regarding the efficacy of existing treatments across ethnicity, mental health practitioners and researchers face a quandary. Can empirically validated treatment approaches such as CT generalize to ethnic/minority patients? Should CT or other approaches be culturally adapted, and if so, how?

In this chapter we discuss the conceptualization and assessment of depression, offer treatment recommendations, and examine the current literature regarding CT treatment outcomes for ethnic/minority groups in an attempt to answer these questions and synthesize available information to fill gaps in our knowledge. We focus on CT for depression in African Americans and Latinos, because research to date on adapting CT for depression in other minority groups, such as Asian Americans, has been limited. We use the term "ethnic minorities" and "ethnicity" to describe both African Americans and Latinos; however, we recognize that based on the U.S. Bureau of the Census distinctions, "African American" represents a racial group and "Latino" represents an ethnic group. Existing treatment studies of adult CT and CBT for mood disorders are reviewed. Increasing our understanding of treatment for African American and Latino groups is critical as we face an increasingly ethnically diverse population. We need to expand our ability to provide efficacious mental health services that will be widely utilized.

CONCEPTUALIZATION OF DEPRESSION AND TREATMENT FOR ETHNIC MINORITIES

We often think that major depression and other disorders look the same for all groups of people; however, several researchers have questioned the assumption of universality with regard to psychological distress and symptomatology (Johnson, Danko, Andrade, & Markoff, 1997), arguing that universal diagnostic criteria cannot adequately capture cultural or race-based aspects of emotional distress (Trierweiler & Stricker, 1998). Efforts to enhance the cultural validity of DSM-IV resulted in the inclusion of cultural considerations for diagnostic criteria, an appendicized glossary of culture-bound syndromes, and an outline for cultural formulations (Mezzich et al., 1999). However, these innovations have been criticized as a political compromise rather than a challenge to universalistic, nosological assumptions or true recognition of the importance of contextualizing illness (Mezzich et al., 1999). Therefore, some researchers have concluded that the conceptualization, measurement, and treatment for psychological illness should be culture specific (Mezzich et al., 1999), and that important phenomenological aspects of illness are obscured when mental disorders are considered universal constructs (Kohn & Hudson, 2002).

Unfortunately, the majority of psychopathology literature indicates that symptoms and syndromes of mental illnesses represent universal phenomena, and that measurement and diagnostic criteria are applied broadly, regardless of ethnicity or race (Gotlib & Hammen, 2002). In addition to the use of universal diagnostic criteria, a vast amount of research on psychopathology supports the universality of mental disorders, regardless of race or ethnicity. Much of this research, however, has neither included ethnically diverse samples nor conducted adequate comparisons of psychopathological phenomena across ethnically distinct groups; therefore, it cannot answer the question of whether depression is experienced or expressed similarly.

There are some indications that in comparison to whites, ethnic/minority individuals may present with different symptom profiles or comorbid conditions prior to treatment. These differences could contribute to less accuracy in diagnosis among African Americans and Latinos (Borowsky, et al., 2000). For example, in comparison to European American patients with depression, depressed African American patients may exhibit more severe somatic symptoms, increased psychiatric comorbidity, greater life stress, and differences in perceived physical functioning and health beliefs (Brown, Schulberg, & Madonia, 1996). Compared to European Americans, African Americans with unipolar depression have reported more depressive symptoms relating to worry, muscular tension, general anxiety, and autonomic symptoms (Fabrega, Merrich, & Ulrich, 1988). In another study, Jackson-Triche et al. (2000), found that in comparison to European Americans, Latinos, and Asian Americans, African Americans with depression were less likely to report suicidal ideation and melancholia but more likely to report poor health-related quality of life and greater adverse life events, likely due to greater reported economic disadvantage. In conducting depression treatment groups with African American women (see Kohn et al., 2002) we found that our patients were more likely to report experiencing increased mood irritability (as opposed to melancholia), increased appetite (as opposed to decreased appetite), and hypersomnia (as opposed to insomnia) than non–African American patients. Though systematic investigations of symptom differences in depression are rare, the limited available evidence suggests that clinicians may need to adjust their conceptualization of depression when working with ethnic/minority individuals.

Ethnic differences in worldview or perspective may contribute to differences in how people understand or experience psychological distress. Compared to whites, Latinos are more likely to endorse a more external locus of control, and to believe that their future is fatalistic and dependent upon external natural and supernatural forces. This orientation may explain some Latinos' view that mental illnesses is caused by external factors and express symptoms in physical terms. Thus, Latino patients may report their depression in terms of dizziness, fatigue, headaches, and other physical symptoms (Arce & Torres-Matrullo, 1982). Therefore, clinicians should assess differences in pretreatment presentations for African Americans and Latinos, and take premorbid functioning and life context into account when planning treatment.

Acculturation, history, and migration differences may also be important in the conceptualization of depression among Latinos. Guarnaccia, Angel, and Worobey (1989) found evidence for a pattern of depressive symptom expression among Latinos that emphasizes a combined somatic and affective dimension rather than differentiated factors, suggesting that physical and emotional aspects may be unified. Guarnaccia et al. believe that Latinos may strategically choose to highlight somatic symptoms in clinical settings due to the stigma of being *loca,* or crazy. Furthermore, among three groups of Latinos—Puerto Ricans, Mexican Americans, and Cuban Americans—interesting cultural and gender differences emerged. Specifically, level of acculturation influenced the conceptualization of depression for Mexican American men such that those who were English-speaking differentiated between primarily affective and primarily physical symptoms. English-speaking Mexican American women, however, appeared similar to Spanish-speaking women in expressing combined affective and somatic problems. Puerto Ricans expressed a greater level of symptoms of loneliness and demoralization, perhaps related to their long history of social dislocation in the United States. A predominant theme for symptom expression among Cuban Americans was isolation, perhaps as a community characterized by homeland migration and an insulated language and culture. These differences indicate that clinicians should include acculturation, gender, and social history in the conceptualization of distress among ethnic/minority patients. Another study of acculturation and depression diagnoses found that physicians were more likely to classify Latinos with higher acculturation status as depressed in comparison to classification based on a self-report measure of depressive symptoms (Chung et al., 2003). To avoid diagnostic bias, careful assessment of depression for ethnic/minority patients is warranted.

ASSESSMENT OF DEPRESSION
FOR ETHNIC MINORITIES

Although several instruments for assessing depressive symptoms and major depression exist, some measures may not adequately or appropriately include symptom patterns or idioms that characterize the illness for ethnic/minority patients. Improved understanding of possible racial or ethnic variations in the manifestation of depressive symptoms will increase diagnostic accuracy (Ayalon & Young, 2003) and lead to better characterization and detection of disorders across distinct groups. Clinicians should use the combination of a standardized assessment tool and individualized assessment of social history, acculturation, physical symptoms and functioning, and atypical symptom expression.

Some studies have found that measures of depressive symptomatology are invariant across race and ethnic groups; therefore, they may be seen as universally valid indicators of distress. Aneshensel, Clark, and Frerichs (1983) used confirmatory factor analysis to determine whether variance in factor patterns of various depressive symptom scales existed in a community sample of European, African Americans, and English-speaking and Spanish speaking Latinos. They did not find any significant differences for the depression factor. Similarly, Hepner, Morales, Hays, Orlando, and Miranda (2005) did not find evidence for item bias or item performance differences between African American and European American women for the mood module of the Primary Care Evaluation of Mental Disorders (PRIME-MD), a widely used primary care assessment tool for screening depression. These findings suggest that standardized instruments may be helpful for assessment of ethnic/minority patients.

A number of other studies, however, have found group differences in the measurement of depressive symptoms. One study found differences in the patterns of depressive symptoms across four groups: whites, blacks, and English- and Spanish-speaking Hispanics (Aneshensel et al., 1983); other researchers have found evidence for variance in depression symptoms among Latinos (Posner, Stewart, Marín, & Pérez-Stable, 2001). Still other studies have found evidence for ethnic differences in the meaning and diagnostic utility of depression, anxiety, and somatic symptoms in ethnic/minority groups. In our study of race differences in the factor structure of the

Center for Epidemiologic Studies—Depression (CES-D) Scale (Radloff, 1977), we found variance in the factor structure of symptoms between European American and African American national survey respondents (Kohn-Wood, Banks, Ivey, & Hudson, 2007). Specifically, African Americans were significantly less likely to endorse three items, "I enjoyed life," "I felt full of energy," and "I felt people cared for me." Colea, Kawachib, Mallerd, and Berjman (2000) utilized item response bias analyses to conclude that two CES-D items ("people are unfriendly" and "people dislike me") were biased by race towards higher endorsement among elderly African Americans in comparison to elderly Whites, possibly due to being confounded with perceptions of racial prejudice. Similarly, in Ayalon and Young's (2003) examination of depressive symptomatology on the Beck Depression Inventory (BDI), a measure similar to the CES-D, 4 of 21 items, including self-dislike, sleep disturbance, loss of appetite, and loss of libido, were significantly more likely to indicate depression severity for African Americans than for European Americans. These studies point to the importance of understanding the comparability of measurement instruments across populations. Are we measuring the same thing across different groups? Given the limited evidence for symptom pattern differences, it is critically important to supplement standardized measures with individualized information. Other than linguistic translations of existing standardized instruments, the field generally lacks available ethnic-specific assessment instruments such as the CES-D-K, recommended for use with Korean populations (Noh, Avison, & Kaspar, 1992).

TREATMENT OF AFRICAN AMERICANS AND LATINOS

A key element in the effective treatment of African American and Latino patients in psychotherapy is to maintain a firm grasp of the basic principles that elevate cultural competence. Increasing ethnic awareness is the key to competence cultivation among practicing clinicians; it is requisite that they become increasingly knowledgeable about commonly shared ethnic/minority experiences and perspectives that are often quite different from their own. Working with ethnic/minority patients highlights the great need for clinicians to remain cognizant of their patients' personal beliefs and assumptions. More importantly, clinicians must resist the harmful tendency to make evaluative judgments, which may have major implications for the overall effectiveness of psychotherapy and treatment with a diverse clientele.

CT with African Americans

Ethnic awareness requires the recognition of potentially large differences in values and experiences between patient and clinician. Interdependence, spirituality, and discrimination are consistently cited markers of cultural difference between mainstream and ethnic/minority populations (Hall, 2001). Despite mounting evidence of the importance of cultural competence in working with ethnically diverse patients, clinicians often make the mistake of overlooking or misunderstanding these constructs as they operate among ethnic/minority patients.

African Americans are likely to differ from the dominant culture regarding conceptualization of self, valuing sociocentrism rather than egocentrism (Randall, 1994). Sociocentrism emphasizes the importance of role fulfillment and interdependence within the social network as opposed to autonomy and individuation. This lack of desire for complete independence can be misinterpreted as passivity or weakness and dependence, resulting in a negative evaluation of an engrained cultural value and the erroneous assumption of a necessity for drastic change. Aside from obvious differences in core values and beliefs, it is also quite possible for seemingly similar values to gain varied expression based on ethnicity. Spirituality provides a prime example; the same religion is often practiced in radically different ways (Hall, 2001). Assumptions of similarity in behavioral expression without consideration for culturally mediated differences are ripe for producing instances of extreme misunderstanding. Likewise, symptoms of psychological disorders may have significantly different manifestations across cultures. Indeed, it is not uncommon for African Americans to express intense irritability as an indicator of depressed mood rather than the prototypical sadness typically associated with depression (Kohn, Oden, Munoz, Robinson, & Leavitt, 2002).

Discrimination is perhaps the most pervasive construct, with particular relevance to therapy with African American patients. By and large, all African Americans share the experience of discrimination, and in multiple domains. Perceived discrimination is likely to have a large impact on therapy wherein possible reasons for early termination may include therapist mistrust and cultural insensitivity (Carter, 1999). Consequently, it is important that clinicians not only recognize the significance of discrimination as it is uniquely perceived by each African American patient but also highlight the contribution of sociopolitical, historical factors to the experience of psychological distress to circumvent misattribution of blame directed toward the patient (McNair, 1996). Maintaining open acceptance of an African American patient's reality further promotes ethnic awareness and offsets the tendency toward hasty (often negative) evaluation in lieu of considering the potentially adaptive functions of culturally mediated thoughts and behaviors. However, although the possibility of minimizing distressing phenomena among African Americans exists, circumstances that might differentially predict either over- or underpathologizing have yet to be investigated (Sue, Zane, & Young, 1994).

In addition to discrimination, it may be important to adapt other constructs. Randall (1994) indicates the likely impact of differing time orientations on therapeutic goals. Failure to recognize ethnic differences in time orientation can lead to misinterpretations of lateness and appointment inconsistency as resistance or lack of motivation. These would be inept conclusions in reference to individuals for whom time is not necessarily an economic commodity that is scheduled well into the future, but perhaps a resource well spent in the present. For many African Americans, the past may hold paramount importance for their present lives, rendering an orientation toward the future as essentially meaningless. Traditional therapeutic goals such as "planning ahead" and adhering to strict assignment schedules may have less relevance for African American patients.

Unfortunately, research on the adaptation of psychotherapy to meet the particular needs of African American patients is sparse. To date, few studies have reported on the outcome of culturally adapted therapy tailored specifically for African Americans. Our study of applied structural (process-based) and didactic (content-based) adaptations to CBT interventions with depressed, low-income African American women indicated that ethnic-specific changes to CBT may be useful (Kohn et al., 2002). Our structural adaptations included closed group therapy sessions within only African American women, language modifications negotiated by the group, and the use of culturally derived anecdotal examples. Didactic adaptations included therapeutic foci on issues relevant to African American women's lives, including healthy relationships, spirituality, family, and African American female identity. Results demonstrated that culturally adapted CBT was more efficacious than traditional CBT in lowering reported levels of depressive symptom intensity. Therefore, greater effectiveness of culturally adapted therapy suggests that traditional CBT may become less effective as groups differ from the original intended population of the intervention.

Other adaptations have been proposed for work with African American patients based on associated cultural values and experiences, though these have not been empirically demonstrated in terms of outcome. Specific to CT, Randall (1994) encourages prudent use of reattribution as a therapeutic technique given that explanations of events may be culturally relative.

In therapy with an African American patient, it may indeed be more useful to openly accept reality as it is perceived and presented rather than to challenge the patient's ability to assess the current milieu appropriately (McNair, 1996).

Group psychotherapy has been cited as a useful approach for working specifically with African American women, for whom a promoted sense of sisterhood may help to combat common feelings of alienation, loneliness, and daily stress (Boyd-Franklin, 1987). It is suggested that combining the collective benefits of an intensive support group and the psychotherapeutic treatment goal of behavior change, results in a therapeutic support group hybrid that allows black women to address a variety of problems including anxiety, symptoms of depression, and low self-esteem. Furthermore, pervasive burdens associated with managing family responsibilities, maintaining healthy relationships, and contending with workplace discrimination are also addressed. African American women's groups should include six to eight members to promote an atmosphere of intimate sharing, while also allowing for periodic absences.

In contrast to the larger adaptations proposed by some researchers, others suggest that practical and relatively minor enhancements to current psychotherapy interventions are also likely to have a beneficial impact on treatment effectiveness for African American patients. Addendums as simple as bolstering the plan of assessment with additional measures based on possible confounding factors likely relevant among African Americans may go a long way in improving quality of therapeutic intervention (Carter, 1999). For example, the inclusion of medical evaluations, as well as acculturation and racial identity scales, may explain a great deal in terms of variance introduced by the extensive within-group heterogeneity of the African American community. Another relatively simple yet extremely useful enhancement is the implementation of immediate symptom relief strategies (e.g., behavioral activation, relaxation training) to help decrease high rates of attrition among African American patients.

However, some cultural enhancements that are proposed to be efficacious require more than minimal effort by clinicians. These pertain to the necessity of environmental intervention to ensure that conditions for therapy are met at the very basic level of access to social services and emergency assistance (Randall, 1994). Such an enhancement highlights the critical relevance of increased clinician knowledge of current public policy for treatment effectiveness. Pertinent public policy issues for many African Americans include boundaries to adequate treatment (e.g., managed care disparities) that extend beyond patients' immediate control into sociopolitical realms and require proactive professional assistance (Boyd-Franklin,

2003). Although worthwhile recommendations have been offered for the apparent benefit of these proposed enhancements, evidence-based outcome research based on successful implementation of the aforementioned treatment improvements has yet to appear in the literature.

Finally, it is important to recognize the considerable within-group heterogeneity of the African American community. Individual differences often play a larger role than presumed cultural norms in expressed values and behaviors. Furthermore, almost nothing is known about gender differences among African Americans' response to treatment. Thus, as with all patients, it is necessary to address directly and negotiate values and goals in therapy with African American patients to ensure clarity and the maintenance of respect for both cultural and individual differences (Boyd-Franklin, 2003). Open negotiation has the added benefit of increasing sense of empowerment, an area of intervention that can be particularly useful in therapy with African American patients (Carter, 1999).

CT with Latinos

As clinicians, embracing cultural dimensions enhances the ways we diagnose, conceptualize, and treat patients within Latino populations (Martinez-Taboas, 2005). Latinos are not a monolithic group; therefore, cultural awareness begins with an acknowledgment and appreciation for the group's culture and diversity. Furthermore, it is also important to understand that acculturation issues can impact mental health among Latinos (Fitzpatrick, 1971). Acculturation can influence the way Latinos embrace traditional Latino principles, with the possibility of acculturated Latinos embracing more principles valued by the American majority such as individualism (Elliot, 2000). All of these variables must be acknowledged within the context of therapy given that demographic, historical, political, socioeconomic, and psychological conditions are culturally unique across subgroups of Latinos (Casas, Vasquez, & Ruiz de Esparza, 2002).

There are many beneficial aspects of CT approaches that can be effective for Latino patients. Brief therapy that provides immediate symptom relief, advice, guidance, and problem-solving strategies is important for traditional Latino patients (Arce & Torres-Matrullo, 1982). These variables are also significant for treatment of low-income patients (Torres-Matrullo, 1982). Time spent in "role preparation" is also important, in that it allows patients to learn about the treatment process and how CBT can help them (Organista & Muñoz, 1996). Role preparation has been found to decrease premature dropout for Latino (Delgado, 1983) and low-income patients (Orlinsky & Howard, 1986). Use of psychoeducation, manuals, and homework helps to eliminate the stigma associated with utilization of mental services (Organista & Muñoz, 1996). Also, ethnic matching is associated with better treatment outcome and lower dropout rates among Latinos with low levels of acculturation (Sue, Fujino, Hu, Takevichi, & Zane, 1991).

Relevant themes that have been found to be significant among many Latino patients include marital and familial interpersonal conflicts, and traditional gender role issues (Comas-Díaz, 1985). These cultural dimensions are clinically relevant given that researchers have found cognitive and behavioral differences between depressed Puerto Rican women who embrace traditional gender roles and those who do not (Comas-Díaz, 1985). Traditional gender roles of *marianismo* and *machismo* may influence presentation issues; therefore, processing the adaptive and maladaptive aspects of these roles is important for therapy (Organista & Muñoz, 1996).

Within treatment, it is important to emphasize the links between patients' current thoughts, feelings, and behaviors and to help patients to think alternatively (Arce & Torres-Matrullo, 1982). However, the traditional ABCD cognitive model (activating events, beliefs, consequences, and dispute of irrational beliefs; Ellis & Grieger, 1977) may not be beneficial for Latino patients. Consequently, Organista and Muñoz (1996) outlined different ways that Latino patients can benefit from embracing the underlying foundation of positive and negative thinking. These researchers suggest reframing thoughts as "helpful" or "unhelpful." Also, therapists can help patients challenge their distortions with "Yes, but . . . " statements, which reframe thoughts from "half-truth" negative statements to "whole-truth" positive statements. This can be particularly helpful with ethnic/minority patients who may habitually subscribe to a fatalistic perspective.

Religion is an important aspect in the lives of many ethnic/minority individuals. Organista and Muñoz (1996) have discussed ways to incorporate cognitive and behavioral therapeutic activities within a religious context, such as helping patients to be more proactive in their prayers. Time spent in prayer or religious activities can be framed as a positive activity and conceived as behavioral activation for depressed patients. Therapy itself can be viewed through a religious lens. For example, when working with a religious African American patient who felt that therapy was counterindicated by her faith and that the only thing she should need was prayer, one of us (L. K.-W.) invoked the well-known (and variously told) religious parable about the man who was drowning in a flood. The man waited for God to answer his prayers. He ignored would-be rescuers in a boat and helicopter by saying that God would save him. When he died and went to heaven he asked why God did not answer his prayers. God replied that He had sent a boat and a helicopter. Therapy could be characterized as a vehicle provided by God and/or prayer to help an individual get well and live life to his/her fullest spiritual potential.

Issues of treatment accessibility and acceptance are important in treating linguistic minorities. As the nation becomes more diverse, clinicians must strengthen their cultural competence skills effectively to treat patients for whom English is not the primary language (Casas et al., 2002). Having bicultural and bilingual staff available for patients is likely to promote culturally sensitive, and more effective, treatment (Arce & Torres-Matrullo, 1982).

There is disagreement about the best way to use CBT to help Latino patients; some researchers recommend integrating patients' cultural beliefs into treatment (Martinez-Taboas, 2005), whereas others suggest challenging the functionality of certain beliefs (Castro-Blanco, 2005). This important distinction to some extent reflects a debate in the field about how best to serve ethnic/minority patients who may hold beliefs that influence mental health or compromise treatment response. Those who recommend integration of cultural beliefs feel that this is the best way to respect diversity and to improve treatment effectiveness. The lack of cultural integration or adaptation is thought to contribute to the lack of treatment seeking, less treatment compliance, and premature termination among ethnic/minority patients. Those who advocate challenging cultural beliefs suggest that because some specific beliefs are deleterious to mental health and contribute to depression, they should be considered depressogenic cognitions in need of therapeutic alteration. For example, cultural beliefs about the importance of suffering and sacrificing may contribute to depressive symptomatology among Latinas. A therapist might opt to incorporate these beliefs by acknowledging the importance of self-sacrifice but emphasizing that one can best help others by being one's best (mentally healthy) self. Alternatively, a therapist might challenge a patient's idea that he/she must suffer as a distorted cognition that should be refuted to improve mental health. Religious beliefs about the spiritual sanctity of marriage may influence a patient's decision to remain in a difficult marriage, contributing to depression. A therapist might attempt to reduce depressive symptoms in the context of the marriage or challenge the notion that God would want the person to remain in an unhealthy situation. Unfortunately, there has been no empirical comparison of these alternative approaches to therapy. Regardless, many therapists have found useful ways to bring cultural components into their work with Latino patients. In general, clinicians must strive for cultural competence by approaching their patients in sensitive ways that embrace and integrate the cultural context, yet challenge distorted beliefs that affect patients' ability to effectively manage their mood.

CASE ILLUSTRATION

Gabrielle, a 35-year-old woman, currently identifies herself as African American but states that she was born and raised in Germany by parents of Jamaican descent. She moved to the United States in her early 20s, married an African American man, and has a young child. After receiving a 2-year training certificate in web programming from a local community college 9 years ago, she began working for a large company as a programmer. She entered therapy at the behest of her husband, after experiencing several symptoms that increased in severity over the past year. Specifically, Gabrielle described an increase in appetite that has led to a weight gain of over 40 pounds. She described a pattern of increased need for sleep and increased irritability, alternating with periods of sadness and hopelessness. She also described a lack of energy and motivation so extreme that her husband had to rouse her from bed to come to her therapy appointment, set out clothes for her to wear, and prod her to shower and dress. Gabrielle stated that she experiences difficulty concentrating and becomes paralyzed when faced with even the simplest decisions, such as what to make for dinner. Although Gabrielle denied suicidal feelings, because "that would be a sin," she did admit that she sometimes wished she would never wake up from sleep or that a car would hit her while she was driving, resulting in a fatal accident. Her symptoms had become so bad that Gabrielle stopped working but she was also pursuing a Department of Labor and Industry claim to pay for mental health treatment for what she described as the escalating pattern of racial discrimination she experienced at work. For the past 3 years, since a change in supervisors at her job, Gabrielle described incidences of race-based harassment and intimidation directed toward her, the only African American programmer in her workplace. She described racial slurs and jokes told in her presence, said that her competence was questioned despite having achieved excellent evaluations during the first 6 years of employment, and said that because of her race she was given the worst assignments and schedule by her supervisor.

Initial treatment for Gabrielle involved a psychiatry referral for a medication evaluation to determine whether an antidepressant was warranted in addition to CT. After a brief interview the psychiatry resident conducting the medication evaluation contacted the referring psychologist to suggest immediate hospitalization. The resident, a young white male, had interpreted Gabrielle's discussion of racial discrimination at work as delusional and felt that her beliefs about racial harassment, along with the depressive symptoms, were indicative of major depression with possible psychotic features. He stated that it was impossible "in this day and age" for someone actually to experience the kinds of incidents Gabrielle described. The referring psychologist, an African American woman, considered the possibility of delusional beliefs but held the perspective that racial discrimination can and does happen, although it is possible that depression may contribute to the interpretation and reaction to particular events. Without pursuing medication, the psychologist embarked on a course of treatment that utilized CT to change Gabrielle's specifically depressogenic beliefs about herself as flawed and the world as malevolent, and utilized behavioral activation to increase positive activities. Cultural adaptations included an explicit discussion of discrimination and Gabrielle's reaction to events at work based on her unique history as a woman of Afro-Caribbean descent who emigrated from another country. Instead of challenging Gabrielle's experience of racial discrimination, the therapist helped Gabrielle work through proactive responses to her situation at work, acknowledging the harm caused by her experiences but helping her increase daily functioning.

REVIEW OF EFFICACY RESEARCH

Empirical validation of treatment approaches is determined based on outcome studies of efficacy and effectiveness. Efficacy studies are based on randomized controlled trials that adhere to strict guidelines for determining identified outcomes related to specific treatment modalities provided by trained experts. Efficacy studies answer the question of whether or not a specific treatment works for a specific disorder. For example, the National Institute of Mental Health Treatment of Depression Collaborative Research Program (NIMH TDCRP) documented the relative efficacy of CT and interpersonal therapy (IPT) in comparison to antidepressant medication (Elkin et al., 1989). In this study, both CT and IPT were found to be effective for reducing symptoms of unipolar depression (Depression Guideline Panel, 1993); however, too few ethnic/minority patients were included in the randomized sample, and differential outcomes by ethnicity were not analyzed. In general, with the few exceptions reviewed in the following section, efficacy studies of CT and CBT have not included enough ethnic/minority individuals to permit analyses of outcomes for African American and Latino populations.

Effectiveness studies differ from efficacy studies in that they apply empirically validated (efficacious) treatments to settings outside controlled laboratory conditions. Therefore, these studies can be important in determining treatment outcomes for diverse groups, because effectiveness research can answer the question of whether a treatment is efficacious in a particular setting or for a particular population. In addition, effectiveness research expands the evaluation of treatment outcomes beyond alleviation of disorder symptoms by including issues such as the feasibility, acceptability, length or cost of treatment, or the degree to which a specific treatment is adequate for the setting or population. We review the available data from available efficacy and effectiveness studies of CT and CBT for depression in African Americans and Latinos, as well as data from studies using cognitive-based interventions for the prevention of depression.

Despite increased research attention paid to the efficacy of treatments for depression since the NIMH Collaborative Study in the 1980s, no available efficacy studies have examined CT or CBT for depression across ethnic groups. This is unfortunate, because empirically validated treatment approaches are increasingly valued in clinical settings and medical insurance policy guidelines. However, there is promising evidence for the utility of cognitive approaches with ethnic/minority patients based on different kinds of studies in the literature. In addition to a few studies with small comparative samples, that tested differences in CT outcome between ethnic/minority and white patients, a handful of within-group studies have tested outcomes for African Americans or Latinos. Also, some studies have examined CT outcomes with specialized populations (e.g., HIV patients with depressive symptoms), and others have tested outcomes of treatment with enhancements to psychotherapy for ethnic/minority patients. These studies have begun to establish the efficacy of cognitive approaches for ethnic/minority patients, particularly those studies with specific adaptations to service delivery and attention to cultural issues.

An early, randomized controlled trial compared group CT therapy and group behavioral therapy (BT) for depression in a small sample of Puerto Rican women (Comas-Díaz, 1981). The 25 participants were randomized to three treatment conditions (CT, BT, and control) and outcomes were determined by self-report and clinical and behavioral ratings. The intervention was conducted over 4 weeks and included five, 1.5-hour treatment sessions. Both therapy groups showed a reduction in depressive symptoms in comparison to the control group, and there were no significant differences between CT and BT groups. At a 5-week follow-up, however, participants in the BT group showed slightly improved outcomes in comparison to the CT group. A nonrandomized study of 175 low-income and minority medical patients, including mostly African Americans and Latinos, showed moderate reductions in depressive symptoms after individual and group treatment with a manualized CBT intervention (Organista, Muñoz, & Gonzalez,

1994). There were no differences in treatment outcome among African American, Latino, and European American patients, although ethnic/ minority patients were more likely to terminate treatment prematurely (a finding similar to that of Sue et al., 1994).

More recent studies with specific groups have shown mixed results for CT and CBT treatment for ethnic/minority patients. It is difficult, though, to draw conclusions due to the inability to analyze differential outcomes in small samples and the ability of results to generalize beyond special populations. For example, an exploratory randomized study of CBT versus supportive psychotherapy versus combination treatment (medication and supportive psychotherapy) was conducted with 101 HIV-positive patients experiencing depressive symptoms (Markowitz, Speilman, Sullivan, & Fishman, 2000). African Americans receiving CBT reported significantly poorer outcomes in comparison to Latino and European American patients. The findings, however, are based on the four African American patients in the CBT condition, out of a total of 18 African Americans in the study sample. Alternatively, in a small exploratory study of depressed, low-income African American women, Kohn et al. (2002) found that participants in a group therapy intervention of culturally adapted CBT reported greater decreases in depressive symptomatology after 16 weeks of treatment in comparison to demographically matched women participating in a nonadapted CBT group.

In an effort to engage and to maintain depressed ethnic/minority patients in therapy and improve functioning, Miranda, Azocar, Organista, Dwyer, and Arean (2003a) examined the impact of including clinical case management as a supplement to standard CBT. The supplemental intervention was intended to work toward resolving environmental stressors (e.g., housing, employment, recreation, relationships) that contribute to distress. Patients receiving case management attended more CBT sessions and were less likely than those without the supplemental intervention to drop out of the intervention. There were no differences in treatment response to CBT between African American and Latino patients. African American patients (41% of the sample) with supplemental case management surprisingly reported more depressive symptoms and worse functioning than those treated with CBT alone. Also, there was no impact of the supplemented therapy on the posttreatment functioning of African American patients, in contrast with Latino patients. African Americans receiving CBT alone showed greater improvement than African Americans receiving supplemental case management with CBT. Though these findings seemingly downplay the importance of environmental stressors for African American treatment outcomes, the researchers explained that the unexpected findings may have resulted from unintended differences in case management delivery. Specifically, posttreatment review of the data revealed that Latino patients received more home visits than African American patients. Greater number of home visits suggests that Latino patients may have received more case management and/or more personalized case management that could have resulted in better treatment outcomes.

Another outcome study provided enhancements to treatment by fulfilling basic needs to promote participation in treatment for depression with African American women and Latina immigrants (Miranda et al., 2003b). The purpose of the study was to assess the impact of appropriate care (i.e., paroxetine or bupropion antidepressant medication, or CBT vs. control) on depressed minority women by reducing accessibility barriers. Enhancements consisted of pretreatment education meetings about depression and treatment, cultural adaptations to guideline-based medication and CBT, intensive outreach and routine follow-up, reimbursement for child care and transportation costs, flexible scheduling, language modifications, and culturally sensitive professionals. Cumulatively, these accommodations helped circumvent barriers and ensured accessibility of appropriate care to a population at risk for receiving inadequate community care. Whereas medication treatment produced superior 6-month outcomes over CBT, patients receiving either type of appropriate care reported improved functioning and significant decreases in depressive symptoms in comparison to the control condition. There were no posttreatment differences in depressive symptoms between African American and Latina patients. Miranda and colleagues (2003c) have noted that minor accommodations, including translated materials for patients, culturally relevant training materials for service providers, and use of ethnic/minority treatment experts, yield particularly large clinical benefits for ethnically diverse patients. Thus, practical modifications and enhancements of traditional CBT delivery appear to benefit depressed ethnic/minority patients by increasing the utilization of appropriate care.

In addition to treating depression effectively, CT approaches have been found to be effective in reducing the risk of major depression. To our knowledge, however, only one preventive intervention trial of CBT with ethnic/minority adults has been conducted. Muñoz, Ying, and Bernal (1995) conducted a randomized controlled trial of a manualized CBT group intervention with 150 low-income, predominantly minority adults at risk for depressive disorder based on symptom levels (but not yet meeting criteria for diagnosis) in a primary care setting. Results indicated that the intervention significantly reduced depressive symptoms in the CBT group compared to the control group. Group CBT has also been found to be effective in reducing risk for depression among low-income urban Latinos who have just migrated to the United States (Arce & Torres-Matrullo, 1982). The groups provided patients support for processing ways to communicate their emotions and approaching their conflicts within a new culture, therefore reducing risk for depression and other disorders. In general, however, more research is needed to understand the potential of CT for reducing risk and preventing the onset of depression.

CONCLUSIONS

Ethnic differences in the experience of psychopathology and the related manifestation of varied symptomatology necessitate that clinicians adopt a broader conceptualization of what it means to be depressed in African American and Latino communities. Furthermore, the unique and multifaceted context in which individual patients experience psychological distress must also be taken into account in light of considerable within-group heterogeneity. Thus, the proper conceptualization and treatment of depression within ethnic/minority populations is intimately linked to the competent practice of thorough assessment protocol. More comprehensive assessment (including both standardized measures and individualized assessment information) is sorely needed to gauge the extent to which acculturative, socioeconomic, and discrimination-related factors, for example, may influence the clinical picture, as well as the resultant treatment plan.

As with any applied (nonmedical) intervention, CT for depression relies not only on the expertise of trained clinicians but also on their sensitivity to issues of racial and ethnic difference. Mental health professionals must take care to be aware of the interface between their own worldviews and those of patients. Culturally competent clinicians are adept at recognizing the point at which effective treatment may require deferral of expertise to the localized experiences of individual patients.

The available, if sparse, literature on ethnic/minority treatment outcomes indicates that cognitive-based intervention approaches are effective for mood disorders experienced by African American and Latinos, particularly when cultural adaptations or enhancements are included and potential barriers are addressed. The limited evidence for treatment outcomes among ethnic/minority patients suggests CT may be effective. However, it remains critically important that future treatment studies include substantial proportions of ethnic/minority participants to establish an evidence base from which more substantive conclusions may be drawn.

REFERENCES

Aneshensel, C. S., Clark, V. A., & Frerichs, R. R. (1983). Race, ethnicity, and depression: A confirmatory analysis. *Journal of Personality and Social Psychology, 44*(2), 385–398.

Arce, A., & Torres-Matrullo, C. (1982). Applications of cognitive behavioral techniques in the treatment of Hispanic patients. *Psychiatric Quarterly, 54,* 230–236.

Ayalon, L., & Young, M. A. (2003). A comparison of depressive symptoms in African Americans and Caucasian Americans. *Journal of Cross-Cultural Psychology, 34,* 111–124.

Borowsky, S. J., Rubenstein, L. V., Meredith, L. S., Camp, P., Jackson-Triche, M., & Wells, K. (2000). Who is at risk of nondetection of mental health problems in primary care? *Journal of General Internal Medicine, 15,* 381–388.

Boyd-Franklin, N. (1987). Group therapy for black women: A therapeutic support model. *American Journal of Orthopsychiatry, 57,* 394–401.

Boyd-Franklin, N. (2003). *Black families in therapy: Understanding the African American experience* (2nd ed.). New York: Guilford Press.

Brown, C., Schulberg, H. C., & Madonia, M. J. (1996). Clinical presentations of major depression by African Americans and whites in primary medical care practice. *Journal of Affective Disorders, 41,* 181–191.

Carter, M. M. (1999). Ethnic awareness in the cognitive behavioral treatment of a depressed African American female. *Cognitive and Behavioral Practice, 6,* 273–278.

Casas, J. M., Vasquez, M. L., & Ruiz de Esparza, C. A. (2002). Counseling the Latina/o: A guiding framework for a diverse population. In P. B. Pedersen, J. G. Draguns, W. J. Lonner, & J. E. Trimble (Eds.), *Counseling across populations* (5th ed., pp. 133–158). Thousand Oaks, CA: Sage.

Castro-Blanco, D. R. (2005). Cultural sensitivity in conventional psychotherapy: A comment on Martinez-Taboas (2005). *Psychotherapy: Theory, Research, Practice and Training, 42,* 14–16.

Chung, H., Teresi, J., Guarnaccia, P., Meyers, B. S., Holmes, D., Bobrowitz, T., et al. (2003). Depressive symptoms and psychiatric distress in low income Asian and Latino primary care patients: Prevalence and recognition. *Community Mental Health Journal, 39,* 33–46.

Colea, S. R., Kawachib, I., Mallerd, S. J., & Berjman, L. F. (2000). Test of item–response bias in the CES-D scale: Experience from the New Haven EPESE Study. *Journal of Clinical Epidemiology, 53,* 285–289.

Comas-Díaz, L. (1981). Effects of cognitive and behavioral group treatment on the depressive symptoms of Puerto Rican women. *Journal of Consulting and Clinical Psychology, 54,* 639–645.

Comas-Díaz, L. (1985). Cognitive and behavioral group therapy with Puerto Rican women: A comparison of content themes. *Hispanic Journal of Behavioral Sciences, 7,* 273–283.

Delgado, M. (1983). Hispanics and psychotherapeutic groups. *International Journal of Group Psychotherapy, 33,* 507–520.

Depression Guideline Panel. (1993). *Depression in primary care: Vol. 1. Detection and diagnosis* (AHCPR Publication No. 93-0550, Clinical Practice Guideline, No. 5). Rockville, MD: U.S. Department of Health and Human Services, Public Health Service, Agency for Health Care Policy and Research.

Elkin, I., Shea, M. T., Watkins, J. T., Imber, S. D., Sotsky, S. M., Collins, J. F., et al. (1989). National Institute of Mental Health Treatment of Depression Collaborative Research Program: General effectiveness of treatments. *Archives of General Psychiatry, 46,* 971–982.

Elliot, K. A. (2000). *The relationship between acculturation, family functioning, and school performance of Mexican American adolescents.* Unpublished doctoral dissertation, University of California, Santa Barbara.

Ellis, A., & Grieger, R. (1977). *Handbook of rational emotive therapy.* New York: Holt, Rinehart & Winston.

Fabrega, H., Mezzich, J., & Ulrich, R. F. (1988). African American–white differences in psychopathology in an urban psychiatric population. *Comprehensive Psychiatry, 29,* 285–297.

Fitzpatrick, J. P. (1971). *Puerto Rican Americans.* Englewood Cliffs, NJ: Prentice-Hall.

Goldstein, A. P. (1971). *Psychotherapeutic attraction.* New York: Pergamon.

Gotlib, I. H., & Hammen, C. L. (2002). *Handbook of depression.* New York: Guilford Press.

Guarnaccia, P. J., Angel, R., & Worobey, J. L. (1989). The factor structure of the CES-D in the Hispanic Health and Nutrition Examination Survey: The influences of ethnicity, gender and language. *Social Science Medicine, 29,* 85–94.

Hall, G. N. (2001). Psychotherapy research with ethnic minorities: Empirical, ethical, and conceptual issues. *Journal of Counseling and Clinical Psychology, 69,* 502–510.

Hepner, K. A., Morales, L. S., Hays, R. D., Orlando, M., & Miranda, J. (2005, May). *Screening for depression among black and white women in primary care.* Poster presented at the annual American Psychological Society Conference, Los Angeles, CA.

Hohmann, A. A., & Parron, D. L. (1996). How the new NIH guidelines on inclusion of women and minorities apply: Efficacy trials, effectiveness trials, and validity. *Journal of Consulting and Clinical Psychology, 64,* 851–855.

Jackson-Triche, M. E., Sullivan, J. G., Wells, K. B., Rogers, W., Camp, P., & Mazel, R. (2000). Depression and health-related quality of life in ethnic minorities seeking care in general medical settings. *Journal of Affective Disorders, 58,* 89–97.

Johnson, R. C., Danko, G. P., Andrade, N. N., & Markoff, R. A. (1997). Intergroup similarities in judgments of psychiatric symptom severity. *Cultural Diversity and Mental Health, 3,* 61–68.

Kohn, L. P., & Hudson, K. M. (2002). Gender, ethnicity and depression: Intersectionality and context in mental health research with African American women. *African American Research Perspectives, 8,* 174–184.

Kohn, L. P., Oden, T., Munoz, R. F., Robinson, A., & Leavitt, D. (2002). Adapted cognitive behavioral group therapy for depressed low-income African American women. *Community Mental Health Journal, 38,* 497–504.

Kohn-Wood, L. P., Banks, K. H., Ivey, A., & Hudson, G. (2007). *Factor variability of depressive symptoms in African Americans and white Americans.* Manuscript submitted for publication.

Markowitz, J. C., Speilman, L. A., Sullivan, M., & Fishman, B. (2000). An exploratory study of ethnicity and psychotherapy outcome among HIV-positive patients with depressive symptoms. *Journal of Psychotherapy Practice and Research, 9,* 226–231.

Martinez-Taboas, A. (2005). Psychogenic seizures in an *espiritismo* context: The role of culturally sensitive psychotherapy. *Psychotherapy: Theory, Research, Practice and Training, 42,* 6–13.

McNair, L. D. (1996). African American women and behavior therapy: Integrating theory, culture, and clinical practice. *Cognitive and Behavioral Practice, 3,* 337–349.

Mezzich, J. E., Kirmayer, L. J., Kleinman, A., Fabrega, H., Parron, D. L., Good, B. J., et al. (1999). The place of culture in DSM-IV. *Journal of Nervous and Mental Disease, 187,* 457–464.

Miranda, J., Azocar, F., Organista, K. C., Dwyer, E., & Arean, P. (2003a). Treatment of depression among impoverished primary care patients from ethnic minority groups. *Psychiatric Services, 54,* 219–225.

Miranda, J., Chung, J. Y., Green, B. L., Krupnick, J., Siddique, J., Revicki, D. A., et al. (2003b). Treating depression in predominantly low-income young minority women: A randomized controlled trial. *Journal of the American Medical Association, 290,* 57–65.

Miranda, J., Duan, N., Sherbourne, C., Schoenbaum, M., Lagomasino, I., Jackson-Triche, M., et al. (2003c). Improving care for minorities: Can quality improvement interventions improve care and outcomes for depressed minorities?: Results of a randomized, controlled trial. *Health Services Research, 38,* 613–630.

Muñoz, R. F., Ying, Y., & Bernal, G. (1995). Prevention of depression with primary care patients: A randomized controlled trial. *American Journal of Community Psychology, 23,* 199–222.

Noh, S., Avison, W. R., & Kaspar, V. (1992). Depressive symptoms among Korean immigrants: Assessment of a translation of the Center for Epidemiologic Studies—Depression Scale. *Psychological Assessment, 4*(1), 84–91.

Organista, K. C., & Muñoz, R. F. (1996). Cognitive behavioral treatment with Latinos. *Cognitive and Behavioral Practice, 3,* 255–270.

Organista, K. C., Muñoz, R. F., & Gonzalez, G. (1994). Cognitive-behavioral therapy for depression in low-income and minority medical outpatients: Description of a program and exploratory analyses. *Cognitive Therapy Research, 18,* 241–259.

Orlinsky, D. E., & Howard, K. I. (1986). Process and outcome in psychotherapy. In S. L. Garfield & A. E. Bergin (Eds.), *Handbook of psychotherapy and behavior change* (3rd ed., pp. 311–381). New York: Wiley.

Posner, S. F., Stewart, A. L., Marín, G., & Pérez-Stable, E. J. (2001). Factor variability of the Center for Epidemiological Studies Depression Scale (CES-D) among urban Latinos. *Ethnicity and Health, 6*(2), 137–144.

Radloff, L. S. (1977). The CES-D Scale: A self-report depression scale for research in the general population. *Applied Psychological Measurement, 1,* 385–401.

Randall, E. J. (1994). Cultural relativism in cognitive therapy with disadvantaged African American women. *Journal of Cognitive Psychotherapy: An International Quarterly, 8,* 195–207.

Snowden, L. R., & Yamada, A. (2005). Cultural differences in access to care. *Annual Review of Clinical Psychology, 1,* 143–166.

Sue, S., Fujino, D. C., Hu, L., Takeuchi, D. T., & Zane, N. (1991). Community mental health services for ethnic minority groups: A test of the cultural responsive hypothesis. *Journal of Consulting and Clinical Psychology, 59,* 533–540.

Sue, S., Zane, N., & Young, K. (1994). Research on psychotherapy with culturally diverse populations. In A. E. Bergin & S. L. Garfield (Eds.), *Handbook of psychotherapy and behavior change* (4th ed., pp. 783–817). New York: Wiley.

Torres-Matrullo, C. (1982). Cognitive therapy of depressive disorders in the Puerto Rican female. In R. M. Becerra, M. Karno, & J. I. Escobar (Eds.), *Mental health and Hispanic Americans* (pp. 101–113). New York: Grune & Stratton.

Trierweiler, S. J., & Stricker, G. (1998). *The scientific practice of professional psychology.* New York: Plenum Press.

U.S. Department of Health and Human Services. (1999). *Mental health: A report of the Surgeon General.* Rockville, MD: U.S. Department of Health and Human Services, Substance Abuse and Mental Health Services Administration, Center for Mental Health Services, National Institutes of Health.

U.S. Department of Health and Human Services. (2001). *Mental health: Culture, race, and ethnicity. A supplement to mental health: A report of the Surgeon General.* Rockville, MD: U.S. Department of Health and Human Services, Substance Abuse and Mental Health Services Administration, Center for Mental Health Services, National Institutes of Health.

16

LESBIAN, GAY, AND BISEXUAL WOMEN AND MEN

Christopher R. Martell

Decades of research have demonstrated that lesbian, gay, and bisexual (LGB) sexual orientations are not symptomatic of psychopathology. In her pioneering research, Evelyn Hooker (1957) was the first to report that gay men were no more pathological than heterosexual men on measures considered acceptable at that time. Literature on lesbian and gay couples demonstrates that same-sex relationships are as happy and healthy as those of heterosexual couples (Kurdek, 1992, 1998). Children of lesbian and gay parents fare as well as children from heterosexual homes, and differences that have been reported are due to children living in single-parent homes (regardless of the sexual orientation of the parent) rather than two-parent households (Flaks, Ficher, Masterpasqua, & Joseph, 1995; Golombok & Tasker, 1996; Wainright, Russell, & Patterson, 2004). By all accounts, being lesbian, gay, or bisexual is not a symptom of any underlying pathology or failure of development (Gonsiorek, 1991). Yet, LGB people exist in a different context than that of their heterosexual counterparts—one that is often invalidating and stressful. Societal values shift between prohibition and acceptance of homosexual or bisexual identity and same-sex partnerships. There are dramatic differences in the treatment of LGB people, and their ability to live openly in their communities, depending on the geographic area in which they live. Within religious denominations there are progressive voices that call for the open reception of LGB people in the congregation and there are vocal, intolerant, condemning attitudes that promote religiously directed prohibition of LGB people.

The stressors begin early in life for LGB people. LGB youth face increased harassment and victimization (D'Augelli, 1998), and have higher rates of attempted suicide than their heterosexual counterparts. Some clinicians within the field of clinical psychology have recommended treating gay or lesbian people who want to change their sexual orientation (Adams, Tollison, & Carson, 1981), whereas others recognize that such self-denigrating desires result from living as part of an oppressed group. Treating LGB people to change their sexual orientation has been criticized on ethical grounds (Davison, 1976; Schroeder & Shidlo, 2001); its treatment effectiveness has been challenged (Haldeman, 1994, 2002) and so-called "conversion therapy" has been rejected or discouraged by most professional mental health organizations (e.g., American Psychiatric Association, 2000; American Psychological Association, 1998). The idea that gay or bisexual men and lesbian or bisexual women are able to change their sexual orientation with help persists, couched in the guise of allowing patient autonomy in decision making. Such an argument overlooks the enormous pressure to be heterosexual that is placed on LGB people from birth forward. The pressure is greatest in families that hold strong religious opinions proscribing same-sex, intimate relationships, and many LGB individuals from such backgrounds experience emotional conflicts (Schuck & Liddle, 2001).

EMPIRICAL RESEARCH ON DEPRESSION WITH LGB WOMEN AND MEN

It is difficult to determine rates of depression in the LGB population, because definitions of sexual orientation are inconsistent and/or unsophisticated in published reports. Many studies that define participants as lesbian or gay according to their self-reported sexual histories indicate higher rates of major depression (Cochran & Mays, 2000a, 2000b; Gilman et al., 2001; Sandfort, de Graaf, & Schnabel, 2001) and other acute psychological disorders. However, use of sexual behavior as a definition of sexual orientation is problematic (Cochran, Sullivan, & Mays, 2003). Consider the possible difference in reports of psychological distress between a man who is heterosexually married but has secret, frequent sexual contact with men and an openly gay man with a loving, accepting family. The former is not likely to identify himself as a gay man, but he would be so classified in research that uses sexual history as the defining factor. Furthermore, the heterosexually married man is more likely to have psychological distress about his hidden sexual life than is the openly gay man, yet his data would be included in the sample of gay men, subsequently increasing the rates of distress. Interpretation of such data is murky at best.

In response to this dilemma, Cochran et al. (2003) evaluated data from the MacArthur Foundation National Survey of Midlife Development in the United States (MIDUS; Brim et al., 1996). The MIDUS survey asked respondents to report whether their sexual orientation was heterosexual, gay, lesbian, or bisexual. To increase power in their analyses, Cochran and colleagues grouped gay and bisexual men and lesbian and bisexual women into two groups and compared them to heterosexual respondents. They report that gay and bisexual men were three times more likely to meet criteria for major depression than were heterosexual men, and that a large proportion of gay or bisexual men meeting criteria for one disorder were comorbid for two or more Axis I disorders. Higher rates of depression were not reported for lesbian or bisexual women, although higher rates of generalized anxiety disorder were reported, and they were more likely to be comorbid for two or more disorders than were heterosexual women meeting criteria for one disorder. The authors cites literature on the impact of stress and adversity on psychopathology as a possible explanation for these findings. Increased rates of certain psychological problems have been observed in LGB populations and are likely due to the stresses of being members of a marginalized group. Meyer (2003) also proposed a model of minority stress to account for the increased rates of psychological problems experienced by LGB individuals.

Although the report of higher rates of depression and anxiety in the Cochran et al. (2003) study is cause for concern about appropriate treatment of LGB people, it cannot be overlooked that more than half of the LGB sample (58%) in the MIDUS study did not meet criteria for any of the five disorders assessed, suggesting that most LGB individuals successfully form positive self-identity and live contented, "normal" lives. Those who do not internalize negative views about being LGB. This has been referred to as "internalized homophobia" (Malyon, 1981–1982); some behavioral psychologists prefer the term "homonegativity" to "homophobia," because disapproval or prejudice against a particular group may not qualify as a phobia per se, although it remains a socially undesirable behavior (Bernstein, 1994). It is unclear how rates of depression and anxiety are correlated to internalized homonegativity.

The impact of social environment on LGB adults often begins prior to adulthood. Several studies have looked at rates of suicidality in LGB youth. Although suicidality does not always indicate depression, the higher rates of suicide and attempted suicide in LGB (and most likely transgender) youth

(Remafedi, French, Story, Resnick, & Blum, 1998) are cause for concern. In a study of 350 LGB youth in a sample from the United States, Canada, and New Zealand, D'Augelli, Hershberger, and Pilkington (2001) found that 25% of the youth reported having seriously thought of suicide in the past year, and 22% of those said that the suicidal thoughts were related to their sexual orientation. Those youth who scored higher on measures of homonegativity, those whose parents did not know about their sexual orientation, and those whose parents rejected them were more likely to have attempted suicide. Safren and Heimberg (1999) compared a sample of LGB and heterosexual youth on factors related to depression, hopelessness, and suicidality. Initially they found group differences between the LGB youth and their heterosexual counterparts on these factors. However, when the investigators did further analyses, it appeared that the differences in the two groups were better accounted for by the effects of stress, social support, and coping through acceptance than by sexual orientation.

Hershberger and D'Augelli (1995) found a relationship between victimization and mental health problems in LGB youth. Family support and self-acceptance mediated the impact of victimization on mental health. D'Augelli (2002), in a study of 542 youth from community settings, found that over 33% of LGB youth reported a past suicide attempt, 75% had been verbally abused, and 15% reported having been physically attacked because of their sexual orientation. More symptoms were related to their parents not knowing about their sexual orientation or to both parents having a negative reaction to their child disclosing an LGB sexual orientation.

Harassment does not necessarily end for LGB people when they leave adolescence behind. In adults, experiencing heterosexism in the workplace is associated with higher levels of depression. Smith and Ingram (2004) found that reports of heterosexism in the workplace were infrequent, although they were related to emotional distress when they occurred. Just as social support has been shown to mediate emotional distress in LGB youth (Safren & Heimberg, 1999), being "out" or open about being lesbian or bisexual and participating in a lesbian or bisexual community has been associated with greater emotional well-being (Morris, Waldo, & Rothblum, 2001). Others have suggested that having a positive gay identity, being more "out," and being connected to an LGB community may be a protective factor for all LGB people when facing heterosexism (Smith & Ingram, 2004).

In summary, the literature suggests that most LGB youth and adults are well adjusted and manage to cope effectively with the stresses of being members of a sexual minority. Nevertheless, LGB youth are at greater risk for depression and suicidality, and LGB adults are at greater risk of depression and anxiety disorders than their heterosexual counterparts. It appears that mediating factors other than sexual orientation significantly contribute to this finding. LGB patients who receive more social support from family and community are better protected from depression and other emotional difficulties. Family reactions to disclosure of an LGB sexual orientation may be particularly important to LGB youth in both positive and negative ways. In general, it appears that accepting one's sexual orientation and disclosing it openly to others is associated with better emotional well-being. This is not the case with every LGB patient, however. Therapists need to allow patients to determine how they identify and how public they wish to be about their identity, while supporting those patients who may wish to disclose to others but do not do so out of fear.

CONCEPTUALIZATION OF DEPRESSION WITH LGB WOMEN AND MEN

Therapists working with LGB patients can readily use the same case conceptualization (Persons, 1989) they would use with non–LGB patients. Given the impact of minority stress on LGB patients (Meyer, 1995), however, therapists need to consider carefully the social context in which their patients live. Therapists should consider not only the social support the patient receives but also the social stress under which the patient lives (Smith & Ingram, 2004). Patient presentation is likely to vary dramatically depending on the patient's identification with a particular ethnic group, the geographic region in which therapy is taking place, the degree to which the patient is public about his/her sexual orientation, and his/her spiritual or moral values. Many of these factors will also covary. For example a male, European American middle-class patient from a large, liberal, coastal city may feel completely comfortable being open about his sexual orientation, may work in an environment that includes sexual orientation in antidiscrimination policies, and may have a very supportive gay community in which he participates. In contrast, a Mexican American woman working as an aide in a day care center, who strongly identifies with her family traditions and religion may experience a great deal of conflict over same-sex attractions, may find emotional support from family but not particularly feel supported over her sexual orientation, and may feel overwhelmed with stress about being lesbian or bisexual.

Many therapists see patients who engage in same-sex behaviors but do not identify themselves as lesbian, gay, or bisexual. For example not all African American men who have sex with men identify as gay, and they may in fact primarily identify with the African American rather than the gay community (Mays, Cochran, & Zamudio, 2004). In some cultures, such as Latino culture, men are identified as homosexual only if they are an anal-receptive partner in sex (Zamora-Hernández & Patterson, 1996). Much of the research on coming out and becoming involved in LGB communities has been based on samples of white LGB people, and therapists should expect great variety in the experience of patients from different cultural backgrounds (Smith, 1997).

When patients do not disclose their sexual orientation, there is not yet information that provides guidelines for what therapists might observe that would alert them to the fact that patients may have intimate relations with others of the same gender. Simple questions (e.g., "Do you date or have sex with women and men?") during intake can help. Such questions show the therapist's openness to the issue of patients having sex with people of the same gender or with both genders. Not all patients will see this as an innocuous question, however, and therapists may get an angry or puzzled response from some. Such a response can give the therapist further information about the patient's worldview that may be useful in case conceptualization. Some therapists may feel uncomfortable asking patients such questions in an initial interview. If so, keep in mind that asking questions is not imposing values on a patient; it is just information gathering. Most therapists would not find it embarrassing to ask a gay male patient, for instance, if he has sex exclusively with men. Therapist and patient discomfort with the reverse, asking a straight man if he has sex exclusively with women, comes from living in a society that has consistently represented homosexuality as deviant. In reality, the question is no different than asking someone whether they sleep 8 hours a night, and whether they wake during the night. It is information that therapists need to understand their patients fully.

A standard cognitive therapy (CT) case conceptualization is useful with LGB patients. Several specific areas of concern need to be addressed, however, that may not be considered with all patients presenting for therapy. It is important, for reasons I stated previously, to know how public the patient is about his/her sexual orientation and what descriptors the patient uses for self-definition. If the patient has "come out," then the age at which he/she did so may be relevant for a number of reasons. A patient who only recently has begun to acknowledge that he/she is LGB may still have conflict about his/her sexual orientation. Patients who have been out a long time may be well integrated into an LGB community, celebrate their sexual orientation, and be completely comfortable in their own skin. Given the homonegative environments in which most LGB people are raised, however, there may be residual negative beliefs. A common example is when a gay male patient specifies that he doesn't like "effeminate" men, or when a bisexual woman says she is not attracted to "butch dykes." They may be self-conscious about their own behavior and hold rigid beliefs about proper gender expression.

Case-conceptualization with LGB individuals is based on the method proposed by Persons (1989). In formulating a problem list to address in therapy, it is a good idea for the therapist to assess for problems in several specific areas. Following are some of the areas that should be considered in formulating the treatment plan.

Level of Openness about Sexual Orientation

It cannot be repeated enough that not all patients who engage in same-sex behaviors identify themselves as LGB. Often this is based on multicultural differences within this population (Trujillo, 1997). Therefore, a therapist should not assume that a patient's lack of identification with an LGB community or self-reference as such means that he/she is "in the closet" or harboring negative beliefs about the self. On the other hand, literature suggests that those individuals who self-identify as LGB fare better when they are connected to an LGB community (DiPlacido, 1998). "Coming out," the public acknowledgment of one's sexual orientation, can be an ongoing process for LGB many people. Furthermore, people may be "out" in certain settings and not others. It is common to encounter individuals who are very open about their sexual orientation among close friends and family. They include partners in family holidays and are comfortable attending some community events for LGB people. Yet these same individuals may remain closeted at work for fear of losing their job or being overlooked for promotions. LGB employees who perceive greater discrimination based on sexual orientation report fewer promotions than their heterosexual coworkers or LGB employees who do not perceive such discrimination (Ragins & Cornwell, 2001). Remaining closeted at work is adaptive for many patients (Badgett, 1996). However, it is not without cost. Partners cannot be invited to company picnics or holiday gatherings. Men and women may frequently be asked why they are not "hitched" in a heterosexual relationship, which forces them either to lie about the gender of their partner or to remain silent about the issue. Such complications can exacerbate a patient's depression if he/she feels like a fraud on the job or that employment necessitates being untrue to him/herself and loved one.

Level of Acceptance of or Resistance to Negative Societal Views about Homosexuality

Nearly all LGB individuals have developed within a culture that openly denigrates LGB people. They have been exposed either to open hostility or to subtle innuendo about gender-atypical behavior. Male–male sexuality has even been blamed for incurring cataclysmic events such as punishment from a deity (Carden, 2004). Many LGB people reject such negative society views and develop a healthy sense of self. Others, however, develop schemas that incorporate these negative views, resulting in self-denigration and other negative emotions.

Stage of "Coming Out"

The several stage models of the "coming out" process that have been identified include recognizing oneself to be LGB, identifying oneself to others as LGB, and, finally, integrating oneself into an LGB community. Although such a stage model makes intellectual sense, it is problematic to assume that every LGB patient will go through a typical stage process. The most glaring problem with the stage models is that they have been based predominantly on white, male samples and may not apply at all to women, to people of color, or to individuals from other than western European cultures (Smith, 1997). Nevertheless, the process experienced by a particular patient is important to understand. For many men, coming out is often a rapid process, and they move quickly from recognizing themselves as gay or bisexual to engaging in sexual or romantic relationships with other men, and telling others about their sexual orientation. This can be a time full of self-doubt, confusion, and distress for many men (DiPlacido, 1998). Women tend to come out more gradually, and sexual orientation may be less fixed for women than it is for men (Kinnish, Strassberg, & Turner, 2005); that is, whereas most men do not experience their sexual orientation as fluid and changeable, many women do. There is evidence that LGB people are better adjusted when they accept their sexuality and become integrated into an accepting environment (DiPlacido, 1998), although this may not be true for people from all cultures (Dworkin, 1997; Greene, 1994). Thus, if the patient is open about his/her sexual orientation, has loving and accepting friends and family, and is comfortable in most settings in which he/she lives, it is likely that being gay or lesbian is not an issue for discussion in therapy.

Problems of Therapeutic Bias

Two particular therapeutic errors that are made with LGB patients require therapists to understand fully the context in which their patients live. Although several errors resulting from therapeutic bias have been identified, the two of primary concern are (1) overemphasizing sexual orientation as a concern in therapy when it is not a concern, and (2) ignoring sexual orientation as a concern when, indeed, it is of concern to the patient (Garnets,

Hancock, Cochran, Goodchilds, & Peplau, 1991). The first of these two errors occurs most frequently with therapists who are not used to working with LGB individuals. Cultural stereotypes suggest that it is very difficult to live as openly LGB persons, and therapists may assume that the problems associated with being members of a sexual minority always cause distress. In other cases therapists may still hold negative homosexual biases that lead them to suggest there is something wrong with being LGB, or to express judgment or open hostility to lifestyle decisions that are culturally acceptable within LGB communities but may not fit a heterosexual norm. Many LGB patients come to therapy with the same concerns as heterosexual patients—concerns about work, relationships, loss of loved ones, social anxieties, general depression, and so on. In many cases a therapist sees a depressed patient who just happens to be LGB. In a few cases, a therapist sees a patient who is depressed about being LGB. It is essential to differentiate between the two, and not to impose one's own agenda on the patient.

In summary, case conceptualization with LGB depressed patients consists of standard CT techniques. However, it is important to consider contextual factors, such as the impact of being a member of a sexual minority, the patient's definition of his/her sexual identity, how public he/she is about sexual orientation, his/her history of having been subjected to negative bias or abuse, and breadth of social support. All of these factors may influence the patient's beliefs about self, world, and others. Most LGB people are not depressed, and therapists need to understand that emotional distress is not a logical by-product of being LGB, although it can be a response to living in an unsupportive, invalidating, or abusive environment.

ASSESSMENT OF DEPRESSION WITH LGB WOMEN AND MEN

Patient verbal self-report and written self-report measures are standard in clinical practice. Although standard self-report measures are useful, clinicians need to review their customary forms for heterosexist content. For example some questionnaires ask about social anxiety around people of the opposite sex. The assumption is that heterosocial anxiety will complicate the individual's establishing intimate relationships. However, simply rephrasing the question to ask whether the patient experiences anxiety around someone he/she finds romantically attractive assesses the same problem and includes same-sex attractions.

Standard measures of depression tend to be gender-neutral and are useful with LGB patients. Conducting an interview with the Hamilton Rating

Scale for Depression (HRSD; Hamilton, 1960) provides the best place to start in assessing the patient's depression. Given the high rate of overlap between depression and anxiety, therapists should also assess for anxiety with either the Hamilton Scales of Anxiety or a measure such as the Anxiety Disorders Interview Schedule for the DSM-IV (ADIS-IV; Brown, Di Nardo, & Barlow, 1994). Clinicians should keep in mind the literature suggesting that gay men are more likely than heterosexual men to meet criteria for major depressive disorder (MDD), whereas lesbian and bisexual women are more likely to meet criteria for generalized anxiety disorder (GAD; Cochran et al., 2003). Although generalizations from the literature are of limited value to the individual case, this research suggests initial, testable hypotheses given the gender of the patient coming to therapy. The Beck Depression Inventory–II (BDI-II; Beck, Steer, & Brown, 1996) and the Beck Hopelessness Scale (BHS; Beck & Steer, 1988) are good measures to use from session to session as a brief assessment of improvement during treatment. Adolescent versions of these scales can be used when working with LGB youth.

TREATMENT OF DEPRESSION WITH LGB WOMEN AND MEN

Standard CT for depression (Beck, Rush, Shaw, & Emery, 1979; J. S. Beck, 1995) includes behavioral components to activate patients, to conduct experiments, and to increase approach behaviors, as well as cognitive restructuring techniques to evaluate patient beliefs. Sessions are structured and include setting an agenda collaboratively with the patient, reviewing between-session homework, summarizing frequently throughout the session, determining homework for next session, and gathering feedback from the patient. The collaborative nature of CT makes it a useful technique with LGB patients, especially for those who fear being told to change or who have had bad therapy experiences previously.

Very little is needed to adapt CT for LGB patients. Padesky (1989) demonstrated the compatibility of CT with feminist therapy, which stresses an egalitarian patient–therapist relationship. Padesky posited that the collaborative nature of CT, use of the Socratic method to nudge patients to use their own knowledge to evaluate beliefs, exemplifies egalitarian therapy. Kuehlwein (1992) presented CT as a structured alternative to the haphazard process that gay men typically undergo when coming to terms with their sexual orientation.

Combining the research on LGB persons with the cognitive-behavioral therapy literature, Martell, Safren, and Prince (2004) developed an LGB-

turally competent therapy, therapists need to recognize their own blind spots or biases toward people different than themselves. This is especially important when a therapist holds negative beliefs about a patient. Therapists who believe that the only normal variant of human sexual behavior is heterosexual are likely to express that bias with LGB patients either overtly (offering a "cure") or covertly (ignoring conversation about same-sex sexual behaviors). On the other hand, therapists may assume that there are no differences at all between their LGB and their heterosexual patients, erring on the side of overconfidence in their skill in working with sexual minority patients.

Second, therapists need to assess how the patient's sexual orientation fits into the case conceptualization. This is extremely important to prevent the therapist from assuming that sexual orientation is a major factor in the patient's presenting problem when it is not, or alternatively, not seeing a relationship between the patient's sexual orientation and his/her presenting problem when clearly there is one. For example in the case of a male patient having unsafe sex with multiple male and female partners both sexual orientation and sexual behavior may be important considerations in the case conceptualization. On the other hand, in the case of a male patient in a long-term relationship who is open and "out" to his family, friends, and coworkers, and who presents with reactive depression following the death of his father, sexual orientation may play a negligible role in the case conceptualization.

The third recommendation is that therapists need to acknowledge the impact of societal norms on the negative beliefs a patient may hold about same-sex sexual attraction. This can become complicated for the therapist who wishes to work collaboratively with patients without promoting his/her own agenda. For example, a patient may hold negative beliefs about his or her sexual attractions because of deeply held religious beliefs. Although the therapist would not attempt to question the religious beliefs, it would still be important to understand that, apart from the societal proscriptions, the patient might be quite happy being attracted to persons of the same sex. The imposed societal norms and mandatory heterosexuality may be at the heart of the problem. Fourth, it is important for therapists to assess the extent of social support the patient receives.

CASE ILLUSTRATION

Primarily, adaptation of CT for LGB patients consists of the therapist being self-aware about his/her biases and aware of contextual factors that contribute to the patient's depression. Sexual orientation is often not an issue for patients. However, as the following case illustrates, a patient may have a long and arduous struggle reconciling sexual orientation with opposing values. The patient held a negative view of himself as a gay man, and his belief that he would never find true love or happiness resulted in behavior that exacerbated his depression. He had developed a self-defeating pattern of engaging in anonymous sexual encounters that were immediately reinforcing but ultimately confirmed his self-effacing beliefs.

The patient, Lance, represents someone struggling to reconcile his sexual orientation with his religious upbringing. Lance, a 27-year-old male, was referred for CT by his primary care physician, who thought that he needed treatment for depression or possible dysthymic disorder. Lance was gainfully employed in the computer industry and lived alone in a small condominium that he owned. The youngest of four children, Lance's parents were still married and were regular church attendees in a conservative Christian denomination, as were his three older siblings. All of his older siblings were married with children. None of his family lived in the same city as Lance. He was in regular communication with his parents and kept in contact with his nieces and nephews by sending birthday, Easter, and Christmas gifts. Lance did not feel particularly close to any of his siblings, and he reported that his relationship with his father was better than that with his mother. He had told his parents about his sexual orientation, and whereas his father had told Lance that he loved him "no matter what," his mother said, "I don't want to know these things, and I'll pray for you. The Lord will heal you." Neither response felt particularly comforting to Lance, although he thought his father was certainly more accepting than his mother had been.

Another contextual factor affecting Lance's case was that his mother had apparently been depressed during a period of Lance's youth. He stated that when he was in the seventh or eighth grade, she had stopped attending church for about a year, spent most of her days lying on the couch, and was very irritable with the four children. He recalled his father telling the children that she was "ill," and he and his siblings made a special effort to be quiet and well behaved. Because his parents never talked openly about such things, Lance could not be sure whether his mother was depressed but he thought she very well might have been.

Lance almost married a woman to whom he was engaged for 1 year, when he was 24 years old. His decision to tell her that he needed to break the engagement because he was gay prompted his coming out to his parents. Notably, his siblings were still unaware of his sexual orientation, and Lance did not tell them because he feared they would not let him be in contact with his nieces and nephews. He believed his parents were keeping his disclosure to them confidential. Lance identified as gay. He said that he used to believe that everyone was heterosexual, and that some people were simply heterosexual and ill. After trying to change his sexual orientation and to become erotically attracted to women through a variety of methods, including prayer and counseling, Lance recognized that his sexual orientation was a part of him and that his efforts to change had been in vain. It was at this point that he broke his engagement with his fiancée and told his parents that he was gay.

From this account it is clear that significant public pressure to be heterosexual and a history of subjection to negative bias played a role in Lance's beliefs about himself. Lance wanted to have a fulfilling relationship and grieved over not having a family and children. He believed that men did not really love one another, rather, they used one another for their own gratification. He occasionally had anonymous sex with men for physical release but never dated. He felt extreme guilt after every sexual encounter. Lance had considered committing suicide. He had a BHS score of 18 when he began therapy and a BDI-II score of 42. He denied a plan or intent to commit suicide and stated that for religious reasons he would not kill himself.

In this case it was important that the therapist not only take an affirming and nonjudgmental stance, but also that Lance's struggles over his sexual orientation be considered an important part of the case conceptualization. Therapists can err by either colluding with a patient in pathologizing nonheterosexual sexual orientation or by being overly affirming and invalidating the patient's struggle. The therapist used a case formulation approach that included developing a problem list (Persons, 1989), as well as a cognitive conceptualization (J. S. Beck, 1995).

The problem list included frequent absences from work due to depression, negative beliefs about self, anonymous sexual encounters, and feelings of guilt, shame and social isolation.

The cognitive conceptualization included:

Core belief: "I am defective."
Intermediate beliefs: "Because I am gay, I will always be alone. I should be heterosexual."

Samples of automatic thoughts were as follows:

Situation: A man gives Lance his telephone number at the gym.
Automatic thought: "He thinks I am just interested in sex."
Feeling: Sad, anxious.

Situation: Lance's nephew calls to tell him that he was selected for the little league team.

Automatic thought: "I'll never have a family."

Feeling: Sad, despondent.

In spite of the distress Lance experienced over his sexual orientation, one of his stated therapy goals was to be comfortable as a gay man. This was an essential goal for the therapist to understand. Some patients experience tension between religious beliefs, cultural allegiance, and sexual orientation. The patient's goals for therapy help the therapist to understand how best to assist in resolving this tension. Lance did not believe the tenets of his religious upbringing, although he expressed a desire to regain a sense of spirituality. His shorter-term goals were to feel less depressed, to reengage with life, and to maintain consistent work performance, so that his job would not be jeopardized.

The therapist first worked on behavioral activation strategies to break the patterns of avoidance that were developing. Lance scheduled routine activities such as cleaning his condominium, calling his parents, and attending mandatory meetings at work. His inertia and avoidance regarding work were complicated by the fact that he was allowed to work remotely from home in his company and frequently used this as an excuse to remain in his pajamas all day long, occasionally responding to e-mail but doing very little else. Thus, the activity scheduling included actually going to the office, regardless of how he felt or whether he could successfully work from home.

Lance was also keeping data about his general activities and using thought records to record automatic thoughts. He began to make a connection between his belief that he was defective and would never have a family, and his anonymous sexual encounters that left him feeling guilty. The first belief that he began to test was that men did not have loving relationships with one another. His therapist recommended a book on male couples, and Lance agreed to do a behavioral experiment to locate and interview men who were in couples. He was to ask how long they had been together, what their living situation was like, and what they believed was positive about their relationship. A small dinner party hosted by a lesbian friend provided the opportunity for Lance to do the experiment, because there were two male couples in attendance.

A second behavioral experiment was attempted to assist Lance in reclaiming his "spiritual self." It had been his belief that all Christian churches condemned LGB people or, alternatively, those that did not were not really Christian. His assignment was to locate and attend churches that were openly affirming of LGB members. Some of the churches he attended had predominantly LGB members, and others were mainline denominations that publicly expressed inclusivity. Lance discovered that several churches were similar to the church in which he had been raised but included LGB people as active members of the congregation. He decided to attend one in particular and joined a Bible Study class that met once a month at the home of one of the gay male church members. Attending such a group, according to Lance, was a complete contradiction of his belief that it was impossible to be gay and spiritual.

Lance completed therapy after 25 sessions. His BDI scores had dropped significantly over the course of therapy, and by Session 25, his scores had been below 9 consistently for three sessions. He still had not met a partner, and wished to do so. He had begun to develop close friendships with several men and women from his church. He was making better choices about sexual behavior, getting acquainted with men prior to becoming sexual, and felt much less guilt about his choices. He had begun to integrate sexuality as an important part of his life and stated to his therapist, "It is time for me to claim my right to have a full life, and I think that I can finally enjoy this life that I've got."

REVIEW OF EFFICACY RESEARCH

A therapist can practice LGB-affirmative CT by understanding the different developmental experiences of LGB patients from the dominant culture, by considering the negative impact of negative societal views on the belief system of the patient, by attending to his/her own biases or lack of knowledge, and by being willing to help the patient do concrete problem solving about negotiating through a world in which one is marginalized. No randomized clinical trials of CT for depression have focused primarily on an LGB population. It is probable that LGB individuals have participated in such clinical trials, but sexual orientation was not considered as a demographic variable, and data that could inform the treatment in regard to sexual orientation of the patient were not gathered. Anecdotally, as a research therapist working in randomized clinical trials, I have firsthand knowledge that LGB individuals were research participants. The next step is actually to collect and evaluate relevant data on a sufficient sample. The simplest way to do this is to include sexual orientation as a demographic variable in predicting outcome following standard CT for depression. If sexual orientation differences are associated with differences in treatment outcome, the next step is to determine whether the modifications suggested by LGB-affirmative practitioners do indeed improve CT with this population.

CONCLUSIONS

Therapists may not always know that the sexual orientation of the patients with whom they work. This is particularly true if questions are asked about sexual orientation rather than behavior. Many patients may engage in intimate sexual or emotional relationships with partners of the same sex without identifying as LGB. This is particularly relevant when cultural backgrounds and customs preclude such labeling. The emphasis on behavioral analysis and specificity in CT makes it an ideal therapeutic orientation for this population of people. Those who identify as LGB can also benefit from CT. The impact of bias, intolerance, and open hostility predispose sexual minority populations to anxiety, depression, and stress reactions. These are the very disorders for which CT has demonstrated efficacy. Treating LGB depressed patients is not so very different than treating heterosexual patients. Cognitive therapists who work with this population need to be aware of their own biases, the pressures from the cultural milieu in which patients exist, and the impact of the internalization of negative beliefs that may have shaped the perceptions and behaviors of men and women in a sexual minority.

REFERENCES

Adams, H. E., Tollison, C. D., & Carson, T. P. (1981). Behavior therapy with sexual deviations. In S. M. Turner, K. S. Calhoun, & H. E. Adams (Eds.), *Handbook of clinical behavior therapy* (pp. 318–346). New York: Wiley.

American Psychiatric Association. (2000). *American Psychiatric Association Commission on Psychotherapy by Psychiatrists Position Statement on therapies focused on attempts to change sexual orientation (reparative or conversion therapies).* Washington, DC: Author.

American Psychological Association. (1998). Resolution on appropriate therapeutic response to sexual orientation: Proceedings of the American Psychological Association, Incorporated, for the Legislative Year 1997. *American Psychologist, 53,* 934–935.

Badgett, L. (1996). Employment and sexual orientation: Disclosure and discrimination in the workplace. *Journal of Gay and Lesbian Social Services, 4,* 29–52.

Beck, A. T., Rush, A. J., Shaw, B. F., & Emery, G. (1979). *Cognitive therapy of depression.* New York: Guilford Press.

Beck, A. T., & Steer, R. A. (1988). *Manual for the Beck Hopelessness Scale.* San Antonio, TX: Psychological Corporation.

Beck, A. T., Steer, R. A., & Brown, G. K. (1996). *Manual for the BDI-II.* San Antonio, TX: Psychological Corporation.

Beck, J. S. (1995). *Cognitive therapy: Basics and beyond.* New York: Guilford Press.

Bernstein, G. S. (1994). A reply to Rowan. *Behavior Therapist, 17*(8), 185–186.

Brim, O. G, Baltes, P. B., Bumpass, L. L., Cleary, P. D., Featherman, D. L., & Hazzard, W. R. (1996). *National Survey of Midlife Development in the United States (MIDUS), 1995–1996.* Retrieved April, 2001, from Harvard Medical School website: *http://midmac.med.harvard.edu.researchhtml.*

Brown, T. A., Di Nardo, P. A., & Barlow, D. H. (1994). *Anxiety Disorders Interview Schedule for DSM-IV (ADIS-IV): Clinician's manual.* Albany, NY: Graywind.

Carden, M. (2004). *Sodomy: A history of a Christian biblical myth.* London: Equinox.

Cochran, S. D., Sullivan, J. G., & Mays, V. M. (2003). Prevalence of mental disorders, psychological distress, and mental health services use among lesbian, gay, and bisexual adults in the United States. *Journal of Consulting and Clinical Psychology, 71*(1), 53–61.

D'Augelli, A. R. (1998). Developmental implications of victimization of lesbian, gay, and bisexual youths. In G. M. Herek (Ed.), *Stigma and sexual orientation: Understanding prejudice against lesbians, gay men, and bisexuals* (pp. 187–210). Thousand Oaks, CA: Sage.

D'Augelli, A. R. (2002). Mental health problems among lesbian, gay, and bisexual youths ages 14 to 21. *Clinical Child Psychology and Psychiatry, 7*(3), 433–456.

D'Augelli, A. R., Hershberger, S. L., & Pilkington, N. W. (2001). Suicidality patterns and sexual orientation-related factors among lesbian, gay, and bisexual youths. *Suicide and Life Threatening Behavior, 31*(3), 250–265.

Davison, G. C. (1976). Homosexuality: The ethical challenge. *Journal of Consulting and Clinical Psychology, 44,* 157–162.

DiPlacido, J. (1998). Minority stress among lesbians, gay men, and bisexuals: A consequence of heterosexism, homophobia, and stigmatization. In G. M. Herek (Ed.), *Stigma and sexual orientation: Understanding prejudice against lesbians, gay men, and bisexuals* (pp. 138–159). Thousand Oaks, CA: Sage.

Dworkin, S. H. (1997). Female, lesbian and Jewish: Complex and invisible. In B. Greene (Ed.), *Ethnic and cultural diversity among lesbians and gay men* (pp. 63–87). Thousand Oaks, CA: Sage.

Flaks, D. K., Ficher, I., Masterpasqua, F., & Joseph, G. (1995). Lesbians choosing motherhood: A comparative study of lesbian and heterosexual parents and their children. *Developmental Psychology, 31*(1), 105–114.

Garnets, L., Hancock, K. A., Cochran, S. D., Goodchilds, J., & Peplau, L. A. (1991). Issues in psychotherapy with lesbians and gay men: A survey of psychologists. *American Psychologist, 46*(9), 964–972.

Gilman, S. E., Cochran, S. D., Mays, V. M., Hughes, M., Ostrow, D., & Kessler, R. C. (2001). Risk of psychiatric disorders among individuals reporting same-sex sexual partners in the National Comorbidity Survey. *American Journal of Public Health, 91,* 933–939.

Golombok, S., & Tasker, F. (1996). Do parents influence the sexual orientation of their children?: Findings from a longitudinal study of lesbian families. *Developmental Psychology, 32*(1), 3–11.

Gonsiorek, J. (1991). The empirical basis for the demise of the illness model of homosexuality. In J. Gonsiorek & J. Weinrich (Eds.), *Homosexuality: Research implications for public policy* (pp. 115–136). Newbury Park, CA: Sage.

Greene, B. (1994). Lesbian women of color: Triple jeopardy. In L. Comas-Díaz & B. Greene (Eds.), *Women of color: Integrating ethnic and gender identities in psychotherapy* (pp. 389–427). New York: Guilford Press.

Haldeman, D. C. (1994). The practice of sexual orientation conversion therapy. *Journal of Consulting and Clinical Psychology, 62,* 221–227.

Haldeman, D. C. (2002). Gay rights, patient rights: The implications of sexual orientation conversion therapy. *Professional Psychology: Research and Practice, 33*(3), 260–264.

Hamilton, M. A. (1960). A rating scale for depression. *Journal of Neurology, Neurosurgery, and Psychiatry, 23,* 56–61.

Hershberger, S. L., & D'Augelli, A. R. (1995). The impact of victimization on the mental health and suicidality of lesbian, gay, and bisexual youths. *Developmental Psychology, 31*(1), 65–74.

Hooker, E. (1957). The adjustment of the male overt homosexual. *Journal of Projective Techniques, 21,* 18–31.

Kinnish, K. K., Strassberg, D. S., & Turner, C. W. (2005). Sex differences in the flexibility of sexual orientation: A multidimensional retrospective assessment. *Archives of Sexual Behavior, 34*(2), 173–183.

Kuehlwein, K. T., (1992). Working with gay men. In A. Freeman & F. M. Dattilio (Eds.), *Comprehensive casebook of cognitive therapy* (pp. 249–255). New York: Plenum Press.

Kurdek, L. A. (1992). Relationship stability and relationship satisfaction in cohabiting homosexual and heterosexual men and women. *Sex Roles, 17,* 549–562.

Kurdek, L. A. (1998). Relationship outcomes and their predictors: Longitudinal evidence from heterosexual married, gay cohabiting, and lesbian cohabiting couples. *Journal of Marriage and the Family, 60,* 553–568.

Malyon, A. K. (1981–1982). Psychotherapeutic implications of internalized homophobia in gay men. *Journal of Homosexuality, 7*(2–3), 59–69.

Martell, C. R., Safren, S. A., & Prince, S. E. (2004). *Cognitive-behavioral therapies with lesbian, gay, and bisexual clients.* New York: Guilford Press.

Mays, V. M., Cochran, S. D., & Zamudio, A. (2004). HIV prevention research: Are we meeting the needs of African American men who have sex with men? *Journal of Black Psychology, 30*(1), 78–105.

Meyer, I. H. (1995). Minority stress and mental health in gay men. *Journal of Health and Social Behavior, 36,* 38–56.

Meyer, I. H. (2003). Prejudice, social stress, and mental health in lesbian, gay, and bisexual populations: Conceptual issues and research evidence. *Psychological Bulletin, 129*(5), 674–697.

Morris, J. F., Waldo, C. R., & Rothblum, E. D. (2001). A model of predictors and outcomes of outness among lesbian and bisexual women. *American Journal of Orthopsychiatry, 71*(1), 61–71.

Padesky, C. A. (1989). Attaining and maintaining a positive lesbian self-identity: A cognitive therapy approach. *Women and Therapy, 8*(1–2), 145–156.

Persons, J. B. (1989). *Cognitive therapy in practice: A case formulation approach.* New York: Norton.

Ragins, B. R., & Cornwell, J. M. (2001). Pink triangles: Antecedents and consequences of perceived workplace discrimination against gay and lesbian employees. *Journal of Applied Psychology, 86*(6), 1244–1261.

Remafedi, G., French, S., Story, M., Resnick, M. D., & Blum, R. (1998). The relationship between suicide risk and sexual orientation: Results of a population-based study. *American Journal of Public Health, 88*(1), 57–60.

Safren, S. A., & Heimberg, R. G. (1999). Depression, hopelessness, suicidality, and Related factors in sexual minority and heterosexual adolescents. *Journal of Consulting and Clinical Psychology, 67*(6), 859–866.

Safren, S. A., & Rogers, T. (2001). Cognitive-behavioral therapy with gay, lesbian and bisexual patients. *Journal of Clinical Psychology, 57*(5), 629–643.

Sandfort, T. G., de Graaf, R., & Schnabel, P. (2001). Same-sex sexual behavior and psychiatric disorders. *Archives of General Psychiatry, 58,* 85–91.

Schroeder, M., & Shidlo, A. (2001). Ethical issues in sexual orientation conversion therapies: An empirical study of consumers. In A. Shidlo, M. Schroeder, & J. Drescher (Eds.), *Sexual conversion therapy: Ethical, clinical and research perspectives* (pp. 131–166). New York: Haworth Medical Press.

Schuck, K. D., & Liddle, B. J. (2001). Religious conflicts experienced by lesbian, gay, and bisexual individuals. *Journal of Gay and Lesbian Psychotherapy, 5*(2), 63–82.

Smith, A. (1997). Cultural diversity and the coming-out process: Implications for clinical practice. In B. Greene (Ed.), *Ethnic and cultural diversity among lesbians and gay men* (pp. 279–300). Thousand Oaks, CA: Sage.

Smith, N. G., & Ingram, K. M. (2004). Workplace heterosexism and adjustment among lesbian, gay, and bisexual individuals: The role of unsupportive social interactions. *Journal of Counseling Psychology, 51*(1), 57–67.

Trujillo, C. M. (1997). Sexual identify and the discontents of difference. In B. Greene (Ed.), *Ethnic and cultural diversity among lesbians and gay men* (pp. 266–278). Thousand Oaks, CA: Sage.

Wainright, J. L., Russell, S. T., & Patterson, C. J. (2004). Psychosocial adjustment, school outcomes, and romantic relationships of adolescents with same-sex parents. *Child Development, 75*(6), 1886–1898.

Wolfe, J. L. (1992). Working with gay women. In A. Freeman & F. M. Dattilio (Eds.), *Comprehensive casebook of cognitive therapy* (pp. 257–265). New York: Plenum Press.

Zamora-Hernández, C. E., & Patterson, D. G. (1996). Homosexually active Latino men: Issues for social work practice. In J. F. Longres (Ed.), *Men of color: A context for service to homosexually active men* (pp. 69–91). Binghamtom, NY: Harrington Park.

17

ADOLESCENTS

Mark A. Reinecke
John F. Curry

Depression among children and adolescents is an important social and clinical concern. Epidemiological studies indicate that, at any given time, approximately 1–3% of children and 5–7% of adolescents meet criteria for major depressive disorder (MDD; Essau & Dobson, 1999). Depression during childhood and adolescence is associated with impaired social and academic performance, and places young people at risk for alcohol and substance abuse. Many youth who meet criteria for MDD also meet criteria for additional psychiatric disorders. In a national sample of adolescents with major depression (Treatment for Adolescents with Depression Study [TADS] Team, 2005), half met formal criteria for one or more comorbid disorders.

Of particular concern is the fact that depression places adolescents at increased risk for suicidal ideation, attempts, and completions (Brent, 1995; Shaffer et al., 1996). Depression also places youth at risk for adult depression and psychosocial impairment (Weissman et al., 1999).

Depression among youth is often chronic and persistent. Kovacs, Obrosky, Gatsonis, and Richards (1997), for example, reported that the median duration of a major depressive episode in a sample of 8- to 13-year-olds was 9 months, and that the median duration of dysthymic disorder was

3.9 years. The median duration of depressive episodes at baseline among youth enrolled in the TADS was 40 weeks and the mean was 71 weeks (TADS Team, 2005). At the same time, depression among children and adolescents tends to be recurrent. Rao and colleagues (1995) reported a 7-year recurrence rate (i.e., emergence of depressive symptoms after a period of sustained recovery from a depressive episode) of approximately 70% among depressed youth.

Taken together, these findings suggest that early-onset depression might be viewed as a chronic, recurring disorder. How, though, shall we define "chronic"? Several approaches have been proposed. One might note the duration of a depressive episode, with episodes exceeding a particular length being defined as "chronic" or "persistent." Alternatively, one could count the number of episodes an individual has experienced (an index of recurrence), or note whether an individual has failed to respond favorably to a trial of treatment. There is little consensus, however, as to the definition of chronic depression; how duration of episode, recurrence, and treatment response are related to one another; or how these guide treatment planning for youth.

How, then, are we to understand chronic depression among youth? In one sense, childhood depression might not be seen as a chronic disorder. Inasmuch as children are, most often, experiencing their first depressive episode, one correctly hesitates to presume that it will become a chronic condition. As we have seen, however, early-onset major depression can be a pernicious disorder, whether persistent or recurring. We propose, then, that early-onset depression may in certain cases be viewed as a particularly malignant subtype of MDD and may be conceptually similar to chronic depression among adults. Like early-onset diabetes or cystic fibrosis, it may follow a fluctuating course and may not spontaneously remit. Early-onset depression may usefully be conceptualized as a chronic disorder and treated accordingly. Childhood depression is an important concern in that evidence suggests that each subsequent episode of depression may increase the likelihood that an individual will experience additional episodes in the future. Studies with depressed adults suggest that the brain may become sensitized when exposed to repeated episodes of depression, reducing the threshold for activation of subsequent episodes (Kendler, Thornton, & Gardner, 2000).

Although important advances have been made during recent years in understanding and treating depression during childhood and adolescence, these disorders continue to present a challenge for clinicians. Over one-fourth of clinically depressed children and adolescents do not respond to treatment with either psychotherapy or medications, and many of those who do respond do not experience a full or complete amelioration of their symptoms. Moreover, relapse and recurrence rates after discontinuation of antidepressant medications are unacceptably high.

More effective strategies for managing treatment-resistant depression and chronic depression among youth, then, are needed. A number of factors appear to be associated with long-term outcomes. Among adults, chronicity and severity of previous episodes of depression are among the most consistent predictors of long-term outcome (Simon, 2000). Research is ongoing into predictors and moderators of adolescent treatment response. Little is known, however, about characteristics of recovered children or adolescents that may predict relapse or recurrence. Existing treatment strategies might be refined, so that they are more effective with these very challenging cases, and approaches based upon research in developmental psychopathology (Reinecke & Simons, 2005) should be developed.

In this chapter we discuss contemporary cognitive-behavioral therapy (CBT) approaches for conceptualizing and treating depression among adolescents, and briefly discuss evidence for the efficacy and effectiveness of these approaches. We conclude with a discussion of possible areas for research and clinical innovation.

ASSESSMENT OF COMPLEX DEPRESSION
IN ADOLESCENTS

The clinical assessment of depression in adolescents requires a careful diagnostic interview, supplemented by self-report measures, and by observations of parents and other collateral sources of information, such as teachers. For a thoughtful discussion of the assessment literature, please see Klein, Dougherty, and Olino (2005). We provide examples of instruments or methods within each major domain required for assessment.

Diagnostic Interview

In the assessment of complex adolescent depression, the diagnostic interview is necessary both to establish the diagnosis and to assess for comorbid psychiatric conditions. The most common comorbid conditions are anxiety disorders, substance use disorders, and disruptive behavior disorders (TADS Team, 2005). Clinicians assessing MDD will also need to assess for possible manic, hypomanic, or psychotic symptoms, since these features will be present in a minority of seriously depressed teens, and have implications for treatment.

An example of a diagnostic instrument is the K–SADS (Schedule for Affective Disorders and Schizophrenia for School–Age Children). A recent version, developed by Kaufman and her colleagues (1997), has several advantages over earlier forms of the instrument. Kaufman's edition, the K–SADS-PL, covers both present episode and worst lifetime episode of various disorders. It includes a Screen Interview with key symptom items from all diagnostic domains to determine the probability that various categories of diagnoses need to be assessed further. In addition to the screen interview, modules cover Affective Disorders, Anxiety Disorders, Substance Use Disorders, Disruptive Behavior Disorders, Tic Disorders, and Eating Disorders. Impairment ratings are completed to ensure that the diagnosis is given only if symptoms are accompanied by functional impairment. We recommend that the interviewer also assess age of onset of mood disturbance, age of first episode, and number of prior episodes of MDD.

The interviewer reviews symptoms separately with the adolescent and with the parent, thus ensuring that both internal states and behavioral observations are taken into account. The diagnostician then synthesizes the information to determine the diagnosis. Psychometric properties of the K–SADS-PL, based on a small sample study, are acceptable (Kaufman et al., 1997).

Discriminating unipolar and bipolar depression can be an important challenge when treating a depressed or dysphoric child. The K–SADS-PL is a widely accepted instrument for diagnosing bipolar disorder in children and adolescents. Augmenting this interview with a parent-report screening instrument, such as the Parent Version of the Young Mania Rating Scale (Gracious, Youngstrom, Findling, & Calabrese, 2002), can help to avoid both false-negative and false-positive diagnoses (Youngstrom et al., 2004).

Clinician-Administered Severity Scales

Diagnostic interviews are valuable for identifying target disorders and accompanying comorbid conditions. However, the range of severity assessed by such interviews is somewhat limited and the time frame relatively broad. Moreover, given their length, these instruments can be cumbersome to readminister. For assessment of change during or after treatment, therefore, clinician rating scales that focus more intensively on target symptoms can be quite helpful.

One such scale, the Children's Depression Rating Scale—Revised (CDRS-R; Poznanski & Mokros, 1995), is a 17-item scale, three items of which are observational ratings by the clinician (Depressed Facial Affect, Listless Speech, and Hypoactivity). The remaining 14 items are assessed in interviews with the adolescent or child and a parent or other observer. We recommend that the adolescent be interviewed first and the parent second, with the clinician then completing summary ratings based on both interviews. For younger children it is usually preferable to interview the parent first to establish the time frame for symptom onset and duration. CDRS-R items are arranged to proceed from less intrusive symptoms (e.g., the effect of depression on schoolwork) to more intrusive or sensitive items (e.g., suicidal ideation). The clinician may modify the order of items to follow spontaneous comments by the respondent.

Self-Report Severity Scales

Self-report scales are valuable indices of change, as well as supplemental indices of severity, in working with depressed teenagers. Some adolescents are more comfortable acknowledging distress in the relative privacy of a self-rating situation than in the interactive interview, although the reverse pattern also occurs. We recommend, at a minimum, administering self-report scales at the beginning, midpoint, and endpoint of acute intervention. Many cognitive-behavioral therapists administer a self-report scale prior to each session as a way to monitor changes in the patient's mood over the course of treatment. Repeated use of the same scale, however, can threaten the validity of the self-report, because some adolescents adopt an all-or-none approach to the items on relatively long self-report scales. For this reason, we suggest informally assessing mood on a weekly basis, always inquiring about suicidal thoughts or behavior, and administering formal scales intermittently over the course of treatment.

An example of a psychometrically strong measure of adolescent depression is the Reynolds Adolescent Depression Scale (RADS). Although it has recently been revised, the original RADS (Reynolds, 1987) is a 17-item self-report instrument. In the TADS study (TADS Team, 2004) the pattern of results based on the RADS was very similar to that on the CDRS-R, suggesting that the RADS may be a reliable and valid measure with clinically depressed youth (Reynolds & Mazza, 1998).

TREATMENT OF DEPRESSION AMONG ADOLESCENTS

Adaptations of Standard Cognitive Therapy

Three CBT protocols have been developed for use with depressed adolescents. The first of these is based on the "standard model" of cognitive therapy (CT) for depression developed by Aaron Beck and his colleagues (Beck,

Rush, Shaw, & Emery, 1979). Based upon cognitive diathesis–stress para-
digms, this model emphasizes the importance of changing automatic
thoughts, maladaptive tacit beliefs or schemas, and other cognitive products
or processes associated with depression as a means of bringing about behavioral and emotional change. Brent and Poling (1997) adapted Beck's CT
protocol for use with adolescents. Based on the core principles of CT,
their approach emphasized identifying and modifying negative automatic
thoughts, dysfunctional attitudes, and maladaptive beliefs. Behavioral interventions, such as activity scheduling, are of value with more impaired
depressed teens who are withdrawn or passive. These techniques are viewed,
however, chiefly as methods for eliciting and testing the validity of negative
cognitions. An emphasis is placed on identifying and rationally disputing
teens' maladaptive thoughts that occur spontaneously during sessions.

CT for teens is delivered in an individual psychotherapy format, and
parents are encouraged to participate in psychoeducational sessions. The
length of acute treatment is 12–16 weeks, with sessions held on a weekly
basis. As in adult CT, the adolescent's depression is assessed before each session with a self-report scale. Teens are also asked to generate goals for their
treatment, and these are used as reference points over the course of treatment.

As in adult CT, emphasis is placed on maintaining a positive, supportive
therapeutic rapport, characterized by collaborative empiricism. Adolescents
are taught to adopt the role of a "personal scientist" as they work with the
therapist to understand how negative thoughts and maladaptive beliefs or
schemas are maintaining their depressed state. Teens are encouraged to participate actively in constructing an agenda for each session. In contrast to
CT with depressed adults, the Brent and Poling (1997) model places relatively less emphasis on between-session homework assignments. Like its
adult counterpart, however, the model utilizes frequent summaries of main
session points. As therapy proceeds, adolescents assume a greater responsibility for directing the treatment process. They learn to set the agenda for the
session, to explore key cognitions, and to summarize the session. Through
this process the adolescent learns how to become his/her own therapist
(Brent & Poling, 1997).

Although CT does not explicitly focus on developing social or behavioral competencies, it remains to some degree a skills-based treatment. To
the extent that they are introduced, specific behavioral or cognitive skills or
techniques are directed toward assisting the adolescent to identify and modify key cognitions. The same techniques used in adult CT are used to modify adolescents' cognitions, including Socratic questioning, role-playing, and
the analysis of "pro" and "con" arguments supporting or challenging the

utility of holding certain beliefs. Cognitive restructuring in CT focuses on developing more adaptive and flexible thoughts, attitudes, beliefs, and expectations. Therapists typically do not suggest specific alternative thoughts. Attention is paid to issues of adolescent autonomy and the impact that developmental tasks may have on the family and peer relationships. A relatively greater emphasis is placed on helping teens to learn problem-solving methods than is typical with adults. Social skills training may be included.

The most significant modification made in adapting Beck's CT for work with adolescents, however, centers on the role of the family. A major emphasis is placed on psychoeducation and on including parents in the treatment process. Brent and Poling (1997) recommended providing caregivers with information about the nature of depression and the process of CT. An objective of psychoeducation is to help parents to understand that depression is an illness, and to counter potentially maladaptive parental beliefs such as "My child is doing this on purpose," or that he/she could "snap out of it."

A second variant of CBT for depressed adolescents is Clarke and Lewinsohn's Coping with Depression (CWD) course (Lewinsohn, Clarke, Hops, & Andrews, 1990). This treatment is based on Lewinsohn's model of depression, which posits that depression is a function of inadequate positive reinforcement, especially social reinforcement. Depression is characterized by decreased behavioral activity, reduced social interaction, and negative thinking. Lewinsohn and Clarke view mood, cognition, and behavior as transactionally related aspects of human functioning that influence one another as the individual adapts to his/her environment. To alleviate depression, a person can make changes in cognition, behavior, or environment.

In contrast to CT, the CWD course places equal emphasis on learning new behaviors and on learning new, more adaptive ways of thinking. A wide range of skills is taught, including goal setting, mood monitoring, increasing pleasant activities, relaxation, social interaction skills, communication, and interpersonal problem solving. A group format is used. The method of delivery is more similar to that of a classroom than to that of an individual psychotherapy session, thus reducing stigma and taking advantage of the teens' sense of familiarity with the process. Homework assignments are emphasized, and group time is highly structured. Therefore, there are relatively few opportunities for tailoring the treatment to the needs of particular individuals. Treatment typically lasts 7–8 weeks, with sessions held twice per week. Parents may be seen in psychoeducational groups once per week, where they discuss the skills their teens are learning, as well as ways to help them implement these skills at home. More recent versions include conjoint parent–adolescent problem-solving sessions.

CWD maintains a clear focus on developing cognitive, social, and behavioral skills to rectify social and cognitive deficiencies associated with depression. Mood is monitored daily on a brief self-report form, and teens learn how activity levels and cognitions influence their mood. Much as Beck and colleagues (1979) encouraged each patient to become a "personal scientist," the CWD course endeavors to help adolescents appreciate how their actions and thoughts influence their mood, and to develop relapse prevention plans that build upon these observations.

More recently a third CBT approach for treating clinically depressed youth, the TADS protocol, has been developed. By the late 1990s a completed body of controlled outcome research supported the acute treatment efficacy of the CT and CWD approaches, as well as medication management with fluoxetine, for treating adolescent depression (Emslie et al., 1997b; Reinecke, Ryan, & DuBois, 1998). CBT and medication had never been compared, however, in a placebo-controlled trial with clinically depressed youth. With this in mind, the TADS was initiated to test the relative and combined effectiveness of CBT and fluoxetine in the acute and continuation treatment of adolescent major depression. TADS treatment was manualized for use across multiple sites by clinicians with varying levels and types of CBT training, and for adolescents typical of clinical samples (Curry & Wells, 2005).

The CBT protocol used in the TADS study represents an amalgam of the two models reviewed above. Borrowing from the Brent and Poling's (1997) CT protocol, TADS CBT utilizes an individual psychotherapy mode of delivery and includes parent and teen psychoeducation about depressive disorder. It emphasizes the importance of maintaining a collaborative therapeutic relationship and incorporating the full array of CT strategies and techniques developed by Beck, including agenda setting, summaries, assignment of homework, and rational disputation of dysfunctional attitudes and thoughts. Like Clarke and Lewinsohn's CWD approach, the TADS CBT protocol places equal emphasis on changing behaviors and cognitions, and requires that all teens receive training in a set of core cognitive and behavioral skills. Additional skills training is optional (Curry & Wells, 2005).

As Curry and Reinecke (2003) noted, TADS CBT uses an individualized, "modular" approach to treatment. After an adolescent has been exposed to the core skills, therapist and patient have a degree of latitude to select skills or modules that best meet the teenager's needs. Unlike the CWD course, the TADS CBT protocol can be tailored to address a teen's specific concerns. All treatment sessions, nonetheless, are relatively structured and follow a general format of agenda setting, homework review, skills training, working on the agenda items, formulation of a homework assignment for the upcoming week, and review. The use of modules permits the therapist to modify the treatment based on the specific needs of the teen, or of the parents, and the selection of treatment targets based on the case formulation.

Mandatory or "core" modules in TADS CBT include Psychoeducation, Goal Setting, Mood Monitoring, Increasing Pleasant Activities, Problem Solving, and Cognitive Restructuring. At the conclusion of therapy, all adolescents participate in one or more sessions during which they summarize and synthesize the material discussed over the course of treatment, and develop strategies for coping with stressful events that might occur in the future. As in CT with depressed adults, active attempts are made to provide teens with skills for preventing relapse. Optional modules include training in Relaxation, Affect Regulation, Assertion, and Social Interaction Skills. All parents receive two sessions of psychoeducation about the nature of major depression and their child's treatment. Optional parent–adolescent sessions center on family communication, problem solving, adjusting parental expectations, and providing appropriate consequences.

Modifications in Timing, Presentation, and Implementation of Interventions

For complex childhood or adolescent depression, modifications of CBT often are needed. These are reflected in the case formulation, which may be modified as treatment progresses (Rogers, Reinecke, & Curry, 2005), as illustrated in three examples.

Consider first the "cognitively immature" adolescent. Cognitive immaturity may be reflected in a lack of self-reflection or insight; poor verbal abstraction skills; an inability to identify and label emotions, and to appreciate relationships between one's thoughts and feelings; or delays in the development of hypotheticodeductive reasoning and problem-solving skills. This may be a function of age, delayed intellectual functioning, or a learning disability. As a general rule, CBT proceeds more slowly for cognitively immature teens than for other teens, and places a relatively greater emphasis on behavioral interventions.

Quite often emphasis during early sessions is placed on developing affect recognition and labeling skills, and on assisting the patient to appreciate how life events, thoughts, and emotions influence one another. Techniques such as attending to physiological changes and somatic experiences associated with anger, tension, and happiness, may prove helpful in this regard. Once these fundamental skills are developed, Mood Monitoring, Behavioral Activation, and Rational Disputation modules are introduced. As behavioral strategies are introduced, more immature teens may benefit from active modeling by the therapist or by interactive games within sessions. These serve to illustrate connections between activity level and mood, and can be helpful in maintaining a positive therapeutic rapport.

When cognitive techniques are introduced, it is helpful for therapists to take a more directive stance. Many young adolescents find rational disputation and cognitive restructuring difficult. Techniques that adults and older adolescents find useful, such as the three-column technique, are simply unhelpful. Under such circumstances therapists may want to present teens with a brief list of alternative "adaptive" thoughts that may lead to more positive affect, and ask them to choose the ones they feel are most sensible. They then practice repeating these "adaptive self-statements," much like a mantra, when they become anxious or depressed.

A second type of modification is needed for young people who experience labile affect. Clinically depressed youth often manifest difficulties in regulating negative moods. Affect regulation skills that develop over the course of childhood and adolescence have been implicated in the development of psychopathology among youth (Bradley, 2000). Several cognitive-behavioral theories of depression emphasize the role of early experience in the acquisition of these capacities, and focus on teens' development of these skills over the course of treatment (Spence & Reinecke, 2003). For emotionally volatile or explosive youth, training in cognitive and behavioral strategies for regulating affect need to be introduced early in course of treatment, shortly after mood monitoring. Otherwise, treatment may be disrupted by behavioral outbursts, self-cutting, or suicidal gestures that occur with little apparent provocation. Both Brent's CT and the TADS CBT protocol used a method developed by Rotheram (1987). After the adolescent becomes familiar with monitoring moods with an "emotions thermometer," he/she is asked to designate a point on the subjective thermometer where emotions reach a "boiling point"—the point at which he/she perceives a loss of control. Then the teen is asked to go back down the thermometer to identify a "choice point," where he/she is still able to control the reactions. The teen then works with the therapist to identify and practice coping strategies (e.g., relaxation, distraction, taking a walk, talking with a parent, adaptive self-statements, shooting baskets) that can be implemented at the "choice point." These are rehearsed in session, and potential triggers for losing control are identified. Strategies for coping with rapid shifts in emotion are reviewed with the parents, who support their child's attempts to use them at home.

A third type of complex depression occurs with adolescents who lack necessary support systems. Such teens may have parents who are impaired by a psychiatric or substance use disorder, or who suffer from severe socio-economic disadvantage. For these teens, it can be quite difficult to partici-pate in psychotherapy on a regular basis, and their parents may be unable to assist them with practicing cognitive-behavioral skills at home. They may come from chaotic homes and communities, and frequently miss sessions or "disappear" from treatment for weeks at a time. The therapist, therefore, will want to order treatment so that the most important elements are covered first. It is inadvisable in such cases to use a skills-sampling approach, because of the adolescents' inconsistent attendance. A small number of key skills should be introduced, with an emphasis on instilling a sense of hope and personal control. At the same time, sessions with parents may focus on understanding and rectifying their beliefs, attitudes, expectations, and attri-butions that may reduce their motivation for participating in treatment. They may believe, for example, "We've tried everything. Therapy won't work," "They're just seeking attention with their suicide talk. We should just ignore it," "This is just blaming the parents, telling us it's our fault," or "It's just a phase, she'll grow out of it." Beliefs such as these, as well as the percep-tion that the therapist does not fully appreciate their perspective about their child's difficulties, can undermine parents' support for the treatment.

The therapist uses psychoeducation, Socratic questioning, and empathic listening to address these beliefs and to give parents a sense that their chil-dren's difficulties are both understandable and resolvable. CT endeavors to give parents, as much as their children, a feeling of being understood and supported, and a sense of hopefulness. At the same time, the therapist attempts to resolve practical issues (e.g., work schedules, cab fare) that may interfere with attendance.

Supplementing Standard CT

Supplements to standard CBT include an array of methods used in clinical child and adolescent psychology, as well as medications prescribed by child psychiatrists. Four commonly used psychosocial supplements include neo-behavioral techniques, school-based interventions, family-based interven-tions, and extended family or community interventions.

Neobehavioral techniques are derived from more recent models of treatment, including dialectical behavior therapy (DBT), and mindfulness- and acceptance-based models. DBT techniques, for example, are often helpful when working with adolescents who engage in self-damaging behavior, such as cutting. Self-soothing techniques that focus on emotion regulation and distress tolerance, such as guided imagery, distraction, and controlled breathing (Linehan, 1993), can be quite helpful in this regard. Acceptance-based interventions focus on recognizing and observing with detachment depressive, anxious, or suicidal thoughts and emotions (Teasdale, 2004). Patients are taught to disengage from maladaptive thoughts and to limit rumination. Unlike standard CT, which focuses on changing the content of thoughts, mindfulness-based approaches emphasize the value of "decentering" from maladaptive thoughts (i.e., viewing them as objects, and not as central to one's sense of self) and of accepting them (rather than actively challenging their validity or endeavoring to escape or avoid them). This permits greater awareness that these are "just thoughts" (not reality) that can be tolerated and will pass.

Reciprocal relations exist between school performance and mood among children and adolescents. Depression can impair academic performance, and a significant percentage of depressed adolescents meet criteria for a comorbid learning disability. School-based interventions, including consultations with teachers, administrators, and school counselors, as well as classroom observations of the student, can be quite helpful in developing a comprehensive treatment program. CBT with children and adolescents attends to not only their intrapsychic experience but also the contexts in which they live, their school and home environments. Depression can have a debilitating effect on academic work and on relationships with classmates. In many cases, explaining to parents and school personnel the nature of the teen's disorder, and of the consequent necessity for adjusted expectations during the recovery period, is of significant benefit. In this regard it is important to convey to school personnel and to parents the anticipated duration of a depressive episode, and the fact that even good response to treatment does not quickly translate into recovery of normal functioning.

Depressed teens are often seen by others as sullen, withdrawn, and apathetic, and their relationships with other family members are often tense and conflicted. Evidence indicates that family conflict is both a cause and a consequence of depression among youth (Kaslow, Deering, & Racusin, 1994). With this in mind, family-based interventions may be a useful supplement to individual or group CBT. Adolescents whose depression is rooted in negative thoughts about self in relation to family, for example, may benefit from family sessions in which a more secure and supportive parent–adolescent attachment is rekindled. Parents whose teenagers' depression is intertwined with oppositional behavior may benefit from parent training about clear communication, monitoring, and providing appropriate consequences. In some cases, the therapist needs to determine whether it is preferable to rely on the family for support in the therapeutic process or to facilitate adolescent independence from the family. The latter option may be considered when family-based interventions exacerbate the adolescent's depression.

Extended family or community interventions engage a broader network of support in assisting depressed teens. For adolescents who live with an extended family, the therapist wants to understand dimensions of affection, caring, control, and authority in the family, as well as the expectations, attributions, attitudes, and beliefs held by other family members. For depressed adolescents who are involved in the judicial or foster care system, community interventions may include meetings with probation officers, court counselors, foster parents, or case managers. In such cases it may be helpful to share the principles of CBT, including the importance of positive reinforcement, limit setting, and the development of realistic, positive beliefs and expectations. It is critical that the therapist engaging in family-, school-, or community-based interventions have a clear case conceptualization and a sense of the role that the wider family and social systems play in maintaining the adolescent's depression. The focus of treatment remains on alleviating the teen's depression, not on effecting broader systemic change. Put another way, the identified patient remains the adolescent and the identified problem remains the depression.

Medications

Emslie et al. (1997) were the first to demonstrate that an antidepressant medication (fluoxetine) was superior to placebo in the treatment of childhood and adolescent MDD. Later studies suggest that other selective serotonin reuptake inhibitors (SSRIs) might be efficacious in treating depression among youth (Whittington et al., 2004). A comprehensive discussion of antidepressant medications for adolescent MDD is beyond the scope of this chapter. However, it is important to note that the combination of fluoxetine and CBT was the most effective treatment for the moderately to severely depressed adolescents in the TADS study (TADS Team, 2004). Therefore, we generally recommend such a combination treatment for teens with this level of depressive severity. There remains the possibility that CBT alone may be efficacious for moderately to severely depressed adolescents, if conducted over more than a 12-week period, or in a manner that differs from the TADS acute treatment model.

Concerns have been raised during recent years about the safety of SSRIs for treating depressed youth. Although the absolute risk is low, there is evidence of treatment-emergent suicidal ideation and behavior among flict at home. When asked if these occurred in his family, Jason noted that his parents often lectured and nagged, and that he ignored them or simply walked out of the room. His parents concurred. Together, we discussed the importance of understanding each other's thoughts and feelings. During the session Jason was able to identify specific emotions he felt when his parents discussed his grades, and he practiced expressing his thoughts and feelings to his parents in a direct, and honest manner.

Session 11: Acting Assertively, Taking Stock, and Summing Up

During this session we discussed what Jason had learned over the course of therapy, what he had found helpful, and what he felt might be useful in the future. Jason noted that the Problem Solving, Pleasant Activities, Social Activities, and Cognitive Restructuring modules had been particularly helpful.

Booster Session: Preparing for the Future

At the conclusion of treatment Jason was asymptomatic, and his academic performance had begun to improve. He was engaged in extracurricular activities after school (theater) and, for the first time, had begun to create a vision for his future. Jason's eye contact was much improved and he was better able to describe emotions.

An explicit goal in CBT is to prepare patients for challenges they may encounter in the future. We began by discussing events in Jason's past, then considered potentially upsetting events in his future and "worst case scenarios" (e.g., failing his calculus class). As Jason noted, "Now if these things happened, I *know* I could solve them." We helped Jason to develop a list of "challenges ahead." These included final exams, end of the school year, job search, problems at work, and maintaining motivation for summer school. We reviewed the skills he had learned and identified which "tools" would be most helpful.

Three months later Jason reported that he continued to do well. He noted that he was not depressed, that he been working part time, and that he regularly went to the movies with a group of friends. He reported that, with the exception of one class, he was doing well academically. He now readily acknowledged that the class "was a problem" and that he "needed to fix it now." Jason had learned over the course of therapy to approach life in a new manner. He was able to reflect on problems, to generate solutions, and to tolerate negative emotions.

children and adolescents treated with these medications relative to youth receiving pill placebo (Hammad, Laughren, & Racoosin, 2006). Although results of TADS study confirmed that during acute treatment there is a statistically nonsignificant increase in the rate of suicidal ideation among youth receiving fluoxetine relative to those receiving placebo, it is important to note that the occurrence of suicidal ideations declined among youth receiving each of the active treatments. Moreover, findings from the TADS study suggest that the attendant risk of suicidal ideations that accompanies the use of SSRIs *may* be mitigated by the concomitant use of CBT (TADS Team, 2004). CBT, either alone or in combination with fluoxetine, appears to reduce suicidal ideations and behavior among adolescents. CBT may accomplish this by bolstering adolescents' ability to cope with stressful life events, providing them with adaptive skills for managing negative moods, and reducing behavioral impulsivity. However, the combination of CBT and fluoxetine did not negate the risk of serious suicidality in TADS. Therefore, it is necessary that clinicians working with young people who have been prescribed SSRIs monitor carefully for suicidality, even when the medication is combined with CBT.

CASE ILLUSTRATION

Jason, a 17-year-old white male, was referred to us for treatment by his parents due to concerns about his mood and academic performance. Jason, who was in an honors program, had erratic and declining grades, and was in danger of having to repeat the school year. At intake he manifested depressed mood, anhedonia, hypersomnia, and social withdrawal. He had been "dropping all his friendships." He acknowledged feeling lonely but minimized this.

Jason responded to direct questions but did not elaborate upon his answers or spontaneously discuss interests or concerns. Rather, he sat quietly and avoided eye contact, and demonstrated prominent psychomotor slowing. Although he was attentive to our conversation, there were long latencies (30–60 seconds) before he answered questions. He walked with a slow, shuffling gait, with his arms flat at his sides. His parents were concerned that his symptoms might be indices of an emerging psychotic disorder.

Initial Assessment

The results of a K-SADS-PL indicated that Jason met DSM-IV criteria for MDD, recurrent. The CDRS-R yielded a score of 52, which was classified as "severe." Jason showed significant functional impairment on a Global Rating Scale. Self-report questionnaires were uninformative, because he minimized problems.

Case Formulation

A range of factors appeared to be implicated in Jason's distress. As became apparent during later sessions, Jason was intimidated by his brothers' academic success and his parents' achievements. Discrepancies were apparent between Jason's performance and the expectations held by Jason and his family. It quickly became apparent that Jason tended to withdraw, both cognitively and behaviorally, from any thought, event, or situation that elicited a negative mood. He simply shifted his attention away from such stimuli. He approached problems and challenges in a passive, avoidant manner. Although he presented as diffident and disengaged, he was acutely aware of his difficulties and felt powerless to rectify them. He had a number of strengths. He was bright, creative, and empathic, and despite recent isolation, his social skills were good.

Course of Treatment

Jason was seen on 11 occasions over 12 weeks. Using a "modular" approach (Curry & Reinecke, 2003), we selected empirically supported treatment components that would meet Jason's individual needs. These included (1) socialization to the CBT model, (2) developing a shared case formulation, (3) goal setting, (4) mood monitoring, (5) pleasant activities scheduling, (6) social problem solving, (7) cognitive restructuring, (8) social interaction and assertion skills, (9) family communication, and (10) relapse prevention. This is a great deal of work to cover in a short period of time. As a consequence, sessions tended to be active, focused, and flexible. We endeavored to maintain a balance between skills acquisition and empathic support.

Sessions 1 and 2:
Presenting the Model, Case Formulation, Goal Setting

Despite Jason's denial of emotional reactions to his school failure and his difficulty in generating goals, in these sessions we shared the rationale for CBT and an initial case formulation with Jason and his parents, and worked with them to identify goals for therapy. We provided a Teen Workbook describing CBT, and introduced the concepts of mood monitoring and pleasant activities to them.

Session 3: Mood Monitoring, Pleasant Activities Scheduling

Jason's mood had improved slightly, and he agreed that failing his classes might be "something of a problem." Although still disengaged and disinterested, we were able to develop a list of pleasant activities he "might enjoy." These included going to a party, visiting friends, playing basketball, going to a movie, watching a boxing match, biking, and winning a competition.

Sessions 4 and 5: Pleasant Activities Scheduling, Problem Solving

Jason's mood continued to improve, and he began to elaborate upon his thoughts during the session. He reportedly went with a friend to a movie, which was first time Jason had gone out socially in several months. Moreover, he signed up to audition for a play at school. We introduced a social problem-solving technique that he could use across multiple situations. Addressing Jason's lack of goals and his difficulties envisioning the future, we asked, "What would give you a great life?" He responded, "Getting a summer job and . . . doing something important to me, so I'm being the person I am." To build upon these statements, Jason's homework assignment was to prepare a list of possible summer jobs, and to consider what he might like to be like as a person in the future.

Sessions 6–9: Cognitive Restructuring

Jason's mood continued to improve, and he reported that he had (quite unexpectedly) joined a community theater. We used the fact that he would have a monologue in the play as an opportunity to practice labeling and expressing emotions. Inasmuch as Jason continued to deny experiencing negative moods, we focused upon how he would express them in a play. The negative automatic thoughts he experienced while thinking about this offered an opportunity to explore the relations between thoughts and emotions. Jason acknowledged, for the first time, that he used cognitive avoidance as a coping strategy. As he remarked, "When I see something bad happening, I just don't think about it."

Session 10: Family Communication

This module, which involves both the teenager and the caregivers, is used when the therapist becomes aware of negative communication in the family or when there are high levels of "expressed emotion." We began with a discussion of common patterns of communication that can contribute to co

REVIEW OF EFFICACY RESEARCH

Brent and colleagues (1997) compared individual CT to systems behavioral family therapy (SBFT) and nondirective supportive therapy (NST) with 107 adolescents with MDD. Treatment was weekly for 12–16 weeks. "Remission" was defined as at least 3 consecutive weeks of normal scores on self-reported depression and absence of MDD. Remission was higher for CT (60%) than for SBFT (38%) or NST (39%). Parents also perceived CT as more credible than the other treatments.

The results of two controlled outcome studies suggest that Lewinsohn and Clarke's CWD course is efficacious in the treatment of clinically depressed adolescents. Lewinsohn et al. (1990) treated 40 teens with MDD or dysthymia in a 7-week, 14-session program, with 19 adolescents serving as a waiting-list control group. Almost half of the treated adolescents, but only one of the waiting-list adolescents, were below diagnostic threshold after treatment. Parents of one-half of the treated adolescents participated in a psychoeducational group intervention, but parent intervention did not significantly affect outcome. In a subsequent trial, Clarke, Rohde, Lewinsohn, Hops, and Seeley (1999) randomly assigned 123 depressed adolescents to group CWD or a waiting-list control, with treatment extending to 8 weeks. Improvement rates were higher in this study (65% and 69%, respectively, in the treated conditions). Almost half of those in the wait-list control group also improved. Booster sessions in the 4 months following treatment improved recovery for adolescents who remained depressed after the acute intervention.

More recently, TADS CBT was compared to fluoxetine (FLX), the combination of CBT and fluoxetine (COMB), and clinical management with pill placebo (PBO) over 12 weeks of acute treatment in a 13-site trial with 439 adolescents with MDD. Acute treatment was followed by continuation treatment for 6 more weeks, then maintenance treatment for 18 additional weeks. "Acute treatment response" was defined as an independent evaluator's rating of 1 (*Very much improved*) or 2 (*Much improved*) on the 7-point Clinical Global Impressions—Improvement scale (CGI-I; TADS Team, 2004). At the 12-week assessment point, response rates were 35% (PBO), 43% (CBT), 61% (FLX), and 71% (COMB). CBT did not separate statistically from PBO, but COMB achieved the highest response rate to date for acute intervention with adolescent MDD. COMB also reduced suicidal ideation more than the other interventions. It appears, then, that 12 weeks of individual CBT may be insufficient for moderately to severely depressed youth. CBT appears, however, to be as effective as fluoxetine alone if treatment is continued for a longer period of time. Results of the TADs study indicate that gains were maintained during the continuation and maintenance phases of treatment. At week 36 the remission rates were 60% for adolescents receiving a continuation of CBT and medication, 55% for adolescents receiving fluoxetine alone, and 64% for those receiving CBT alone. Paired comparisons indicate that, by week 24, all three active treatments have equivalent remission rates (The TADS Team, 2007).

This pattern of findings, in which a combination of CBT and medications is superior to CBT alone for the acute treatment of depression (TADS Team, 2004), is similar to that observed in a recent study of the treatment of chronic depression among adults (Keller et al., 2000).

Combining data across studies to date, at least 14 randomized, controlled trials of CBT have been completed with depressed youth. Reviews and initial meta-analyses indicated that the effect sizes obtained are moderate to large and therapeutic gains are maintained over time (Reinecke et al., 1998). The results of a recent meta-analysis by Weisz, McCarty, and Valeri (2006), however, brought into question the strength of the effects observed. They reported a mean acute treatment for CBT effect size of 0.34, which was markedly lower than that found in earlier reviews. This difference appears to stem from several factors, including increasing severity of depression among youth participating in more recent studies, increasingly stringent control groups, and differences in analytic models employed in the meta-analyses (Klein, Jacobs, & Reinecke, 2007).

CONCLUSIONS

On the basis of available evidence, several conclusions regarding depression in adolescents and children can be drawn with some confidence. First, early-onset unipolar depression is often a chronic, recurring condition. It is associated with vulnerability for recurrent depression during adulthood, with impaired social, emotional, and academic functioning. It is a condition that places a burden on families and causes suffering for the child and his/her family. Second, a number of methodologically sound outcome studies have been completed during recent years. As a group, they suggest that CBT can be effective for treating major depression among adolescents. CBT appears to be more effective than no treatment, a wait-list control, or simple support. Although CBT has been found to be more effective than some other forms of psychotherapy (Brent et al., 1997), it has not been found to be as effective acutely as fluoxetine (TADS Team, 2004). Preliminary evidence indicates that, taking risk and benefit into account, the combination of CBT and an SSRI may offer the best chance of rapid clinical improvement and enhanced psychosocial functioning (TADS Team, 2004), and that CBT may be as effective as medication alone over 36 weeks of treatment. On the basis of research regarding course, phenomenology, and response to treatment, we suggest that early-onset major depression may usefully be conceptualized as a chronic disorder, and that it should be treated accordingly.

Looking forward, additional work is needed to make CBT, and other forms of empirically-supported treatment, more available, and to determine which components of the treatment mediate improvement. Although research to date has been fairly consistent in suggesting that CBT can be helpful in treating adolescents with MDD, it is not clear that CBT is uniquely helpful. Interpersonal psychotherapy also appears to be efficacious, although it has not yet been compared to or combined with medication. Work is also needed on the prevention of relapse among depressed children and adolescents, and on the treatment of adolescents who fail to respond to an initial treatment trial. Although we have learned a great deal about early-onset affective disorders during the past 20 years, our work is, in a true sense, only beginning. For these most challenging cases, a great deal of additional work remains to be done.

REFERENCES

Beck, A., Rush, A., Shaw, B., & Emery, G. (1979). *Cognitive therapy of depression*. New York: Guilford Press.

Bradley, S. (2000). *Affect regulation and the development of psychopathology*. New York: Guilford Press.

Brent, D. (1995). Risk factors for adolescent suicide and suicidal behavior: Mental and substance abuse disorders, family environmental factors, and life stress. *Suicide and Life Threatening Behavior, 25*, 52–63.

Brent, D., Holder, D., Kolko, D., Birmaher, B., Baugher, M., Roth, C. et al. (1997). A clinical psychotherapy trial for adolescent depression comparing cognitive, family, and supportive treatments. *Archives of General Psychiatry, 54*, 877–885.

Brent, D., & Poling, K. (1997). *Cognitive therapy treatment manual for depressed and suicidal youth*. University of Pittsburgh, unpublished manuscript

Clarke, G., Rohde, P., Lewinsohn, P., Hops, H., & Seeley, J. (1999). Efficacy of acute group treatment and booster sessions. *Journal of the American Academy of Child and Adolescent Psychiatry, 38*, 272–279.

Curry, J., & Reinecke, M. (2003). Modular therapy for adolescents with major depression. In M. Reinecke, F. Dattilio, & A. Freeman (Eds.), *Cognitive therapy with children and adolescents* (2nd ed., pp. 95–127). New York: Guilford Press.

Curry, J., & Wells, K. (2005). Striving for effectiveness in the treatment of adolescent depression: Cognitive behavior therapy for multisite community intervention. *Cognitive and Behavioral Practice, 12*, 177–185.

Emslie, G., Rush, A., Weinberg, W., Kowatch, R., Hughes, C., Carmody T., et al. (1997). A double-blind, randomized, placebo-controlled trial of fluoxetine in children and adolescents with depression. *Archives of General Psychiatry, 54*, 1031–1037.

Essau, C., & Dobson, K. (1999). Epidemiology of depressive disorders. In C. Essau & F. Petermann (Eds.), *Depressive disorders in children and adolescents: Epidemiology, course and treatment* (pp. 69–103). Northvale, NJ: Aronson.

Gracious, B., Youngstrom, E., Findling, R., & Calabrese, J. (2002). Discriminative validity of a parent version of the Young Mania Rating Scale. *Journal of the American Academy of Child and Adolescent Psychiatry, 41*, 1350–1359.

Hammad, T., Laughren, T., & Racoosin, J. (2006). Suicidality in pediatric patients treated with antidepressant drugs. *Archives of General Psychiatry, 63*, 332–339.

Kaslow, N., Deering, C., & Racusin, G. (1994). Depressed children and their families. *Clinical Psychology Review, 14*, 39–59.

Kaufman, J., Birmaher, B., Brent, D., Rao, U., Flynn, C., Moreci, P., et al. (1997). Schedule for Affective Disorders and Schizophrenia for School-Age Children— Present Episode and Lifetime Version (K-SADS-PL): Initial reliability and validity data. *Journal of the American Academy of Child and Adolescent Psychiatry, 36*, 980–988.

Keller, M., McCullough, J., Klein, D., Arnow, B., Dunner, D., Gelenberg, A., et al. (2000). A comparison of nefazodone, the cognitive behavioral-analysis system of psychotherapy, and their combination for the treatment of chronic depression. *New England Journal of Medicine, 342*, 1462–1470.

Kendler, K., Thornton, L., & Gardner, C. (2000). Stressful life events and previous episodes in the etiology of major depression in women: An evaluation of the "kindling" hypothesis. *American Journal of Psychiatry, 157*, 1243–1251.

Klein, D., Dougherty, L., & Olino, T. (2005). Toward guidelines for evidence-based assessment of depression in children and adolescents. *Journal of Clinical Child and Adolescent Psychology, 34*, 412–432.

Klein, J., Jacobs, R., & Reinecke, M. (2007). Cognitive-behavioral therapy for adolescent depression: A meta-analytic investigation of chagnes in effect size estimates. *Journal of the American Academy of Child and Adolescent Psychiatry, 46*(11), 1403–1413.

Kovacs, M., Obrosky, D., Gatsonis, C., & Richards, C. (1997). First-episode major depressive and dysthymic disorder in childhood: Clinical and sociodemographic factors in recovery. *Journal of the American Academy of Child and Adolescent Psychiatry, 36*, 777–784.

Lewinsohn, P., Clarke, G., Hops, H., & Andrews, J. (1990). Cognitive-behavioral treatment for depressed adolescents. *Behavior Therapy, 21*, 385–401.

Linehan, M. (1993). *Skills training manual for treating borderline personality disorder.* New York: Guilford Press.

Poznanski, E., & Mokros, H. (1995). *Children's Depression Rating Scale—Revised (CDRS-R)*. Los Angeles: Western Psychological Services.

Rao, U., Ryan, N., Birmaher, B., Dahl, R., Williamson, D., Kaufman, J., et al. (1995). Unipolar depression in adolescents: Clinical outcome in adulthood. *Journal of the American Academy of Child and Adolescent Psychiatry, 34,* 566–578.

Reinecke, M., Ryan, N., & DuBois, D. (1998). Cognitive-behavioral therapy of depression and depressive symptoms during adolescence: A review and meta-analysis. *Journal of the American Academy of Child and Adolescent Psychiatry, 37,* 26–34.

Reinecke, M., & Simons, A. (2005). Vulnerability to depression among adolescents: Implications for cognitive-behavioral treatment. *Cognitive and Behavioral Practice, 12,* 166–176.

Reynolds, W. (1987). *Reynolds Adolescent Depression Scale manual.* Odessa, FL: Psychological Assessment Resources.

Reynolds, W., & Mazza, J. (1998). Reliability and validity of the Reynolds Adolescent Depression Scale with young adolescents. *Journal of School Psychology, 36,* 295–312.

Rogers, G., Reinecke, M., & Curry, J. (2005). Case formulation in TADS CBT. *Cognitive and Behavioral Practice, 12,* 198–208.

Rotheram, M. (1987). Evaluation of imminent danger for suicide among youth. *American Journal of Orthopsychiatry, 57,* 102–110.

Shaffer, D., Gould, M., Fisher, P., Trautman, P., Moreau, D., Kleinman, M., et al. (1996). Psychiatric diagnosis in child and adolescent suicide. *Archives of General Psychiatry, 53,* 339–348.

Simon, G. (2000). Long-term prognosis of depression in primary care. *Bulletin of the World Health Organization, 78,* 439–445.

Spence, S., & Reinecke, M. (2003). Cognitive approaches to understanding, preventing, and treating child and adolescent depression. In M. Reinecke, & D. Clark (Eds.), *Cognitive therapy across the lifespan: Evidence and practice* (pp. 358–395). Cambridge, UK: Cambridge University Press.

Teasdale, J. (2004). Mindfulness-based cognitive therapy. In J. Yiend (Ed.), *Cognition, emotion, and psychopathology: Theoretical, empirical and clinical directions* (pp. 270–289). Cambridge, UK: Cambridge University Press.

Treatment for Adolescents with Depression Study (TADS) Team. (2004). Fluoxetine, cognitive-behavioral therapy, and their combination for adolescents with depression: Treatment for Adolescents with Depression Study randomized controlled trial. *Journal of the American Medical Association, 292,* 807–820.

Treatment for Adolescents with Depression Study (TADS) Team. (2005). The Treatment for Adolescents with Depression Study (TADS): Demographic and clinical characteristics. *Journal of the American Academy of Child and Adolescent Psychiatry, 44,* 28–40.

The TADS Team (2007). The Treatment for Adolescents with Depression Study: Long-term effectiveness and safety outcomes. *Archives of General Psychiatry, 64*(10), 1132–1144.

Weissman, M., Wolk, S., Goldstein, R., Moreau, D., Adams, P., Greenwald, S., et al. (1999). Depressed adolescents grown up. *Journal of the American Medical Association, 281,* 1707–1713.

Weisz, J., McCarty, C., & Valeri, S. (2006). Effects of psychotherapy for depression in children and adolescents: A meta-analysis. *Psychological Bulletin, 132,* 132–149.

Whittington, C., Kendall, T., Fonagy, P., Cottrell, D., Cotgrove, A., & Boddington, E. (2004). Selective serotonin reuptake inhibitors in childhood depression: Systematic review of published versus unpublished data. *Lancet, 363,* 1341–1345.

Youngstrom, E., Findling, R., Calabrese, J., Gracious, B., Demeter, C., DelPorto Bedoya, D., et al. (2004). Comparing the diagnostic accuracy of six potential screening instruments for bipolar disorder in youths aged 5 to 17 years. *Journal of the American Academy of Child and Adolescent Psychiatry, 43,* 847–858.

18

OLDER ADULTS

Patricia A. Areán
Leilani Feliciano

For many years people over the age of 65 were excluded from psychotherapy research. The assumption that drove this exclusion was that older people are unable to learn new skills, and that mental illness, depression in particular, is a normal consequence of aging. In the early 1980s, this assumption was challenged primarily in research conducted by Drs. Gallagher-Thompson and Thompson, who were able to demonstrate that not only can older people benefit from psychotherapy, but that they can also learn new mood regulation skills, almost as well as younger people (Mackin & Areán, 2005). In addition to this research, emergent neuropsychological research was beginning to show that whereas older people learn differently than younger people, they can in fact *learn*, and that the brain, and all the accompanying cognitive functions, remains relatively plastic (Knight & Satre, 1999). The mental health field's assumption about aging was further confronted by Epidemiologic Catchment Area study data showing that older people have significantly lower rates of current and lifetime depression than younger cohorts (Koenig & Blazer, 1992).

This new research turned the gerontological field on its head, forcing it to move from a palliative model of mental health to a preventive and action-oriented model of mental health. As a result, psychotherapy research with older adults has become far more advanced. Not only are there more data to show that older adults can benefit from psychotherapies, but also we are more familiar with how these therapies should be adapted to fit the needs of current cohorts of older people (Areán, Hegel, & Reynolds, 2002). Cognitive therapy (CT) in particular has made significant advances in gerontology. In this chapter, we discuss assessment and formulation of late-life depression, data in support of CT in late-life depression, and how CT in older cohorts differs from that in younger cohorts. These issues are illustrated with the case of Mr. Z.

CONCEPTUALIZATION OF DEPRESSION IN OLDER ADULTS

Mr. Z is a 75-year-old, widowed man who suffers from macular degeneration and diabetes, which resulted in above-the-knee amputation. He lives on the second floor of a walk-up building and has difficulty leaving his apartment because of his poor eyesight, and because his prosthesis no longer fits his leg since Mr. Z's weight loss of 15 pounds in the past year. His only income is social security, with which he barely makes ends meet. Since his eyesight began to fail and his disability increased, Mr. Z has difficulty sleeping, has little energy, has trouble gaining pleasure from activities that he once enjoyed, has trouble concentrating, and feels that life is not worth living. In addition, his eldest son needed temporarily a place to stay and asked persistently to move in with Mr. Z, a situation, which in the past has led to friction. The San Francisco based Home-Delivered Meals Program referred Mr. Z to the University of California–San Francisco (UCSF) Over-60 Clinic program for assessment of depression and treatment.

Depression in older adults can vary considerably across persons in terms of presentation and etiology. Between 1 and 4% of older adults experience major depression (Waraich, Goldner, Somers, & Hsu, 2004), with 40% of depression in older adults representing a recurrent episode, with the first episode having occurred in young adulthood, and 30% being the very first episode of depression ever (late-onset depression; Blazer, 2003). For many years, researchers felt that depression was an understandable consequence of aging, because older adults are exposed to so many risk factors associated with the onset of depression. It is not uncommon for older adults to complain about sadness related to bereavement, social isolation, caregiver strain, and financial problems—all salient psychosocial risk factors for depression

(Areán & Reynolds, 2005). Furthermore, older adults are exposed to many *medical* conditions that can influence depression directly by their effect on brain chemistry, and indirectly through the onset of disability (Bruce, 2002). Finally, studies have shown that depression in late life may also be influenced by certain *cognitive risk factors*, such as vascular disease and age-related changes in executive functions (Rapp et al., 2005). Despite their increased exposure to depression risk factors, the fact remains that depression is a relatively uncommon condition in older adults (Charney et al., 2003), and according to the Successful Aging Studies (Rowe & Khan, 1997), not all older people who face these stressors become depressed.

The degree to which these negative life events become salient risk factors for late-life depression depends on how undesirable, disruptive, and uncontrollable these events are. What puts people at risk for depression is not age or exposure to the risk factors discussed earlier, but the predisposing vulnerabilities associated with depression. According to this line of research, the chance of becoming depressed when confronted with the negative life events described earlier is a function of *resilience*, which has been found to moderate the negative effects of stress in older adults (Wagnild & Young, 1993). Similar to cognitive theory of depression, late-life resilience is seen as a function of having a balanced view of life, a sense of purpose in life, the ability to function even in the face of failures, acceptance of one's life, and self-efficacy (Wagnild, 2003). Considerable research indicates that in addition to resilience, *behavioral coping* moderates the effect of negative life events in older adults. Older adults who take a more active stance in solving everyday problems tend to be less vulnerable to depression than those who use passive coping strategies, such as avoidance, leaving problem solving to others, and rumination (Denney, 1995; Heidrich & Denney, 1994). Denney and Pearce (1989) found that use of problem-solving skills to deal with life strain is related to better psychological adjustment in late life, and Koenig, George, Titus, and Meador (2004) found that spirituality and active involvement in spiritual endeavors are also related to better psychological well-being in later life.

Based on these findings, late-life depression is a multifaceted problem. Therapists who work with older adults must think multidimensionally about their older patients' problems. Although older adults are faced with a number of potentially adverse events that could each contribute to depression, the fact remains that few older adults suffer from major depression even in the face of these negative events. The research on coping skills and resilience suggests that late-life depression is not solely a function of exposure to negative events but a combination of these life events, cognitive vulnerabili-

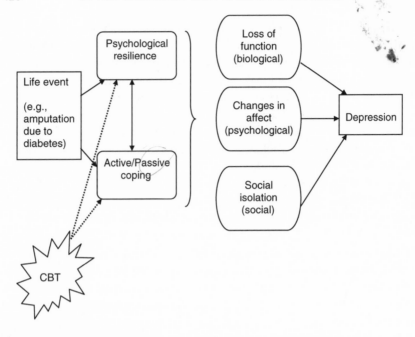

FIGURE 18.1. CBT conceptualization of late-life depression.

ties, and skills deficits. As depicted in Figure 18.1, CT addresses late-life depression by targeting the older person's psychological resilience and coping skills, so that negative life events do not adversely affect his/her mood. How CT works in older adults is discussed in more detail in the section on CT adaptations for late-life depression.

ASSESSING LATE-LIFE DEPRESSION

Mr. Z was seen by one of the Over-60 clinicians for an assessment of depression. In addition to a comprehensive health and mental health history, the clinician also spoke with Mr. Z's doctor to obtain results from a recent physical exam. The clinician administered the 9-item Patient Health Questionnaire (PHQ-9) and the Folstein Mini-Mental Status Exam (MMSE). Based on his symptom count and his score on the PHQ-9, Mr. Z met criteria for major depression. His MMSE was a 26. Mr. Z had lived in the United States for over 30 years, but English was not his first language. Mr. Z reported that he had had symptoms of depression for a year, which coincided with his son's request to move in with him and a recent move to publicly funded senior housing. These symptoms also coincided with an increase in his hemoglobin A1c (a measure of blood glucose). The clinician was left with several issues to consider in managing Mr. Z's depression. First, his hemoglobin A1c could have accounted for several of his symptoms, particularly lack of energy and lack of interest in activities. However, he also had two stressful life events that seemed to contribute to his depression. Although his MMSE was within normal limits, it was on the low side, which could indicate early-stage dementia. Was Mr. Z's depression a result of uncontrolled diabetes, early dementia, or psychosocial stress?

Diagnosing depression in older people can be tricky given the cluster of symptoms that defines the disorder. For instance, research has shown that symptoms of fatigue, trouble concentrating, and lack of enjoyment can be the result of illness or early stages of dementia (Karel, Ogland-Hand, & Gatz, 2002). Some researchers on the assessment of late-life depression has found that somatic symptoms overidentify depression in older community-dwelling adults (Yesavage et al., 1982–1983). Others have found that affective symptoms, particularly feeling sad and depressed, are underreported in older people, particularly older medical patients; thus, late-life depression goes unrecognized (Gallo & Rabins, 1999). This mixed body of research suggests that assessment in older adults must take into consideration physical and cognitive explanations for depressive symptoms. As illustrated with Mr. Z, determining the causes of depressive symptoms in older adults is not a straightforward task. Although Mr. Z presented with several symptoms of depression, many of them could be explained by an exacerbation of his diabetes and potential cognitive impairment.

When assessing an older person's depression, the therapist should keep in mind the following: the biological, psychological, and social risk factors that are contributing to the depression; the degree to which depression is influenced by medical conditions, and in turn the degree to which the management of illness is affected by depression; how cognitively intact the patient is (whether he/she can participate in CT); the patient's ability to take part in activities of daily living (managing self-care, finances, cooking); the extent of the patient's social support; and finally, the patient's past history with regard to previous strengths and weaknesses in handling adversity (Scogin, 2000).

This information is easily obtained by making sure the patient comes to his/her first session with some basic information. At the Over-60 clinic at UCSF, we typically ask patients to bring with them a recent medical report from their primary care physician to rule-out other causes of depression (malnutrition, anemia, thyroid disease, diabetes, hepatitis, cancer). If patients have chronic medical conditions, we ask to have recent lab reports sent to us. In addition, we also ask patients to bring all their medications with them, so that we can investigate issues of polypharmacy (which can contribute to some symptoms of depression; e.g., trouble concentrating, fatigue, and sleeplessness) and to make sure patients are not on medications that can exacerbate depression, such as prednisone, beta-blockers, medications for Parkinson's disease, and interferon (Rodin, Crave, & Littlefield, 1991). When we are concerned that an illness or medication may be contributing to depression, we contact the patient's physician to discuss the possibility of either treating the condition or changing medications.

Brief cognitive screening is typically helpful in determining if an older patient is mentally intact enough to engage in a learning-based therapy such as CT, and if depression is a precursor to an illness that causes dementia. Because some dementias are reversible if caught early, and depression has been identified as a prodrome for dementias (Lyketsos, Rosenblatt, & Rabins, 2004), this assessment is particularly important. The most widely used cognitive screening test, the Folstein MMSE (Folstein, Folstein, & McHugh, 1975), is popular because it covers several areas of cognitive function, such as fund of information, immediate and delayed recall, verbal functioning, visual–spatial functions, and, to some degree, executive functions; it is also easy to administer, taking 5–10 minutes in a cognitively intact patient. It has its limitations, however, in that it is influenced by education (Jones & Gallo, 2001) and must be administered exactly as intended; variations in administration can change the score by as much as 5 points. Most researchers consider an MMSE score of 24 or better to be within the range of normal cognitive functioning for depressed older patients (Scogin, 2000). It is important to note here that mild cognitive impairment is common in late-life depression; 60% of older adults with depression have some form of cognitive impairment; the most common impairment is executive dysfunction (Alexopoulos et al., 2005).

Although physical and cognitive exams give the clinician information about how the patient's body is functioning, it is still important to determine whether the older patient feels that he/she is functioning physically and cognitively as well as before. The Medical Outcomes Study 36-item Short-Form Health Survey (SF-36; Gandek, Sinclair, Kosinski, & Ware, 2004) provides useful information with regard to the degree to which the older patient can complete his/her activities of daily living. This scale provides information about the older patient's ability to complete basic activities, and the degree to which he/she feels that his/her disability is attributed to depression or physical illness.

The cognitive therapist should also ask about older patients' social networks. Although formal assessments of social support do exist, these instruments can be too long and cumbersome for clinical settings. The clinician can assess social support informally by asking patients whether they have friends and family who they feel have been helpful and supportive of them in the past. Social support is an important moderator for treatment outcome in older adults, in that persons with low social support do not respond as well to treatment as those who have good social support (Karel et al., 2002); older adults with good social networks can call upon others in the event that they need help in participating in therapy. As an example, Mr. Z reported that he could not get the news regularly, which contributed to feelings of isolation. In discussing several alternatives for getting up-to-date news, the therapist discovered that Mr. Z's nephew passed his apartment every day on the way to work, and he was able to stop by in the morning and drop off the morning paper. This small gesture on the part of a supportive family member helped Mr. Z to feel more connected with his community and improved his mood considerably.

Therapists should not overlook the possibility of comorbid substance abuse in older patients. Heavy use of alcohol, by far the most common substance of abuse in older populations, is associated with increased morbidity, impaired social functioning, isolation, and poor mental health, including increased suicidality (Finlayson, Hurt, Davis, & Morse, 1998). In assessing alcohol or drug abuse, it is important that the therapist ask directly about the patient's alcohol intake and be very clear about what he/she means by one drink (3 ounces of wine, 12 ounce of beer, or 1 ounce of hard liquor). Many older adults who drink are unaware of the amount that constitutes one alcoholic drink. When assessing for drug abuse, it is also important to ask about prescription drugs, the second most common form of substance abuse among older adults (Blow, Cook, Booth, Falcon, & Friedman, 1992).

In asking about an older patient's experience with mental health care, it is important to note the type of treatment received, when he/she was in treatment, and his/her expectations for this treatment. More often than not, older patients have not had experience with CT and it is important to socialize them about cognitive theory and the process of care. Some people have been exposed only to mental health treatment as it was 30 or 40 years ago, largely inpatient based, and relying on long-term, intensive therapies. Thus, education about the current mental health system is necessary and should be conducted early on in the therapy. Laidlaw, Thompson, Dick-Siskin, and Gallagher-Thompson (2003) suggest that if this education does not occur early on, patients may prematurely terminate therapy.

Finally, older patients should be allowed the opportunity to tell their story. At the UCSF Over-60 Clinic program, we have found that allowing patients the time to talk about their past, previous employment and education history, and family issues contributes to the development of a good therapeutic alliance. Older people have little opportunity to talk about their pasts, despite the fact that this type of narrative is a common developmental process in late life. At the UCSF Over-60 Clinic, we typically guide this narrative by asking the patient to tell us about specific events in their lives. For example, Mr. Z was first asked to talk about his upbringing as a child, the people he looked up to most, the important events in his life, what regrets, as well as successes, he might have had.

Symptom Measures

We have found that the best measures for older patients are those that can be administered relatively easily in a short period of time. Several common measures, each of which has its strengths and weaknesses, are briefly discussed here.

Patient Health Questionnaire

The 9-item Patient Health Questionnaire (PHQ; Spitzer, Williams, Kroenke, Hornyak, & McMurray, 2000), known as the PHQ-9, assesses depression symptoms and has been found to be sensitive and selective in detecting depression in older adults. The patient indicates the degree to which he/she has experienced symptoms over the course of 2 weeks, and each item is scored on a Likert scale from 0 to 4. A score of 10 or more is considered the most accurate cutoff for detecting late-life depression (Spitzer et al., 2000). It is highly accurate in tracking change in depression over the course of therapy, which makes it an excellent clinical tool (Lowe, Unutzer, Callahan, Perkins, & Kroenke, 2004).

Geriatric Depression Scale

The 15-item Geriatric Depression Scale (GDS; Yesavage et al., 1982–1983) was created primarily for use with older adults to overcome the potential biases that medical illness may introduce in the detection of depression. This reliable instrument is also quite accurate in detecting late-life depression, using a cutoff score of 4 or more (Van Marwijk, Arnold, Bonnema, & Kaptein, 1993). Most older adults find it an acceptable instrument, with an easy answer format and understandable questions (D'Ath, Katona, Mullan, Evans, & Katona, 1994).

Beck Depression Inventory for Primary Care

The Beck Depression Inventory for Primary Care (BDI-PC; Beck, Guth, Steer, & Ball, 1997) is a seven-item true–false scale that takes 2 minutes to complete. According to Beck et al. the BDI-PC is a reliable instrument with no age or ethnic bias. A cutoff score of 4 best detects depression in older adults (Scheinthal, Steer, Giffin, & Beck, 2001).

Summary of Late-life Depression Assessment

Assessing the causes of depression and its severity in older patients should be done with a holistic mind-set. Older adults come to treatment with long histories and a wealth of experiences that have shaped who they are. These histories provide points of reference for how older patients' functioning is now compared to the recent and far past. In addition, older patients may have several interlinking causes for being depressed, all of which should, and can, be addressed in CT. Therapists should keep in mind medical, neurological, educational, and social factors in making an assessment. Thorough assessments not only help the cognitive therapist understand the causes of depression and the patient's goals for change but also assist in determining the potential problems that could influence the therapeutic process when treatment begins. We discover what these problems are and how they may be addressed in the following section.

ADAPTING CT FOR THE OLDER PATIENT

After compiling a thorough examination of Mr. Z's physical, cognitive, and environmental risk factors, his therapist determined that in addition to working with Mr. Z's physician to help get his diabetes under control and linking Mr. Z to some much need social services, he would be an appropriate candidate for CT. Although his MMSE score was low, it was within normal limits; thus, the therapist determined that some modifications to the treatment would be helpful. Based on the results of the MMSE and observations during the intake, Mr. Z's therapist decided to begin the therapy by first introducing Mr. Z to all the concepts he would learn in CT: affect regulation strategies, activity scheduling, and communication skills. To facilitate learning, the therapist illustrated these new concepts using examples from Mr. Z's past, so that the new concepts were linked to well-learned events. Furthermore, Mr. Z was provided both written and audiotaped educational materials as aides in learning the new skills. During sessions, the therapist engaged in "cue and review" techniques that allowed Mr. Z several opportunities to encode the new information. The therapist also took into consideration Mr. Z's physical limitations and offered to provide CT in his home. Finally, the therapist was available to Mr. Z between sessions to reinforce the use the new strategies between sessions.

CT for late-life depression is very similar to CT for other populations, with only a few modifications. There is typically a psychoeducational component to educate the patient about cognitive theory of depression and the process of therapy; a focus on challenging pessimistic thinking; behavioral activation strategies; and other skills-based training as needed (social skills, anxiety management, time management, and problem solving). Therefore, the modifications to CT focus largely on accounting for age-related changes in cognitive functions that impact new learning and attention; accounting for physical disabilities; adjusting the therapeutic frame to allow for disability and the numerous demands that older people have on their time and energy; and a consideration of cohort beliefs. Thus, CT content does not change; rather, the means by which it is presented and the speed at which information is acquired are different for older patients. Table 18.1 summarizes this

TABLE 18.1. Late-Life Adaptations for CBT

Age-related challenge	CBT process	Adaptation
Disability; time constraints; instrumental barriers	Therapeutic frame; frequency of visits	Home/telephone-based therapy; case management
Learning novel concepts	Overall knowledge acquisition	Tie new information to overlearned and contextual information
Verbal recall	Thought records; differentiating thought from feeling	Simplify terms and forms; avoid jargon
Perceptual speed	Homework; adherence; session time	Increase number of sessions; simple homework; schedule time for homework; telephone support
Attention and focus	Structured tasks; information gathering; weighing the evidence	Redirection
Working memory	Learning new skills	Cue and review; multimodal presentation
Isolation	Termination	Early fading; relapse prevention; booster sessions

section by listing the CT strategy, the age-related challenge in using the strategy, and the modification that address these challenges.

Psychoeducation and the Early Phases of CT with Older Adults

The initial phases of CT typically focus on first ascertaining the patient's reasons for seeking treatment, his/her experience with therapy and expectations, then socializing the patient to CT. Older adults in particular may need considerable education about the expectations of therapy, as well as the structure of CT. Often, older adults' attitudes about their own age group can interfere with effective treatment (Knight, 2004; Laidlaw et al., 2003). Older people often have little exposure to psychotherapy compared to younger adults; thus, they may require information regarding what mental health services are and how therapy is distinct from needing inpatient care or having severe mental illness (being "crazy"), and to learn that although depression is often a common reaction to grief, loss, and transition in social role, it can be treated in late-life. Laidlaw, Thompson, and Gallagher-Thompson (2004) suggest that therapists can encourage attitudinal change by acknowledging that although members of the individual's cohort may share these beliefs, these beliefs are no longer prevalent in today's society given advances in our knowledge about mental health and illness.

In addition to educating older patients about depression and CT, therapists also need to determine any limitations to coming to therapy on a regular basis. For instance, older patients commonly have limited resources with regard to travel and rely on others to get to appointments (Coon & Gallagher-Thompson, 2002). Furthermore, some older patients still work or take care of family members, and have little time for homework, reading new material, or coming to weekly appointments. Some older patients are too disabled to attend regularly, or they may become disabled during the course of treatment and no longer be able to attend as expected. Therapists working with older patients need to remain flexible with regard to the therapeutic frame; by determining these potential limitations early on in treatment; they can prevent problems in starting the therapy process. Some therapists provide initial case management services to link older patients to services that facilitate the use of therapy, such as senior transportation or respite care (Coon & Gallagher-Thompson, 2002). Others arrange to provide home-based therapy, or therapy in a setting that is more convenient for the older patient to access, such as a senior center or a church (Areán et al., 2005; Scogin et al., 2003). Although preliminary, there is also recent evidence to suggest that telephone-based CT is not only effective in treating depression in disabled patients, but results in near perfect attendance and adherence (Mohr, Burke, Beckner, & Merluzzi, 2005).

To illustrate the importance of flexibility in the therapeutic frame, we turn to Mr. Z, who was considerably disabled by his poorly fitting prosthesis and at one point developed a pressure sore that became infected. Because could not leave his house easily, Mr. Z had indicated to the therapist that he would be unable to resume therapy until his leg healed and he was fitted for a new prosthesis. The therapist offered to come to Mr. Z's home while he was healing, which Mr. Z appreciated. This flexibility allowed Mr. Z to continue treatment and make gains despite a setback in his health. Had the therapist simply agreed to meet again when Mr. Z had healed, they would have had a six-week interruption in treatment.

In these initial sessions, therapists also need to attend to any sensory deficits older patients may have. At least 14% of noninstitutionalized older adults have some type of sensory deficit; 35% of older adults age 85 and older have these impairments (Waldrop & Stern, 2003). When conducting therapy with an older adult with visual or hearing problems, the therapist should sit in front of the person in a well-lighted environment when speaking. Although many therapists prefer muted lighting in their offices to instill a calming effect, this may impair an older person's ability to connect to the therapist. Therapists should encourage visually impaired patients to use devices such as magnifying glasses and large-print materials. A therapist may want to consider utilizing other modalities to present therapy modules, such as audiotaping sessions and providing auditory instructions for homework and data collection (e.g., audiotaped thought diaries). Similarly, when conducting therapy with an older adult with a hearing impairment, it is important to use amplifying technology if possible. If the person wears a hearing aid, ensure that it is turned on or working correctly. Even with advances in hearing aid technology, it is often surprising how many older people either do not know how to, or do not *want* to use these aids. We require new clinicians at the Over-60 Clinic program to attend free workshops offered by the Light House and the Center on Deafness to understand better how reading and listening aids work. During sessions, therapists often use gestures or objects to assist with communication (Springhouse, 2001), or bibliotherapy to support the information being taught in session (Coon & Gallagher-Thompson, 2002). Finally, therapists should consider using short sentences, taking care to enunciate words (National Institute on Aging, 2002). These strategies should assist in promoting better communication, therefore facilitating the therapy process.

Teaching CT to Older Patients

CT is largely a learning-based therapy. Much of how we help patients over-come depression is through providing new information about their condition, helping them to learn new strategies for regulating their affect, to try different ways to interact with others, and to look at problems differently than before. Whereas older patients are very capable of learning new material, how they learn and the rate at which they learn is different than the pace and rate at which younger people learn; thus, the therapist must make an extra effort to ensure that older patients attend to, process, and encode the new information accurately. Although the degree to which older and younger patients differ in their learning abilities varies from patient to patient, it is nonetheless important that therapists working with older adults be equipped to handle potential learning challenges that can arise as people age.

The most common age-related neurocognitive changes that affect the process of CT are changes in information processing, language recall, pro-cessing speed, attentional resources, and working memory. Many older peo-ple have subtle changes in these processes; therefore, it is very hard to discern that they are processing information differently than when they were youn-ger. However, depression imparts its own cognitive slowing; thus, these dif-ferences in processing may be more noticeable the more depressed the older adult is (Pearson, Teri, Reifler, & Raskind, 1989).

Enhancing Information Processing and Encoding

Changes in information processing and encoding affect learning the mate-rial in CT, particularly since much of the information taught is relatively novel. Research shows that older adults have greater difficulty learning novel concepts when these concepts are presented the same way they are pre-sented to younger people. However, age differences in learning novel infor-mation virtually disappear when the information has contextual relevance to the older person (Carstensen & Turk-Charles, 1994; Hultsch & Dixon, 1990). Therefore, adapting the content of the material to make use of the individual's own experiences may increase the likelihood that an older adult can learn and retain the new material easily. As an example, when teaching Mr. Z problem-solving strategies, the therapist relied heavily on Mr. Z's past experiences as an engineer. Problem-solving therapy is based largely on engineering principles, and drawing parallels between the therapeutic strat-egy and how Mr. Z would solve engineering problems facilitated his under-standing and use of these strategies.

Language Recall: Letting Go of the Jargon

Many CT manuals are laden with jargon and new terminology that eventually make sense to younger patients but can leave older patients behind. Longitudinal studies indicate that as people age, they begin to show a decrease in the ability to recall new terminology; thus, when working with older patients, therapists should limit their use of jargon (Small, Dixon, & Hultsch, 1999). Difficulties in recall also influence older patients' ability to engage in self-expression and to conduct exercises that require defining an emotional experience in different ways (Knight, 2004). Verbal recall particularly affects the ability to conduct thought records, because patients must first be able to separate mood from thinking, label the depressive thinking to uncover depressive patterns, and then restructure or redefine the thoughts to reflect a different perspective about the triggering event—all activities that rely heavily on language and verbal recall. At the Over-60 Clinic program, we have simplified the thought record to involve only a few categories for the older person to define. Instead of the typical four-column approach—Activating Event, Belief, Cognition, and Dispute—we use simpler terms, such as "What made me feel badly," "What I said in my head," "What I felt," and "Another way of looking at my problem," and the record is in the form of a diary, a recording method with which older patients tend to be more familiar.[1] Although many CT experts have attempted to simplify terms such as "cognitive distortions" into terms that are more meaningful, such as "mental filter," these terms also may be hard for some older people to grasp. Instead, terms such as "helpful thoughts" or "balanced thoughts" have more semantic meaning for older patients and do not require them to learn new terminology.

A topic related to jargon is the use of terms that, because of their emotional meaning to the older patient, can make adherence to the process of CT difficult. We have found that a common distraction for many older patients is the use of the term "homework" or "assignment." For many older adults in the current cohort, or for those with poor educational backgrounds, referring to between-session activities as "homework" can increase the risk of early termination. Instead, we use the term "action plan" to described between-session assignments. Many older adults with chronic illnesses are familiar with this term, which was developed by chronic illness programs and is used extensively in the health fields to describe health

---

[1]Adapted CT materials can be acquired by e-mailing Brandon Brown at *bbrown@lppi.ucsf.edu*; materials are also available at the COPED website *http://psych.ucsf.edu/copedweb/members/ucsf.asp*, and may be downloaded for free.

maintenance behaviors upon which patient and physician agree in managing an illness.

Perceptual Speed: Slowing the Pace of Therapy

Perceptual speed is particularly impaired in older adults with depression (Lezak, 1995). Many older depressed patients tend to need more time in session to understand a new skill. They also need more time to talk about emotional content and are sometimes slow to respond to questions in therapy. Adapting to cognitive slowing involves several changes in therapeutic delivery, including slower pacing, reducing the amount of material covered within a single session and simplifying homework assignments (Coon & Gallagher-Thompson, 2002). Several researchers recommend the use of concrete examples in goal setting and homework assignments, as well as midweek telephone calls to discuss and therefore prompt homework completion, or having patients schedule a daily time for homework to allow more time for both processing written words and writing tasks (Coon & Gallagher-Thompson, 2002; Knight, 2004; Morris & Morris, 1991).

Attention and Focus: Redirection

Decreased attentional resources, particularly selective attention, or the ability to tune out distracting or extraneous stimuli, also present a challenge (McDowd & Birren, 1990). In particular, older patients' ability to focus on discussions in therapy, to conduct structured tasks, and to answer directive questions is affected by their ability to concentrate on the task at hand. Deficits in attention and focus look very much like tangential thinking in the therapy context. As an example, one therapist in training asked a patient to elaborate on how his dietary restrictions contributed to his depression. As the patient began to explain the current problem, he became distracted by additional information about his eating habits, and within a period of 10 minutes, had shifted from answering the therapist's question to talking about a blender he had bought in 1960. The patient then paused and asked, "I'm sorry, what was your question?" The therapist had been so distracted by the conversation that he no longer remembered! This not uncommon occurrence in therapy with older adults can be more upsetting to patients than being redirected by the therapist. Therapists need to become comfortable with redirection to keep the focus of the therapy on the material/activity at hand (Dick & Gallagher-Thompson, 1996). When it is apparent that patients have difficulty focusing in therapy, the therapist can first point out the process as it occurs in the session, then let them know that he/she may need to redirect them back to the initial question or task.

Working Memory: Cue and Review

The decrease in available working memory, or in the ability to hold something in one's mind and manipulate the information, leads to a diminished capacity to conduct and grasp CT tasks. The therapist working with an older adult often relies more heavily on written materials, diagrams, and concrete examples in teaching CT basic skills. In addition, the decrease in working memory may require patience on the part of therapist, because the older adult may require more repetition and review of important concepts. Hegel et al. (2005) use a strategy called "cue and review" to allow for better encoding of new information. In this strategy, a therapist starts by explaining the new skill, such as a thought record, then using a simple, less emotionally laden example to show the patient how to use the thought record. Once the therapist sees that the patient understands the process, he/she has the patient complete the thought record in the session using another simple example. By presenting the new information in this way, the patient has additional exposures and more time to incorporate the information. Then, the therapist can apply the same format as that used in the insession model to out-of-session homework to be completed, utilizing it to encourage the appropriate behaviors.

Termination and Skills Generalization

As it is for any patient, the therapeutic relationship can be very important and special for older patients. Older adults tend to have few opportunities to talk about their problems; whereas the common societal perception of older adults is that they talk freely about their problems (particularly medical ones), many of our patients indicate that they tend *not* to complain, because they are very aware of how continued complaints can turn people away. Some older adults feel embarrassed about needing mental health care, and do not tell friends and family they are feeling depressed. Thus, the therapist is usually the one person to whom they can talk freely about their worries. In addition, older patients have learned many new ways to cope with their moods and problems by the end of treatment, and they tend to feel anxious about their ability to use these new skills on their own. Cognitive therapists who work with older adults must make extra efforts to ensure that older patients feel able to manage these new skills on their own. This requires preparation early on in treatment to ensure that patients understand that they will be using these new skills on their own.

In addition, as soon as older patients grasp the new strategies or skills, therapists should have them begin work on the thought record and activity scheduling forms. Some patients at the Over-60 Clinic program are given the opportunity to attend monthly booster sessions to reinforce the new skills when they no longer feel depressed.

Summary of CT with Older Adults

Although the content of CT for older patients does not differ, the process by which these patients learn and use CT differs because of physical, cognitive, and social factors specific to older adults. Although we have presented several techniques to make CT more amenable for older patients, therapists should keep in mind that not all these strategies need to be employed, and in fact that for a number of older patients, CT need not be modified. As we stated in the assessment section, careful attention to why older patients may not be doing action plans, or appear not to be attending to therapy may help the therapist decide whether and when these modifications are needed. The extra time and effort in working with older adults in this manner is well worth it. As we detail below, resolution of depression results in better mood and quality of life for older patients.

REVIEW OF EFFICACY RESEARCH

After 16 sessions of CT, Mr. Z noticed a considerable decrease in depression and reported that he felt physically better; thus, he was able to engage in social activities he had been avoiding because of his disability and depression. In addition, he was able to provide his son with shelter, but he developed a plan to set limits on his son's behavior and the length of his stay. Through problem solving and behavioral rehearsal, Mr. Z was able to set appropriate limits that his son respected (much to Mr. Z's surprise). CT was a successful treatment for Mr. Z, particularly in the long run. One year after treatment, Mr. Z wrote his therapist to tell her that he was using the cognitive strategies he had learned in treatment, and that he continued to feel happy, productive, and healthy.

The empirical evidence for treatment in older populations is broad, including several small trials, larger randomized clinical studies, and case examples. Recent evidence from the literature suggests that Mr. Z's experience with CT is a common reaction for a majority of older adults treated with this intervention. Not only is there a reduction in depressive symptoms, but patients also report improved health and functioning, and a greater purpose in life. A number of reviews are available in the CT literature on late life depression, and three meta-analyses have been based upon this literature (Engels & Vermey, 1997; Pinquart & Sorensen, 2001; Scogin & McElreath, 1994). For instance, Koder, Brodaty, and Anstey (1996) examined the literature from 1981 to 1994 and reviewed seven empirical examinations of CT in older depressed adults. These studies included comparisons to other types of therapy (e.g., psychotherapy, pharmacotherapy), and the authors computed effect sizes for four of these studies. Results indicated that CT was more effective than psychodynamic therapy, behavioral therapy, and waiting-list control in pre- posttreatment self-reported depression with the BDI (Koder et al., 1996).

In a more recent review, Mackin and Areán (2005) reviewed evidenced-based psychotherapies in older adults with late-life depression, covering the time period of 1840 to 2005. The authors found only 17 studies that met the criteria for an empirically supported treatment using the Chambless and Hollon (1998) criteria, which requires that there be at least 30 participants per treatment arm in the study, and that the intervention be compared to a gold standard, care as usual, or a waiting-list control. Of these, 10 studies evaluated CT in older adults with major depressive disorder, minor depression, or dysthymia. The authors concluded that for all reviewed studies, cognitive therapy resulted in better depression outcomes than did usual care, wait list control, no treatment, and placebo. In addition, several reviews found supporting evidence that treatment gains are maintained over time, for as long as 1-year posttreatment termination (e.g., Koder et al., 1996; Thompson, Coon, Gallagher-Thompson, Sommer, & Koin, 2001), concluding that CT is an evidence-based method for treating late-life depression.

CONCLUSIONS

Depression comprises a combination of somatic and emotional symptoms and affects in all areas of an individual's life (i.e., social, emotional, cognitive, and physical domains). Diagnosing depression in older people can be difficult given the myriad symptoms, both physical and psychological, that can comprise its picture. Accurate identification is key in the successful treatment of depression and prevention of excessive disability. When treating older adults, therapists necessarily need to consider depression within the complex interaction and overlap of sociocultural factors, and physical and cognitive abilities. When working with older adults, therapists must keep in mind the potential confounders of treatment efficacy, such as issues of disability, time constraints, and cognitive changes. Evidence-based data indicate that cognitive therapists who use the adaptations discussed in this chapter will have as much success in treating their older patients as they do in treating younger patients.[2]

REFERENCES

Alexopoulos, G. S., Kiosses, D. N., Heo, M., Murphy, C. F., Shanmugham, B., & Gunning-Dixon, F. (2005). Executive dysfunction and the course of geriatric depression. *Biological Psychiatry, 58*(3), 204–210.

Areán, P. A., Gum, A., McColluch, C., Bolstrom, A., Gallagher-Thompson, D. E., & Thompson, L. (2005). Treatment of depression in low-income older adults. *Psychology and Aging, 20*(4), 601–609.

Areán, P. A., Hegel, M., & Reynolds, C. (2001). Treating depression in older primary care patients. *Journal of Clinical Geropsychology, 7*(2), 93–104.

Areán, P. A., Hegel, M. T., & Reynolds, C. F. (2002). Adapting psychotherapy for older primary care patients. *Journal of Geriatric Psychology.*

Beck, A. T., Guth, D., Steer, R. A., & Ball, R. (1997). Screening for major depression disorders in medical inpatients with the Beck Depression Inventory for Primary Care. *Behaviour Research and Therapy, 35*(8), 785–791.

Blazer, D. G. (2003). Depression in late-life: Review and commentary. *Journals of Gerontology A: Biological Sciences and Medical Sciences, 58,* 249–265.

Blow, F. C., Cook, C. A., Booth, B. M., Falcon, S. P., & Friedman, M. J. (1992). Age-related psychiatric comorbidities and level of functioning in alcoholic veterans seeking outpatient treatment. *Hospital and Community Psychiatry, 43*(10), 990–995.

Bruce, M. L. (2002). Psychosocial risk factors for depressive disorders in late life. *Biological Psychiatry, 52*(3), 175–184.

Carstensen, L. L., & Turk-Charles, S. (1994). The salience of emotion across the adult life span. *Psychology and Aging, 9,* 259–264.

Chambless, D. L., & Hollon, S. D. (1998). Defining empirically supported therapies. *Journal of Consulting and Clinical Psychology, 66*(1), 7–18.

Charney, D. S., Reynolds, C. F., III, Lewis, L., Lebowitz, B. D., Sunderland, T., Alexopoulos, G. S., et al. (2003). Depression and Bipolar Support Alliance consensus statement on the unmet needs in diagnosis and treatment of mood disorders in late life. *Archives of General Psychiatry, 60*(7), 664–672.

Coon, D. W., & Gallagher-Thompson, D. (2002). Encouraging homework completion among older adults in therapy. *Journal of Clinical Psychology, 58*(5), 549–563.

[2]Additional training in conducting CT and PST with older populations may be obtained online at the Over-60 Clinic. For more information, please contact Dr. Heather Bornfeld (*hbornfeld@lppi.ucsf.edu*) or Ms. Maura McLane (*mmclane@lppi.ucsf.edu*), or by visiting our website at *www.coped.lppi.ucsf.edu.*

D'Ath, P., Katona, P., Mullan, E., Evans, S., & Katona, C. (1994). Screening, detection and management of depression in elderly primary care attenders: The acceptability and performance of the 15 item Geriatric Depression Scale (GDS15) and the development of short versions. *Family Practice, 11*(3), 260–266.

Denney, N. W. (1995). Critical thinking during the adult years: Has the developmental function changed over the last four decades? *Experimental Aging Research, 21*(2), 191–207.

Denney, N. W., & Pearce, K. A. (1989). A developmental study of practical problem solving in adults. *Psychology and Aging, 4*(4), 438–442.

Dick, L. P., & Gallagher-Thompson, D. (1996). Late-life depression. In M. Hersen & V. B. Van Hasselt (Eds.), *Psychological treatment of older adults: An introductory text.* New York: Plenum Press.

Engels, G. I., & Vermey, M. (1997). Efficacy of nonmedical treatments of depression in elders: A quantitative analysis. *Journal of Clinical Geropsychology, 3*(1), 17–35.

Finlayson, R. E., Hurt, R. D., Davis, L. J., Jr., & Morse, R. M. (1988). Alcoholism in elderly persons: A study of the psychiatric and psychosocial features of 216 inpatients. *Mayo Clinic Proceedings, 63*(8), 761–768.

Folstein, M. F., Folstein, S. E., & McHugh, P. R. (1975). "Mini-Mental State": A practical method for grading the cognitive state of patients for the clinician. *Journal of Psychiatric Research, 12,* 189–198.

Gallo, J. J., & Rabins, P. V. (1999). Depression without sadness: Alternative presentations of depression in late life. *American Family Physician, 60*(3), 820–826.

Gandek, B., Sinclair, S. J., Kosinski, M., & Ware, J. E., Jr. (2004). Psychometric evaluation of the SF-36 health survey in Medicare managed care. *Health Care Finance Review, 25*(4), 5–25.

Hegel, M. T., Unutzer, J., Tang, L., Areán, P. A., Katon, W., Noel, P. H., et al. (2005). Impact of comorbid panic and posttraumatic stress disorder on outcomes of collaborative care for late-life depression in primary care. *American Journal of Geriatric Psychiatry, 13*(1), 48–58.

Heidrich, S. M., & Denney, N. W. (1994). Does social problem solving differ from other types of problem solving during the adult years? *Experimental Aging Research, 20*(2), 105–126.

Hultsch, D. F., & Dixon, R. A. (1990). Learning and memory in aging. In J. E. Birren & K. W. Shaie (Eds.), *Handbook of the psychology of aging* (3rd ed., pp. 259–274). San Diego: Academic Press.

Jones, R. N., & Gallo, J. J. (2001). Education bias in the Mini-Mental State Examination. *International Psychogeriatrics, 13*(3), 299–310.

Karel, M. J., Ogland-Hand, S., & Gatz, M. (2002). *Assessing and treating late-life depression: A casebook and resource guide.* New York: Basic Books.

Koder, D. A., Brodaty, H., & Anstey, K. J. (1996). Cognitive therapy for depression in the elderly. *International Journal of Geriatric Psychology, 11,* 97–107.

Koenig, H. G., & Blazer, D. G. (1991). Epidemiology of geriatric affective disorders. *Clinics in Geriatric Medicine, 8*(2), 235–251.

Koenig, H. G., George, L. K., Titus, P., & Meador, K. G. (2004). Religion, spirituality, and acute care hospitalization and long-term care use by older patients. *Archives of Internal Medicine, 164*(14), 1579–1585.

Knight, B. G. (2004). *Psychotherapy with older adults* (3rd ed). Thousand Oaks, CA: Sage.

Knight, B. G., & Satre, D. D. (1999). Cognitive behavioral psychotherapy with older adults. *Clinical Psychology: Science and Practice, 6*(2), 188–203.

Laidlaw, K., Thompson, L. W., Dick-Sisken, L. D., & Gallaher-Thompson, D. (2003). *Cognitive behaviour therapy with older people.* West Sussex, UK: Wiley.

Laidlaw, K., Thompson, L. W., & Gallaher-Thompson, D. (2004). Comprehensive conceptualization of cognitive behaviour therapy for late life depression. *Behavioural and Cognitive Psychotherapy, 32,* 389–399.

Lezak, M. D. (1995). *Neuropsychological assessment* (3rd ed.). New York: Oxford University Press.

Lowe, B., Unutzer, J., Callahan, C. M., Perkins, A. J., & Kroenke, K. (2004). Monitoring depression treatment outcomes with the Patient Health Questionnaire–9. *Medical Care, 42*(12), 1194–1201.

Lyketsos, C. G., Rosenblatt, A., & Rabins, P. (2004). Forgotten frontal lobe syndrome or "executive dysfunction syndrome." *Psychosomatics, 45*(3), 247–255.

Mackin, R. S., & Areán, P. A. (2005). Evidenced-based psychosocial interventions for geriatric depression. *Psychiatric Clinics of North America, 28,* 805–820.

McDowd, J. M., & Birren, J. E. (1990). Aging and attentional processes. In J. E. Birren & K. W. Schaie (Eds.), *Handbook for the psychology of aging* (3rd ed., pp. 222–234). San Diego: Academic Press.

Mohr, D. C., Burke, H., Beckner, V., & Merluzzi, N. (2005). A preliminary report on a skills-based telephone-administered peer support programme for patients with multiple sclerosis. *Multiple Sclerosis, 11*(2), 222–226.

Morris, R. G., & Morris, L. W. (1991). Cognitive and behavioural approaches with the depressed elderly. *International Journal of Geriatric Psychiatry, 6,* 407–413.

National Institute on Aging. (2002, September). *AgePage, hearing loss* (U.S. Department of Health and Human Services, Public Health Service, National Institutes of Health). Retrieved on June 6, 2005, from *www.niapublications.org/engagepages/hearing_loss.pdf.*

Pearson, J. L., Teri, L., Reifler, B., & Raskind, M. (1989). Functional status and cognitive impairment in Alzheimer's disease patients with and without depression. *Journal of the American Geriatrics Society, 37,* 1117–1121.

Pinquart, M., & Sorensen, S. (2001). How effective are psychotherapeutic and other psychosocial interventions with older adults?: A metanalysis. *Journal of Mental Health and Aging, 7,* 207–243.

Rapp, M. A., Dahlman, K., Sano, M., Grossman, H. T., Haroutunian, V., & Gorman, J. M. (2005). Neuropsychological differences between late-onset and recurrent geriatric major depression. *American Journal of Psychiatry, 162,* 691–698.

Rodin, G., Craven, J., & Littlefield, C. (1991). *Depression in the medically ill: An integrated approach.* New York: Brunner/Mazel.

Rowe, J. W., & Khan, R. L. (1997). *Successful aging.* New York: Pantheon.

Scheinthal, S. M., Steer, R. A., Giffin, L., & Beck, A. T. (2001). Evaluating geriatric medical outpatients with the Beck Depression Inventory—Fastscreen for medical patients. *Aging and Mental Health, 5*(2), 143–148.

Scogin, F. (2000). *The first session with seniors.* San Francisco: Jossey-Bass.

Scogin, F., & McElreath, L. (1994). Efficacy of psychosocial treatments for geriatric depression: A qualitative review. *Journal of Consulting and Clinical Psychology, 62,* 69–74.

Scogin, F. R., Hanson, A., & Welsh, D. (2003). Self-administered treatment in stepped-care models of depression treatment. *Journal of Clinical Psychology, 59*(3), 341–349.

Small, B. J., Dixon, R. A., & Hultsch, D. F. (1999). Longitudinal changes in quantitative and qualitative indicators of word and story recall in young-old and old-old adults. *Journals of Gerontology B: Psychological Sciences and Social Sciences, 54,* P107–P115.

Spitzer, R. L., Williams, J. B., Kroenke, K., Hornyak, R., & McMurray, J. (2000). Validity and utility of the PRIME-MD Patient Health Questionnaire in assessment of 3,000 obstetric–gynecologic patients: The PRIME-MD Patient Health Questionnaire Obstetric–Gynecologic Study. *American Journal of Obstetrics and Gynecology, 183*(3), 759–769.

Springhouse. (2001). *Diseases* (3rd ed.). Springhouse, PA: Springhouse Corporation.

Thompson, L. W., Coon, D. W., Gallagher-Thompson, D., Sommer, B. R., & Koin, D. (2001). Comparison of desipramine and cognitive/behavioral therapy in the treatment of elderly outpatients with mild-to-moderate depression. *American Journal of Geriatric Psychiatry, 9,* 225–240.

Van Marwijk, H., Arnold, I., Bonnema, J., & Kaptein, A. (1993). Self-report depression scales for elderly patients in primary care: A preliminary study. *Family Practice, 10*(1), 63–65.

Wagnild, G. (2003). Resilience and successful aging: Comparison among low and high income older adults. *Journal of Gerontological Nursing, 29*(12), 42–49.

Wagnild, G. M., & Young, H. M. (1993). Development and psychometric evaluation of the Resilience Scale. *Journal of Nursing Measurement, 1*(2), 165–178.

Waldrop, J., & Stern, S. M. (2003). *Disability status: 2000* (Census 2000 Brief, C2KBR-17). Washington, DC: U.S. Bureau of the Census.

Waraich, P., Goldner, E. M., Somers, J. M., & Hsu, L. (2004). Prevalence and incidence studies of mood disorders: A systematic review of the literature. *Canadian Journal of Psychiatry, 49,* 124–138.

Williams, L. S., Brizendine, E. J., Plue, L., Bakas, T., Tu, W., Hendrie, H., et al. (2005). Performance of the PHQ-9 as a screening tool for depression after stroke. *Stroke, 36*(3), 635–638.

Yesavage, J. A., Brink, T. L., Rose, T. L., Lum, O., Huang, V., Adey, M., et al. (1982). Development and validation of a geriatric depression screening scale: A preliminary report. *Journal of Psychiatric Research, 17*(1), 37–49.

INDEX

439